small animal surgery

The National Veterinary Medical Series for Independent Study

small animal surgery

Joseph Harari, M.S., D.V.M.
Diplomate ACVS
Associate Professor
Department of Veterinary Clinical Sciences
College of Veterinary Medicine
Washington State University
Pullman, Washington

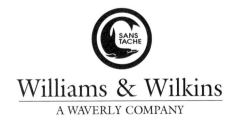

Williams & Wilkins

A WAVERLY COMPANY

BALTIMORE • PHILADELPHIA • LONDON • PARIS • BANGKOK
BUENOS AIRES • HONG KONG • MUNICH • SYDNEY • TOKYO • WROCLAW

1996

Senior Acquisitions Editor: Elizabeth A. Nieginski
Development Editors: Melanie Cann, Rebecca Krumm
Managing Editor: Amy G. Dinkel
Production Coordinator: Danielle Santucci
Editorial Assistants: Beth Goldner, Carol Loyd

The publisher gratefully acknowledges the Professional Examination Service (PES) for providing information about the format and content of the National Board Examination (NBE) for Veterinary Medical Licensing.

Copyright © 1996
Williams & Wilkins
Suite 5025
Rose Tree Corporate Center
Building Two
1400 N. Providence Road
Media, PA 19063 USA

Printed in the United States of America

Library of Congress Cataloging-in-Publication Data

Small animal surgery / [edited by] Joseph Harari.
      p.   cm. — (The National veterinary medical series for independent study)
   Includes bibliographical references and index.
   ISBN 0-683-03910-5
   1. Veterinary surgery—Outlines, syllabi, etc.   2. Veterinary surgery—Examinations, questions, etc.   I. Harari, Joseph. II. Series.
SF911.S5   1995
636.089'7—dc20   95-35809
                               CIP

96 97 98
10 9 8 7 6 5 4 3 2 1

Dedication

For Denise and the brightest stars in our universe, Hannah and Eve

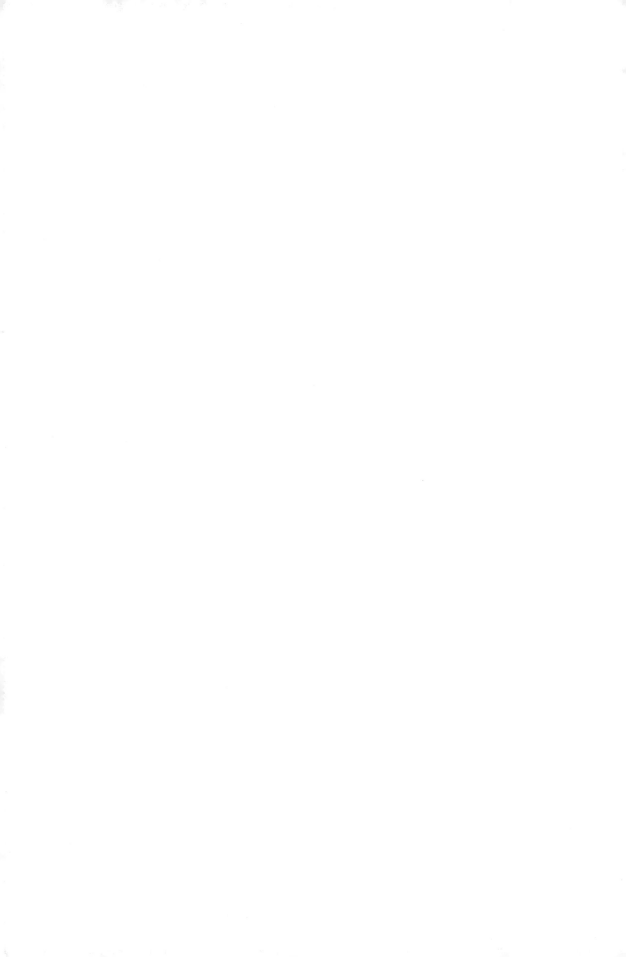

Contents

Part II   Soft Tissue Surgery

Contributors

Rodney S. Bagley, D.V.M.
Diplomate
American College of Veterinary Internal
   Medicine (Neurology, Internal Medicine)
Assistant Professor
Clinical Neurology and Neurosurgery
Department of Clinical Sciences
Washington State University
Pullman, Washington

**Giselle L. Hosgood, B.V.Sc., M.S.,
F.A.C.V.Sc.**
Diplomate
American College of Veterinary Surgeons
Associate Professor
Department of Veterinary Clinical Sciences
Baton Rouge, Louisiana

Spencer A. Johnston, D.V.M., M.S.
Diplomate
American College of Veterinary Surgeons
Assistant Professor
Department of Small Animal Clinical Sciences
Virginia-Maryland Regional College of
   Veterinary Medicine
Blacksburg, Virginia

Robert D. Keegan, D.V.M.
Diplomate
American College of Veterinary
   Anesthesiologists
Associate Professor
College of Veterinary Medicine
Washington State University
Pullman, Washington

Elizabeth J. Laing, D.V.M., D.V.Sc.
Diplomate
American College of Veterinary Surgeons
Surgical Referral Service
Stoughton, Wisconsin

Candace E. Layton, D.V.M., M.S.
Former Associate Professor
Department of Clinical Sciences
College of Veterinary Medicine
Kansas State University
Manhattan, Kansas

James K. Roush, D.V.M., M.S.
Diplomate
American College of Veterinary Surgeons
Associate Professor
Department of Clinical Sciences
College of Veterinary Medicine
Kansas State University
Manhattan, Kansas

Alan J. Schulman, D.V.M.
Diplomate
American College of Veterinary Surgeons
Veterinary Surgical Referral Service
Los Angeles, California

Karen M. Swalec Tobias, D.V.M., M.S.
Diplomate
American College of Veterinary Surgeons
Assistant Professor
College of Veterinary Medicine
Washington State University
Pullman, Washington

Preface

The goal of this *National Veterinary Medical Series* text is to provide students, veterinarians, and technicians with a relevant, concise, and easy-to-read manual describing general principles and treatments in small animal surgery. Contributors were selected based on their professional expertise and diversity in clinical training and practice.

Important perioperative considerations (e.g., anesthesia, nutrition, wound healing, infection, bandages, and physical therapy) are considered first, followed by chapters devoted to surgical treatments of common soft tissue, orthopedic, and neurologic disorders. Material is presented in a narrative outline format and includes brief reviews of applied anatomy, perioperative considerations, diseases treated by surgery, operative procedures, and postoperative care, including complications. In each chapter, illustrations are used to highlight critical points and selected readings are listed as additional references. A comprehensive examination featuring board-like questions and complete explanations appears at the end of the book.

This book is not intended to be all-inclusive, but rather a framework for the reader interested in clinical aspects of small animal surgery. Extensive information regarding surgery, anesthesiology, radiology, medicine, and pharmacology should be reviewed in major reference texts specifically devoted to these fields.

Acknowledgments

The editor gratefully acknowledges the invaluable efforts of Elizabeth Nieginski, who played an integral role in the genesis of this project, and Melanie Cann, who consistently provided focus and clarity to our manuscripts. The individual chapter authors should also be recognized for their excellent contributions to this text. Connie Freudenberg and Mazie Keller deserve credit for typing our manuscripts. Finally, I thank my colleagues and students at Washington State University who have contributed to an enlightening academic atmosphere.

PART I

INTRODUCTION

Chapter 1

Preoperative Considerations

James K. Roush

I. PATIENT ASSESSMENT

A. History. A complete medical history should be collected from the owner of the affected pet.

1. **Signalment** (i.e., weight, breed, age, sex) and **reproductive status** should be determined. Often, careful consideration of patient signalment and history is sufficient to eliminate many diseases.

2. The **animal's overall health and normal habits** (e.g., the frequency of vomiting, diarrhea, urination, and coughing; exercise intolerance; water intake) should be discerned from the owner.

3. **Past medical problems**, including information about the **therapy and outcome** of those conditions, should be noted. If surgery is contemplated, it is necessary to gather **information about prior surgeries, previous blood transfusions, surgical or anesthetic complications, drug reactions,** and **tendencies for increased bleeding**.

4. The animal's **diet** (i.e., the type of food and the frequency of feeding) and **appetite** should be discerned.

5. **Current medications**, including the dose, duration of therapy, and response to medication, should be noted.
   a. All medications should be evaluated for possible adverse pharmacologic interactions or combined toxicity.
   b. A delay in surgery may be necessitated by some drugs, particularly corticosteroids, anticonvulsants, and sedatives.

6. **Characteristics of the animal's normal environment,** including exercise, housing, bedding, and the presence and proximity of other animals should be noted.

7. **Details of the current problem,** including the circumstances associated with its onset and its duration, should be sought.

B. Physical examination

1. **Introduction**
   a. A complete physical examination is necessary to accurately diagnose the problem. If surgery is the treatment of choice, information from the physical examination aids in classifying the animal according to physical status and identifying surgical and anesthetic risk factors (see II B–C).
   b. A complete, systematic evaluation of the animal should be performed, despite a natural inclination to concentrate on the presenting complaint. An exception to this rule is an emergency situation, which requires collection of the data necessary to provide immediate treatment. Once the animal is stabilized, however, a complete physical examination should be performed.

2. **Components**
   a. **Assessment of the general condition of the animal.** The degree of hydration, the nutritional status, and the alertness of the animal, and the degree of care given the animal by the owner should be noted.
   b. **Assessment of the nervous, gastrointestinal, cardiopulmonary, respiratory, urinary, and reproductive systems**
      (1) **Auscultation of the thoracic cavity** is imperative to assess respiratory and cardiac function and to eliminate or identify surgical risk posed by congenital or acquired cardiac abnormalities.

          (2) **Abdominal palpation** is important to identify masses, determine relative organ size, and assess the degree of abdominal discomfort exhibited by the patient.

          (3) **The special senses** (e.g., vision, hearing, proprioception) should be evaluated.

     c. **Evaluation of the affected region and related systems.** For example, a client may bring an animal that has been hit by a car to the veterinarian because of bilateral hind limb dysfunction resulting from pelvic fractures. Urinary bladder and sciatic nerve function should be evaluated because soft tissue and nerve trauma may occur in association with these fractures. **Any animal with possible vehicular trauma should receive an electrocardiogram (ECG) and chest radiographs in addition to routine presurgical screening.**

C. **Secondary diagnostic aids** (e.g., magnetic resonance imaging, computed tomography) may be employed to help the clinician arrive at a definitive diagnosis.

    1. A sound understanding of disease mechanisms and related diagnoses is essential when selecting additional tests. Because of the expense and required expertise associated with many of these tests, secondary diagnostic aids are employed with discretion.

    2. Availability of equipment often limits the tests that may be employed.

II. SURGICAL RISK ASSESSMENT

A. **Introduction.** Surgical risk assessment involves weighing the relative benefits of surgery (e.g., the change in quality of life available from the procedure) versus the potential for harm (Table 1–1). Factors to consider include:

    1. Anesthetic risk (see II B), the invasiveness of the procedure, and the potential for complications

    2. The extensiveness of the procedure (long procedures are associated with more surgical trauma and increased strain on the animal's physical resources)

    3. The animal's age and general condition

    4. The effect of the animal's current physical status on postoperative recovery

B. **Anesthetic risk.** Once existing problems have been identified via a physical examination, a **physical status** is assigned that identifies anesthetic risk and provides general

TABLE 1–1. Assessment of Surgical Risk

Risk	Description
Excellent	No reasonable potential for negative consequences to patient, high probability that surgery will resolve the presenting problem
Good	Low potential for complications resulting from surgery, high probability of successful outcome
Fair	One or more serious but manageable problems, procedure associated with moderate possibility of complications
Poor	Significant chance of major complications leading to unsuccessful outcome

TABLE 1–2. Physical Status Classification

Classification*	Results of Physical Examination	Examples of Physical Examination Findings	Prognosis for Survival
I	Healthy, no underlying disease	No abnormalities	Excellent
II	Geriatric or obese animals, neonates, local disease with mild systemic disturbance	Controlled diabetes, closed fracture	Excellent
III	Disease with moderate systemic signs	Anemia, cachexia, fever, renal disease, cardiac disease	Good
IV	Disease with severe systemic signs	Shock, uremia, toxemia, gastric torsion, colic, hemorrhage	Guarded
V	Moribund or comatose	Advanced disease, solitary or multisystemic organ failure	Poor

* When the procedure is done as an emergency with minimal patient preparation, the letter "E" is written beside the numerical classification.

guidelines for routine or recommended laboratory evaluation of the patient (Table 1–2). **Relative weight** refers to how much emphasis is placed on abnormalities discovered during the physical examination when assigning physical status.

1. **Major emphasis** should be placed on cardiopulmonary, renal, or hepatic abnormalities, or abnormalities in two or more body systems.

2. **Intermediate emphasis** should be given to abnormalities in the gastrointestinal, reproductive, and endocrine systems.

3. **Minor emphasis** is relegated to abnormalities in the peripheral neurologic, musculoskeletal, ophthalmic, integumentary, and lymphatic systems.

C. Surgical risk

1. **Diseases that involve a major organ system or more than one organ system** increase surgical risk.
   a. **Major cardiopulmonary abnormalities** often preclude surgery, except in life-threatening situations. Complications are more frequent in patients with cardiomyopathy, congestive heart failure, conduction abnormalities, and pulmonary edema.
   b. **Renal failure, traumatic bladder rupture,** or **urethral obstruction** render the animal a poor candidate for surgery. Preoperative correction of acid–base disturbances, electrolyte imbalances, or increased serum urea or creatinine concentrations may minimize surgical risk in these patients (see IV).
   c. **Liver disease** often impairs the animal's ability to metabolize drugs, and may impair clotting or wound healing capabilities. Surgical risk in animals with liver disease can be lessened by improving the nutritional status through hyperalimentation, careful fluid therapy, and blood transfusions.
   d. **Endocrine disorders**, primarily hyperadrenocorticism, hypoadrenocorticism, and diabetes mellitus, increase surgical risk. These disorders should be recognized and proper therapy instituted before surgery.
      (1) **Hypoadrenocorticism.** An increase in endogenous cortisol concentrations is necessary to meet the demands placed on the animal by surgery and hospitalization. These stresses can cause an acute crisis in animals with hypoadrenocorticism.

(2) **Diabetes mellitus.** Proper pre- and postoperative management of animals with diabetes mellitus is necessary to reduce impaired wound healing.
  (a) In diabetic animals, food is generally withheld for 12 hours before surgery and half the normal dose of insulin is administered the morning of surgery.
  (b) Administration of dextrose-containing fluids and careful monitoring of blood glucose are important during surgery and recovery.
(3) Because most animals with endocrine disorders are more susceptible to surgical infection, prophylactic antibiotics should be administered to these animals.

2. **Obesity** increases the risk of surgical complications. In obese animals, ventilation is depressed as a result of intrathoracic fat accumulations, wound healing is impaired, and the incidence of infections is increased.

D. **Presurgical screening**
1. **Laboratory tests**
   a. The **absolute minimum database** for young, healthy animals includes the **packed cell volume (PCV)** and **total plasma protein level.**
      (1) This data provides a baseline for monitoring hemorrhage and fluid balance during surgery.
      (2) Table 1–3 details additional tests that are required according to the physical status of the animal.
   b. In areas where the incidence of *Dirofilaria immitis* is high, **Knott's test** or an **occult heartworm test** is recommended. Similarly, when infestation with intestinal parasites is possible, **fecal flotation** is recommended.
   c. Animals with significant liver disease, hypoproteinemia, or other clotting deficiencies should undergo **coagulation testing** (i.e., platelet count, activated clotting time, prothrombin time, thrombin time, partial thromboplastin time, and bleeding time). If there is a significant risk of hemorrhage, the animal's blood should be crossmatched with that of an available donor before surgery.

2. **Additional tests**
   a. An **ECG** and **thoracic radiographs** are indicated in addition to routine presurgical screening for any animal sustaining possible **vehicular trauma** or with a preexisting **cardiac abnormality.**

TABLE 1–3. Recommended Presurgical Tests per Physical Status

Physical Status Classification	Laboratory Tests	
	Minor Procedure*	**Major Procedure†**
I	PCV, TPP, urine specific gravity	CBC, urinalysis, minor panel‡
II	PCV, TPP, urine specific gravity	CBC, urinalysis, complete chemistry profile
III	CBC, urinalysis, minor panel	CBC, urinalysis, complete chemistry profile, ECG
IV	CBC, urinalysis, complete chemistry profile, ECG, blood gas analysis	CBC, urinalysis, complete chemistry profile, ECG, blood gas analysis
V	CBC, urinalysis, complete chemistry profile, ECG, blood gas analysis	CBC, urinalysis, complete chemistry profile, ECG, blood gas analysis

Analysis of PCV, TPP, electrolyte levels and blood gases is advisable in emergency situations. Thoracic and abdominal radiography or ultrasonography may be required for patients classified as physical status IV or V, or trauma patients. CBC = complete blood count; ECG = electrocardiogram; PCV = packed cell volume; TPP = total plasma protein levels.
* Minor procedure: duration < 1 hour and minimal surgical trauma OR patient < 5 years of age.
† Major procedure: duration > 1 hour OR patient > 5 years of age.
‡ Minor panel = blood urea nitrogen (BUN), creatinine, alanine aminotransferase, alkaline phosphatase, electrolytes.

b. An **echocardiogram** is indicated for animals with cardiac abnormalities.

c. **Additional tests may be ordered on the basis of the procedure to be performed.** For instance, oblique and flexed radiographic views of the elbow joint are helpful prior to performing arthrotomy for joint fragments in dogs.

III. **COMMUNICATION WITH THE CLIENT.** Discussions with clients should always be carried out in a candid manner. Important elements of these discussions include:

A. An explanation of the disease or problem

B. Treatment options

C. Prognosis for the animal if no treatment is undertaken and with the recommended course of treatment

D. If surgery is indicated, an explanation of the procedure, including potential complications and postoperative management of the animal

E. An estimate of the immediate and future costs of the surgery

IV. **PREOPERATIVE PATIENT STABILIZATION** is imperative to decrease anesthetic and surgical risks.

A. **Fluid therapy.** Surgical patients require a normal fluid balance before surgery to prevent hypotension caused by peripheral vasodilation during surgery, and to protect against excessive loss of fluid during surgery through hemorrhage or tissue drying.

1. The **volume of fluids administered** is the sum of the **replacement needs, maintenance requirements,** and **estimated future losses.** Fluids (and electrolytes) given for patient stabilization are best **administered intravenously.**

   a. **Replacement needs**
      (1) **Assessment of fluid deficits**
         (a) **Dehydration.** Clinical signs of dehydration include skin "tenting," dry mucous membranes, and sunken eyes.
         (b) **Laboratory test results. PCV** and **total plasma protein levels** can be used to assess fluid balance, but these parameters may be inaccurate in the presence of recent, uncompensated fluid loss.
         (c) **Gross estimation.** Extravascular fluid loss can be estimated grossly by the number of blood- or fluid-soaked surgical sponges (each sponge absorbs approximately 10 ml of fluid), or by measuring the volume of fluid obtained by squeezing the sponge.
      (2) **Replacement needs** can be calculated as follows:

$$\text{Need (L)} = \% \text{ dehydration} \times \text{body weight (kg)} \times 1 \text{ L} \\ + \text{ losses from vomiting, diarrhea}$$

   b. **Maintenance requirements.** The maintenance requirement for normal dogs and cats is approximately 50–70 ml/kg/day. This value increases proportionately as metabolic requirements increase (e.g., during surgery or with systemic disease).

2. The **rate of fluids administered** varies with the condition of the animal. In general, before surgery takes place, the entire fluid deficit should be corrected and maintenance fluids should be administered.

   a. Fluids may be administered at a rate of up to 100 ml/kg/hr to hypovolemic patients that do not have cardiovascular disease.

    b. Replacement over 12–24 hours is preferred when the condition of the animal allows it.

3. The **choice of fluids** depends on the concentration of the fluids lost and the electrolyte status of the animal.

    a. Lactated Ringer's solution is the optimum choice in unknown or emergency situations, because its electrolyte composition closely resembles plasma and because it helps maintain acid–base balance.

    b. Isotonic saline solutions administered intravenously remain within the extracellular fluid compartment and are useful for increasing intravascular fluid volume.

    c. Hypertonic saline solutions (greater than 0.9% sodium chloride) administered intravenously cause rapid relocation of fluids from the interstitial to the intravascular space. Although these solutions rapidly increase the intravascular fluid volume, they do so at the expense of additional peripheral tissue dehydration.

    d. 5% Dextrose and other carbohydrate solutions are hypotonic and essentially supply free water.

4. Reassessment of fluid balance

    a. Urine. With adequate fluid replacement, urine production should reach normal levels (1–2 ml/kg/hr) and the urine specific gravity should become isosthenuric (1.008– 1.017).

    b. The **PCV** and **total plasma protein levels** may reach normal values.

    c. Clinical signs of dehydration should disappear.

B. **Restoring acid–base balance**

1. Specific therapy is only necessary when the pH is less than 7.2 or greater than 7.51. Acid–base disorders should be corrected before anesthesia.

2. In conditions of metabolic acidosis, bicarbonate replacement may be calculated as follows:

$$\text{Needed bicarbonate (mEq)} = 0.3 \times \text{body weight (kg)} \times \text{base deficit}$$

C. **Electrolyte therapy**

1. Sodium and chloride. In most animals, sodium and chloride deficits are rectified during fluid replacement therapy with isotonic electrolyte solutions.

    a. Sodium is the major extracellular cation and the major determinant of serum osmolality. Isotonic saline solutions may be used to replenish sodium levels.

    b. Chloride is the major extracellular anion.

    c. Deficits are calculated as follows:

$$\text{Deficit (mEq)} = 0.3 \times \text{body weight (kg)} \times (\text{desired} - \text{actual})$$

2. Potassium is primarily contained within the intracellular space.

    a. Assessment of potassium levels

        (1) Serum values must be interpreted with caution because severe total body deficits can exist without changes in serum concentration, and several systemic diseases (e.g., hypoadrenocorticism, diabetes mellitus) also affect serum potassium concentration.

        (2) Potassium concentrations increase by 0.3 mEq/L with each 0.1-unit decrease in blood pH.

    b. Potassium supplementation

        (1) Potassium should be supplemented at a rate of 20–30 mEq/L in anorectic animals or animals with restricted food intake in order to replace normal losses through the urine and gastrointestinal tract.

        (2) Rapid rates of potassium administration (i.e., greater than 0.5 mEq/kg/hr) must be avoided. If it is absolutely necessary to administer potassium at rates exceeding 0.5 mEq/kg/hr, simultaneous electrocardiographic monitoring is imperative.

D. **Component and fresh whole blood therapy**

1. **Indications for transfusion**

    a. **PCV less than 25%.** The oxygen-carrying capacity of the blood should be sufficient if the PCV is greater than 25%. Following acute blood loss, representative changes in PCV occur slowly (i.e., within 8–12 hours) because of the time required for fluid compartment equilibration.

    b. **Significant potential for surgical blood loss.** Patients should be transfused preoperatively if the potential for surgical blood loss is significant.

    c. **Coagulopathies.** Component or fresh whole blood therapy is indicated if coagulopathies are detected clinically or during preoperative evaluation.

    d. **Plasma protein levels below 4.5 g/dl or albumin concentrations below 1.5 g/dl.** Plasma transfusions should be administered before surgery to animals with diminished plasma protein or albumin levels to avoid complications associated with low plasma oncotic pressure (e.g., delayed wound healing, diminished protein binding of anesthetic drugs).

2. **Calculating blood or component requirements**

    a. For animals with a PCV of less than 25%, the volume of blood required can be calculated as follows:

    $$\text{Need (ml)} = \frac{[\text{body weight (kg)} \times PCV_{desired}] - [PCV_{patient} \times K]}{PCV_{donor}} \text{ , where}$$

    $$K = 70 \text{ ml/kg (cat) or } 90 \text{ ml/kg (dog).}$$

    b. Alternatively, 2.2 ml whole blood/kg body weight may be administered for each 1% increase in PCV desired, assuming a donor PCV of 40%.

3. **Crossmatching** of patient and donor blood is recommended for all transfusions, particularly when multiple transfusions are required.

E. **Nutritional support** of surgical candidates is discussed in Chapter 5 III.

SELECTED READINGS

Birchard SJ: Patient management. In *Saunders Manual of Small Animal Practice.* Edited by Birchard SJ, Sherding RG. Philadelphia, WB Saunders, 1994, pp 1–12.

Chew DJ: Fluid therapy for dogs and cats. In *Saunders Manual of Small Animal Practice.* Edited by Birchard SJ, Sherding RG. Philadelphia, WB Saunders, 1994, pp 64–76.

Fries CL: Assessment and preparation of the surgical patient. In *Textbook of Small Animal Surgery,* 2nd ed. Edited by Slatter DH. Philadelphia, WB Saunders, 1993, pp 137–147.

Hendrix PK, Raffe MR: Fluid, electrolyte, and acid–base disorders. In *Disease Mechanisms in Small Animal Surgery,* 2nd ed. Edited by Bojrab MJ. Philadelphia, Lea & Febiger, 1993, pp 21–31.

Rentko VT, Cotter SM: Transfusion therapy in dogs and cats. In *Disease Mechanisms in Small Animal Surgery,* 2nd ed. Edited by Bojrab MJ. Philadelphia, Lea & Febiger, 1993, pp 44–48.

Chapter 2

Anesthesia

Robert D. Keegan

I. PREANESTHETIC CONSIDERATIONS

A. **Patient evaluation.** Preoperative evaluation of surgical candidates includes anamnesis, physical examination, and cytologic and chemical blood evaluations (see Chapter 1 I–II).

B. **Restrictions.** Food should be withheld for 12 hours prior to elective surgery and anesthesia. Water is made available at all times to prevent hypovolemia.

C. **Preanesthetic agents** (Table 2–1). Use of preanesthetic agents can facilitate surgery and anesthesia by improving the smoothness of induction and recovery, reducing anxiety, and providing analgesia.

1. **Anticholinergics** (e.g., **atropine, glycopyrrolate**) block muscarinic cholinergic receptors and reduce parasympathetic tone throughout the body. They are useful as preanesthetic agents when reduction of salivary secretions, bronchodilation, or mydriasis is desired, or to counteract parasympathetically induced bradycardia.

2. **Tranquilizers** (e.g., **phenothiazines, butyrophenones, benzodiazepines**) are administered to decrease hyperactivity, reduce doses of intravenous and maintenance anesthetics, and improve the quality of inductions and recoveries. They have no intrinsic analgesic activity but may potentiate the analgesic effects of opioids.
   a. **Acepromazine** is a phenothiazine tranquilizer. Its low cost and predictability make it extremely popular as a preanesthetic in small animal practice.
   b. **Droperidol**, a butyrophenone tranquilizer, is available as a veterinary drug only in combination with fentanyl, an opioid. This preparation is commercially known as **Innovar-Vet**.

3. **Opioids** (e.g., **morphine, oxymorphone, meperidine, butorphanol**)
   a. **Indications.** Opioids are excellent analgesics and provide mild to moderate preanesthetic sedation. Aggressive dogs may be administered an opioid in combination with acepromazine to promote handling of the animal and induction of anesthesia.
   b. **Side effects** include respiratory depression, parasympathetic stimulation, excitement, dysphoria, and histamine release.

4. **α_2-Adrenergic agonists** (e.g., **xylazine, medetomidine**)
   a. **Indications.** These agents have potent sedative and analgesic activity in dogs and cats. Medetomidine is approved for use in Europe, Australia, and Japan, but it is not currently approved for use in the United States. Medetomidine produces profound analgesia and sedation and thereby approaches the definition of a complete anesthetic.
   b. **Side effects. Cardiovascular changes** are profound and include vasoconstriction, bradycardia, and markedly diminished cardiac output.
      (1) Concurrent administration of an anticholinergic corrects the bradycardia.
      (2) Specific reversal agents (i.e., yohimbine, atipamezole) are available.

5. **Benzodiazepines** (e.g., **diazepam, midazolam**) are often referred to as "minor" tranquilizers. In humans, they produce moderate to profound tranquilization and have an antianxiety effect, but in most animals, they are not potent sedatives.
   a. **Indications**
      (1) Benzodiazepines can be used to augment sedation and muscle relaxation in combination with other anesthetics (e.g., ketamine) or analgesics (e.g., opioids).

TABLE 2–1. Dosages of Preanesthetic Agents

Agent	Action	Dosage Dog	Dosage Cat	Comments
Atropine	Anticholinergic	0.04 mg/kg, IV, IM, SQ	0.04 mg/kg, IV, IM, SQ	
Glycopyrrolate	Anticholinergic	0.01 mg/kg, IV, IM, SQ	0.01 mg/kg, IV, IM, SQ	
Acepromazine	Tranquilizer	0.025–0.1 mg/kg, IV, IM, SQ	0.025–0.1 mg/kg, IV, IM, SQ	Maximum total dose = 3.0 mg
Innovar-Vet (fentanyl and droperidol)	Sedative/analgesic	0.1–0.3 ml/dog, IV 0.25–1.5 ml/dog, IM, SQ	Not recommended for use in cats	Administer with an anticholinergic
Oxymorphone	Sedative/analgesic	0.025–0.1 mg/kg, IV, IM, SQ	0.025–0.05 mg/kg, IM, SQ	Administer with an anticholinergic
Meperidine	Sedative/analgesic	2–6 mg/kg, IM, SQ	2–6 mg/kg, IM, SQ	IV administration may cause cardiac depression
Morphine	Sedative/analgesic	0.25–0.5 mg/kg, IM, SQ	0.05–0.1 mg/kg, IM, SQ	Large IV doses may produce histamine release; administer with an anticholinergic
Butorphanol	Sedative/analgesic	0.1–0.2 mg/kg, IV, IM, SQ	0.1–0.2 mg/kg, IV, IM, SQ	Administer with an anticholinergic
Xylazine	Sedative/analgesic	0.2–1.0 mg/kg, IV, IM, SQ	0.2–1.0 mg/kg, IV, IM, SQ	Administer with an anticholinergic
Diazepam	Tranquilizer	0.2 mg/kg, IV	0.2 mg/kg, IV	Usually used in combination with opioids or anesthetic agents
Midazolam	Tranquilizer	0.2 mg/kg, IV	0.2 mg/kg, IV	Usually used in combination with opioids or anesthetic agents

IM = intramuscularly, IV = intravenously, SQ = subcutaneously.

(2) They may provide adequate sedation as sole agents when administered to debilitated animals or neonates.

(3) Midazolam is an excellent sedative in birds when administered intramuscularly.

b. Precautions. Administration to awake, healthy dogs may result in excitation and aggression.

D. **Preemptive analgesia** is the administration of analgesics in anticipation of, rather than in response to, surgical pain. Ideally, animals that are likely to experience pain after a surgical procedure should be administered an analgesic before, during, and after anesthesia.

1. **Basis of surgical pain.** Peripheral and central nervous sensitization occur in response to painful stimuli.
   a. Peripheral sensitization is based on numerous mediators (e.g., prostaglandins, bradykinin) that are released in response to tissue trauma and produce an increase in the transduction mechanism of high-threshold nociceptors. Increased peripheral sensitization results in **allodynia** (i.e., pain resulting from a normally nonpainful stimulus).
   b. Central sensitization results from increased excitability of spinal cord neurons. Nociceptive afferent input triggers the increase in spinal cord excitability, and excitability persists after nociceptive input is decreased.
   c. The **net effect** is twofold:
      (1) Afferent input from mechanoreceptors, which are not normally painful, begins to produce pain.
      (2) The receptive field of spinal cord dorsal horn neurons is increased so that previous subthreshold afferent input is converted into a suprathreshold response, and the magnitude and duration of the response to threshold stimuli increase.

2. **Effects of preemptive analgesia.** If surgical pain can be prevented or reduced, peripheral and central sensitization does not occur.
   a. Animals require a **lower total dose of opioid postoperatively** when preemptive analgesia has been administered.
   b. Much of the **stress response** that occurs postsurgically is also **eliminated.**

3. **Methods of providing preemptive analgesia**
   a. Preoperative infiltration of the surgical site with a local anesthetic blocks transmission of nociceptive inputs along the peripheral nerve.
   b. Preoperative epidural administration of local anesthetics, opioids, α_2-adrenergic agonists, alone or in any combination, blocks transmission of nociceptive input to the brain.
   c. Preoperative administration of systemic antiprostaglandin drugs
   d. Preoperative administration of systemic opioids, α_2-adrenergic agonists, or both

II. INDUCTION OF ANESTHESIA

A. **Intravenous anesthesia** (Table 2–2)

1. **Ultrashort-acting barbiturates**
   a. Thiobarbiturates. The two most commonly used thiobarbiturates are **thiamylal** and **thiopental.**
      (1) Indications
         (a) Induction of short-term intravenous anesthesia
         (b) Induction of general anesthesia prior to inhalational anesthesia
      (2) Administration. Repeated doses of thiobarbiturates saturate redistribution depots and result in longer durations of action.
      (3) Precautions

TABLE 2–2. Dosages of Intravenous Anesthetic Agents

Agent	Class	Dosage Dog	Dosage Cat	Comments
Thiopental	Thiobarbiturate	10–20 mg/kg	10–20 mg/kg	
Thiamylal	Thiobarbiturate	10–20 mg/kg	10–20 mg/kg	
Methohexital	Oxybarbiturate	8–10 mg/kg	8–10 mg/kg	
Propofol	Phenol	5–8 mg/kg	5–8 mg/kg	
Etomidate	Imidazole	1–4 mg/kg	1–4 mg/kg	
Ketamine + diazepam	Cyclohexylamine/ benzodiazepine	2–10 mg/kg 0.2 mg/kg	2–10 mg/kg 0.2 mg/kg	
Ketamine + midazolam	Cyclohexylamine/ benzodiazepine	2–10 mg/kg 0.2 mg/kg	2–10 mg/kg 0.2 mg/kg	
Telazol (tiletamine and zolazepam)	Cyclohexylamine/ benzodiazepine	2–10 mg/kg	2–10 mg/kg	
Oxymorphone	Opioid	0.2 mg/kg	Not recommended for use in cats	Administer with an anticholinergic
Fentanyl	Opioid	0.02 mg/kg	Not recommended for use in cats	Administer with an anticholinergic
Innovar-Vet (fentanyl and droperidol)	Opioid/ butyrophenone	1 ml/25 kg	Not recommended for use in cats	Administer with an anticholinergic

(a) Thiobarbiturates are supplied in a water-soluble alkaline solution that **can cause tissue necrosis if injected perivascularly.**
(b) Barbiturates are highly protein-bound, and a **more intense effect is evident in hypoproteinemic and acidotic animals.**
(c) The **duration of action of thiobarbiturates is significantly longer in sight hound breeds** than in mixed breed dogs, and **recovery from thiobarbiturate induction is often prolonged and rough** in these breeds. Alternative drugs (e.g., methohexital or diazepam and ketamine) for induction of anesthesia in sight hound breeds should be considered.
(d) **Cardiopulmonary effects** include respiratory depression, a short period of apnea following induction of anesthesia, and a dose-dependent depression of cardiovascular function, all of which may lead to ventricular arrhythmia.

b. **Oxybarbiturates.** The only commonly used oxybarbiturate in veterinary anesthesia is **methohexital.**
(1) **Indications**
(a) Methohexital is often used to induce anesthesia in **sight hound breeds.**
(b) Because oxybarbiturates have an even shorter duration of action than thiobarbiturates, they are indicated **when a rapid recovery is desirable.**
(2) **Precautions**
(a) **Induction** is generally smooth, but apnea and excitement may occur following induction of anesthesia.

(b) **Recovery** may be rough (i.e., paddling or vocalizing is common). Poor recoveries are less of a problem if the patient is premedicated with a tranquilizer and general anesthesia is maintained with an inhalant for longer than 30 minutes.

2. **Phenols. Propofol** is a short-acting, nonbarbiturate induction agent.
   a. **Indications**
      (1) Propofol is used for **short-term intravenous anesthesia when rapid recovery is desirable.**
      (2) It is used as an **intravenous induction agent** prior to the induction of anesthesia with an inhalant.
      (3) Infusion of propofol is useful for **maintaining general anesthesia.**
   b. **Induction and recovery**
      (1) **Induction.** Intravenous administration of propofol produces unconsciousness rapidly.
      (2) **Recovery,** even from an infusion or multiple doses, is rapid because of rapid metabolism by the liver.
   c. **Precautions**
      (1) **Respiratory depression.** Apnea after bolus administration is common. Respiratory depression can be minimized by administering the drug slowly to effect.
      (2) **Cardiovascular depression** is similar to that produced by thiobarbiturates.

3. **Imidazoles. Etomidate** is a nonbarbiturate, imidazole-containing compound for induction of anesthesia.
   a. **Indications.** Etomidate is virtually devoid of deleterious cardiovascular effects and is a good choice for intravenous induction in patients with hypertrophic cardiomyopathy.
   b. **Induction and recovery.** Etomidate is water-soluble and produces rapid loss of consciousness and a rapid recovery from anesthesia.
   c. **Precautions**
      (1) Pain on injection and involuntary muscle movements (myoclonus) have been observed during induction of anesthesia.
      (2) Respiratory depression and apnea following intravenous bolus administration have been reported. The incidence and severity of these effects are reduced by administering the drug slowly to effect.

4. **Cyclohexylamines (ketamine, Telazol).** These agents produce **dissociative anesthesia,** a cataleptoid state characterized by poor muscle relaxation, open eyes, profuse salivation, and intense somatic but poor visceral analgesia.
   a. **Ketamine**
      (1) **Administration.** Poor muscle relaxation and stimulation of the central nervous system (CNS) and cardiovascular system necessitate **concurrent administration of a sedative or tranquilizer** (e.g., acepromazine, diazepam, xylazine).
      (2) **Precautions**
         (a) **Cardiovascular effects** include:
            (i) Increased heart rate, frequently in excess of 160 beats per minute
            (ii) Increased arterial pressure
            (iii) Increased cardiac output
            (iv) Increased myocardial oxygen demand
         (b) Animals with **renal insufficiency** may have **prolonged recoveries** because of their inability to excrete active ketamine metabolites. Use of ketamine in these patients should be limited to small intravenous doses.
   b. **Telazol** contains equal amounts of the cyclohexylamine **tiletamine** and the benzodiazepine **zolazepam.**
      (1) The addition of zolazepam improves muscle relaxation and reduces the incidence of CNS excitation.
      (2) The metabolism of tiletamine and zolazepam varies among animals.
         (a) Dogs metabolize the zolazepam more quickly than the tiletamine; therefore, recoveries may be rough.
         (b) Cats metabolize the tiletamine more quickly than the zolazepam; there-

fore, recoveries may be prolonged. Reversal of the zolazepam component with the benzodiazepine antagonist flumazenil may hasten recovery.
  c. **Administration.** Ketamine and Telazol may be administered intravenously or intramuscularly.
    (1) Intravenous administration produces rapid loss of consciousness and rapid recovery.
    (2) Intramuscular administration produces loss of consciousness within 5–10 minutes and a prolonged recovery from anesthesia.

5. **Opioids**
  a. **Indications**
    (1) Large doses of opioids are useful for the induction of anesthesia in patients having a fixed, low cardiac output.
    (2) Opioids may be used to facilitate endotracheal intubation (see II B 2); however, large doses are required, and young, healthy dogs may not be depressed enough by opioids to enable endotracheal intubation.
      (a) Twenty-five percent of the calculated dose of opioid is given and intubation is attempted.
      (b) If intubation is unsuccessful, additional opioid is given until intubation is accomplished.
      (c) If more than the calculated dose of opioid is required to facilitate intubation, small doses of diazepam, midazolam, or acepromazine are preferable to the administration of more opioid.
  b. **Agents. Oxymorphone, fentanyl,** and **Innovar-Vet** are commonly used when large doses of opioids are required because they do not cause histamine release or depress cardiac contractility following administration of the necessary dose.
  c. **Precautions.** Opioids may leave the animal too awake to intubate but too obtunded to protect the airway via pharyngeal and laryngeal reflexes; therefore, animals that have eaten prior to surgery are not good candidates for opioid inductions.
  d. **Side effects**
    (1) Large doses of opioids produce bradycardia. Administration of anticholinergics prior to opioid administration prevents opioid-induced bradycardia.
    (2) Large doses of opioids cause excitement and delirium in cats and are therefore not recommended for this species.
    (3) Opioids produce dose-dependent respiratory depression. Preoxygenation with 100% oxygen for 5 minutes prior to an opioid induction is recommended.

B. **Inhalation anesthesia**

1. **Mask induction**
  a. **Advantages**
    (1) Mask induction allows concurrent administration of 100% oxygen.
    (2) There is minimal reliance on hepatic metabolism and redistribution for recovery from anesthesia.
    (3) Mask inductions usually provide smooth inductions in unpremedicated geriatric or debilitated patients; however, premedication usually results in a much smoother induction in young, healthy patients.
  b. **Precautions.** Intense patient excitation and struggling during a mask induction may result in profound sympathetic stimulation, producing tachycardia and dysrhythmias and increasing myocardial oxygen demand.
  c. **Facilitation of mask induction**
    (1) **Neuroleptanalgesic combinations** (e.g., Innovar-Vet, acepromazine plus oxymorphone) are used to provide sedation prior to mask induction. Administration of an anticholinergic drug prior to sedation with the neuroleptanalgesic is indicated.
    (2) Mask inductions are easily accomplished in a **dark, quiet environment** using inhalant anesthetics of low solubility (e.g., halothane, isoflurane).

2. **Endotracheal intubation** is necessary to maintain a patent airway during anesthesia.
  a. **Endotracheal tubes**

- **(1) Composition.** Endotracheal tubes may be made of medical grade silicone, polyvinylchloride (PVC), or rubber.
- **(2) Style**
  - **(a)** Endotracheal tubes may be **cuffed or noncuffed.**
    - **(i) Cuffed endotracheal tubes** have an inflatable cuff near the patient end of the tube. The cuff provides a seal between the tube and the tracheal wall to prevent leakage of gases or liquids around the tube.
    - **(ii) Noncuffed endotracheal tubes.** When a noncuffed endotracheal tube is used, a tube that is the proper diameter for the animal's airway must be selected to provide a reasonable seal.
  - **(b)** The **Murphy tube** has a hole (the Murphy eye) located near the patient end of the tube to allow flow of gases should the tube lumen become occluded.
  - **(c) Guarded tubes** have a metal or nylon coil embedded within the tube wall to resist kinking.
- **(3) Length.** The endotracheal tube should extend from the thoracic inlet to the incisors.
- **(4) Diameter.** Endotracheal tubes ranging from 3.5–14 mm in diameter are suitable for use in cats and dogs.
  - **(a)** An endotracheal tube that is too small in diameter increases the work of breathing, because the internal diameter of the endotracheal tube is the primary determinant of resistance to airflow.
  - **(b)** An endotracheal tube that is too large in diameter may damage the larynx.
- **b. Intubation techniques.** Tracheal intubation is easily accomplished in dogs and cats.
  - **(1) Preoxygenation.** In patients where a difficult intubation is anticipated, preoxygenation for 5 minutes using face mask administration of 100% oxygen is advisable. Preoxygenation with 100% oxygen delays the onset of hypoxemia should apnea occur after induction of anesthesia.
  - **(2) Visualization of the airway**
    - **(a)** A **laryngoscope,** which combines a light source with a flat blade useful for depressing the tongue, is not essential but facilitates difficult intubations in brachycephalic patients or animals presenting with cervical masses.
      - **(i)** The blade of the laryngoscope is placed at the base of the tongue, ventral to the epiglottis.
      - **(ii)** Depression of the tongue by the tip of the laryngoscope blade pulls the epiglottis forward and exposes the glottis.
    - **(b)** In patients where visualization of the airway is difficult, placement of a **guide tube** before insertion of the endotracheal tube is often indicated.
  - **(3) Passage of the endotracheal tube.** After the airway is visualized, the endotracheal tube is passed **between the arytenoid cartilages and into the trachea.** Cats often experience laryngospasm during intubation, leading to adduction of the arytenoid cartilages.
    - **(a)** Laryngospasm makes intubation more difficult and may result in hypoxemia.
    - **(b)** Topical application of lidocaine prior to intubation reduces the incidence of laryngospasm.
- **3. Anesthetic machines and circuits.** Anesthetic machines deliver carrier gases and anesthetic agents to the breathing circuit.
  - **a. Components of the anesthetic machine**
    - **(1) Gas cylinders** are used for bulk storage of the carrier gases (i.e., oxygen and nitrous oxide).
    - **(2)** The **regulator** is a valve that reduces the pressure of the gases coming from the bulk storage cylinder to approximately 50–60 pounds per square inch (psi).
    - **(3)** The **flowmeter** accepts gas from the regulator at reduced pressure and controls the gas flow.

(4) The **flush valve** diverts 100% O_2 into the breathing circuit.

(5) The **vaporizer** converts the liquid anesthetic agent into a vapor and adds a controlled amount of the vapor to the inspired gas mixture.

    (a) **Precision vaporizers** deliver a precise concentration of anesthetic vapor over a long period of time.

    (b) **Nonprecision vaporizers** deliver a concentration of anesthetic that varies with the ambient temperature and the animal's minute ventilation.

b. Anesthetic circuits

    (1) Functions

        (a) Delivery of oxygen to the patient

        (b) Delivery of the anesthetic gas mixture in controlled concentrations to the patient

        (c) Assisted or controlled ventilation

        (d) Removal of carbon dioxide from the inspired gases

    (2) Types (Table 2–3)

        (a) **Open circuits** include the gauze mask, which consists of an anesthetic-saturated piece of gauze, which is placed near the animal's mouth and nose.

        (b) **Semi-open circuits** include the Bain circuit, the Norman elbow circuit, the Ayres T piece circuit, and the Magill circuit. Semi-open circuits are often used for animals that weigh less than 10 kg.

            (i) These circuits have a reservoir (rebreathing) bag that permits minimal rebreathing of exhaled gases.

            (ii) Elimination of carbon dioxide is accomplished by adjusting the fresh gas flow so that it is greater than or equal to the animal's minute ventilation.

        (c) **Semi-closed circuits** are **circle systems** with a fresh gas flow rate that is 3–5 times greater than the patient's metabolic oxygen demand.

            (i) Semi-closed circuits have a reservoir that permits significant rebreathing of exhaled gases.

            (ii) Elimination of carbon dioxide is accomplished through the use of a chemical absorber (e.g., soda lime).

        (d) **Closed circuits** are **circle systems** with a fresh gas flow rate that equals the patient's metabolic oxygen demand (approximately 10 ml/kg/min).

            (i) Closed circuits are identical to semi-closed circuits, except for the differences in the required rate of fresh gas flow.

            (ii) During the first 5 minutes after induction of anesthesia, the fresh gas flow rate into the closed circuit must be 3–5 times higher than the patient's metabolic oxygen demand in order to remove nitrogen from the patient and the circuit.

TABLE 2–3. Comparison of Breathing Circuits

Type	Advantages	Disadvantages
Open	Minimal equipment	Imprecise delivery of anesthetics; inability to assist ventilation
Semi-open	Lightweight, few movable parts, easy to clean; impart little resistance to airflow	Uses more oxygen and anesthetic; promotes drying of airways and loss of body heat
Semi-closed	Precise calculations of the animal's metabolic oxygen demand are not necessary	Bulky equipment; higher fresh gas flow rate consumes more carrier gases and anesthetic (compared with closed circuit)
Closed	Most economical	Bulky equipment; precise calculations of the animal's metabolic oxygen demand are necessary

4. **Agents** (Table 2–4)
    a. **Introduction**
        (1) Factors affecting delivery of the anesthetic to the lung include the alveolar ventilation and the concentration of the inspired anesthetic.
        (2) Factors affecting the uptake of anesthetic by the pulmonary blood include the solubility of the anesthetic and the patient's cardiac output.
    b. **Methoxyflurane**
        (1) **Advantages.** Methoxyflurane produces good muscle relaxation and may provide analgesia into the recovery period.
        (2) **Disadvantages.** Inductions, recoveries, and changes in depth of anesthesia are slow because of methoxyflurane's high solubility.
    c. **Halothane**
        (1) **Advantages.** Halothane usually produces adequate muscle relaxation for most surgical procedures. It is markedly less soluble than methoxyflurane and produces more rapid induction and recovery and more rapid changes in anesthetic depth.
        (2) **Disadvantages.** Halothane is a potent cerebral vasodilator and greatly increases cerebral blood flow; therefore, it is inappropriate for use in animals with intracranial pathology (e.g., neoplasia).
    d. **Isoflurane**
        (1) **Advantages**
            (a) Isoflurane usually produces good muscle relaxation that facilitates most surgical procedures.
            (b) Isoflurane is advocated for use in animals with intracranial disease or those undergoing intracranial surgery.
            (c) Isoflurane maintains hepatic blood flow better than other potent inhaled anesthetics; therefore, it is advocated for use in patients with hepatic insufficiency.

TABLE 2–4. Properties of Inhalation Anesthetics

Parameter	Halothane	Isoflurane	Methoxy-flurane	Nitrous oxide
Cardiac output	↓↓↓	↓	↓↓	—
Dysrhythmias	↑↑↑↑	↑	↑↑	—
Respiratory depression	↓	↓↓↓	↓↓↓	—
Total peripheral resistance	↓↓	↓↓↓	↓↓↓	↑
Blood pressure*	↓↓	↓↓↓	↓↓↓	↑
Hepatic blood flow	↓↓↓	↓↓	↓↓↓↓	—
Renal blood flow	↓↓	↓↓↓	↓↓↓	—
Cerebral blood flow†	↑↑↑↑	↑↑	↑↑	↑
Muscle relaxation	↑	↑↑	↑↑↑	—
MAC‡	0.87	1.3	0.23	188
Partition coefficient§	2.36	1.41	13	0.47
Vapor pressure‖	243	240	24	39,500
Cost	¢	$$$$	¢	¢

↑ = increase; ↓ = decrease; — = no change; MAC = minimum alveolar concentration.
* The decrease in blood pressure seen with halothane results from depression of cardiac contractility, whereas the decrease in blood pressure seen with isoflurane results from vasodilation.
† The effects of inhalation anesthetics on cerebral blood flow are greatly modified by the arterial carbon dioxide tension.
‡ MAC is the minimum alveolar concentration of the anesthetic that prevents purposeful movement in response to a noxious stimulus, expressed as a percentage. The values given here are for an average-sized dog. The lower the MAC, the more potent the agent.
§ The partition coefficient is an indicator of solubility.
‖ Vapor pressure is a measure of volatility. Anesthetics with higher vapor pressures are more easily converted from the liquid to gaseous state. The values given here are at a temperature of 20°C.

      (d) Isoflurane is the best of the potent inhalants at maintaining cardiovascular function.

      (e) Inductions, recoveries, and changes in anesthetic depth are more rapid with isoflurane than with halothane or methoxyflurane.

    (2) Disadvantages

      (a) Rapid recovery may cause emergence delirium, necessitating resedation.

      (b) Isoflurane is more expensive than the other inhalation anesthetics.

  e. Nitrous oxide

    (1) Advantages

      (a) Although nitrous oxide provides no muscle relaxation, it is an analgesic. Administration of nitrous oxide in combination with a potent inhalant has been advocated for providing improved analgesia during surgery.

      (b) Delivery to, and removal from, the brain is rapid because of nitrous oxide's low solubility.

    (2) Disadvantages. Because of its low potency, large volumes of nitrous oxide must be administered to produce beneficial effects. Concentrations of 50%–66% are used in combination with a potent inhalant.

C. **Intraoperative monitoring** of patients is essential because most general anesthetics produce depression of the cardiopulmonary system.

  1. Blood pressure. Most organs are able to regulate their blood flow to meet their oxygen demands provided that the mean arterial pressure is maintained within the limits of autoregulation.

    a. Monitoring blood pressure

      (1) Direct monitoring of blood pressure involves placement of an arterial catheter connected to a calibrated measuring device (i.e., a pressure transducer or an aneroid manometer).

        (a) Direct monitoring is **accurate at all pressure ranges,** but it is an **invasive procedure.**

        (b) Arteries available for cannulation include the dorsal pedal, lingual, and femoral arteries.

      (2) Indirect methods of measuring arterial pressure include Doppler ultrasound and oscillometry.

    b. Treatment of intraoperative hypotension may necessitate an increased rate of intravenous crystalloid administration, a reduction in anesthetic depth, and administration of a catecholamine.

      (1) A lower vaporizer setting and the administration of an opioid (e.g., fentanyl, oxymorphone) or nitrous oxide may provide adequate anesthesia with less cardiovascular depression.

      (2) Catecholamines used include ephedrine, dobutamine, and dopamine.

  2. Heart rate. Heart rates vary widely during general anesthesia, depending on the anesthetics administered and the surgical procedure performed.

    a. R-wave monitors measure heart rate by recording the number of waves that exceed a preset millivoltage. R-wave monitors do not display a graphical representation of the electrical activity of the heart.

    b. Oscilloscopes display a real-time graph of the electrical activity of the heart in millivolts as a function of time.

      (1) Oscilloscopes permit differentiation of cardiac dysrhythmias.

      (2) Some oscilloscopes contain a pressure channel and permit connection of a pressure transducer.

  3. Heart and lung sounds. Esophageal and **precordial stethoscopes** are used to auscultate the heart and lungs during surgical procedures.

    a. Esophageal stethoscopes are inserted into the esophagus to the level of the base of the heart.

    b. Some brands of esophageal stethoscopes incorporate electrocardiogram (ECG) leads or a microphone that enables the ECG to be displayed or the heart sounds to be amplified.

III. **POSTOPERATIVE CONSIDERATIONS**

A. **Recovery from anesthesia** occurs when brain concentrations of anesthetic are reduced below a certain level.

1. **Inhalant anesthetics** are eliminated predominately via exhalation.

2. **Lipid-soluble injectable anesthetics** are eliminated via redistribution to other tissues and metabolism.

3. **Hypothermia** is a common cause of prolonged recovery from anesthesia. Warming may be accomplished with the use of circulating warm water blankets, warm water bottles, and administration of warm intravenous fluids.

B. **Extubation and airway management.** Animals are usually extubated as laryngeal reflexes return. Brachycephalic patients may require the endotracheal tube to remain in place after laryngeal reflexes return to maintain a patent airway.

1. **Prior to extubation,** the endotracheal tube cuff should be deflated. Animals that have regurgitated during anesthesia may need to have their laryngeal area evacuated prior to extubation. Suction or swabbing the laryngeal area with gauze removes foreign material and reduces the chance of aspiration following extubation.

2. **Following extubation,** the patient should be closely monitored to detect laryngospasm and subsequent hypoxemia.
   a. If laryngospasm is recognized early, the patient may be reanesthetized using a thiobarbiturate or other rapid-acting intravenous anesthetic, intubated, and ventilated with 100% oxygen.
   b. Administration of corticosteroids and furosemide may decrease swelling and recurrence of spasm.
   c. Tracheostomy may be necessary if laryngospasm persists.

C. **Postoperative analgesia.** Recovery from a surgical procedure often includes administration of an opioid analgesic (Table 2–5).

1. **Timing.** Postoperative administration of opioids should be timed to coincide with extubation, prior to the animal becoming fully conscious. Administration of the opioid prior to extubation may decrease the cough reflex and delay extubation.

TABLE 2–5. Dosages of Opioids Used for Postoperative Analgesia

Agent	Dosage	
	Dog	Cat
Morphine	0.25–0.5 mg/kg, IM, SQ	0.05–0.1 mg/kg, IM, SQ
	0.1 mg/kg in 0.25 ml/0.9% saline/kg, EP	
Oxymorphone	0.025–0.05 mg/kg, IV, IM, SQ	0.025–0.05 mg/kg, IM, SQ
	0.05–0.1 mg/kg in 0.25 ml/ 0.9% saline/kg, EP	
Meperidine	2–6 mg/kg, IM, SQ	2–6 mg/kg, IM, SQ
Fentanyl	2–6 μg/kg, IV	Not recommended for use in cats
Butorphanol	0.1–0.2 mg/kg, IM, SQ	0.1–0.2 mg/kg, IM, SQ
Buprenorphine	5–20 μg/kg, IM, SQ	5–20 μg/kg, IM, SQ

A tranquilizer such as acepromazine (0.025–0.05 mg/kg) may be administered concurrently with the analgesic.
Neuroleptanalgesic combinations may be useful if patient overactivity is undesirable.
EP = epidurally; IM = intramuscularly; IV = intravenously; SQ = subcutaneously.

2. **Administration** of postoperative opioids may be intravenous, intramuscular, or epidural.
   a. **Intravenous.** Small incremental doses of oxymorphone can be given intravenously as the animal regains consciousness.
   b. **Intramuscular.** A calculated dose of opioid is administered intramuscularly at the time of extubation. Opioids administered intramuscularly have an onset time of 15–30 minutes.
   c. **Epidural.** Morphine (0.1 mg/kg diluted with 0.25 ml saline/kg) administered into the lumbosacral epidural space is useful for providing analgesia as far cranially as the thoracic limb for 12–24 hours in dogs.

3. **Additional doses.** Administration of additional opioid is on an as-needed basis. Durations of action are 4–6 hours for morphine, oxymorphone, and butorphanol administered intramuscularly; 1–2 hours for meperidine administered intramuscularly; and 20–30 minutes for fentanyl administered intravenously.

4. **Complications** of systemic postoperative opioid administration include cardiorespiratory depression, increased intracranial pressure, and histamine release.

SELECTED READINGS

Hall LW, Clarke KW: *Veterinary Anaesthesia*, 9th ed. London, Baillière Tindall, 1991.

Hansen BD: Analgesic therapy. *Compendium on Continuing Education for the Practicing Veterinarian* 16:868–874, 1994.

Lemke KA, Tranquilli WJ: Anesthestics, arrhythmias, and myocardial sensitization to epinephrine. *J Am Vet Med Assoc* 205:1679–1684, 1994.

Muir WW, Hubbell JAE, Skarda R, Bednarski RM: *Handbook of Veterinary Anesthesia*. St. Louis, CV Mosby, 1995.

Muir WW, Hubbell JAE: *Equine Anesthesia: Monitoring and Emergency Therapy*. St. Louis, Mosby Year Book, 1991.

Short CE: *Principles and Practice of Veterinary Anesthesia*. Baltimore, Williams & Wilkins, 1987.

Chapter 3

Infection Control

James K. Roush

I. FACTORS IN WOUND INFECTION

A. Contamination

1. **Critical level of bacterial contamination.** All wounds are contaminated when the skin barrier is broken (e.g., when an incision is made); however, achievement of a critical level of bacterial contamination (approximately 10^5 **bacteria/g of tissue**) is necessary before wound infection results. When clotted blood, necrotic tissue, or foreign material is present within a wound, the level of bacterial contamination that will result in infection is lower, because normal body defenses are inhibited.

2. **Wound classification** is **based on the degree of contamination** (Table 3–1).
   a. As the level of contamination increases, the postoperative infection rate increases. Clean wounds usually have a postoperative infection rate of less than 2%.
   b. Wound therapy, cleansing, antibiotic use, and surgical closure or nonclosure are best determined in response to the wound classification.

B. Minimization and prevention of contamination

1. **Examination room.** Prevention of infection begins in the examination room, where care should be taken to prevent contamination of open wounds or body tracts with nosocomial hospital organisms.
   a. Open soft tissue wounds that are bandaged on admission should be left covered until the dressings can be removed in an aseptic manner, the wound cleaned, and a sterile dressing reapplied.
   b. Thermometers, ophthalmoscopes, stethoscopes, and otoscopes used in general examination rooms should be cleaned regularly with suitable disinfectants.

2. **Operating room.** Strategies that minimize the incidence of surgical wound infection include:
   a. **Proper patient preparation and maintenance of a sterile operating room**
   b. **Efficient operative techniques.** Longer operations increase the risk of wound infection.
   c. **Anatomic apposition of tissue** minimizes the available space for collection of wound fluid.

TABLE 3–1. Wound Classification

Classification	Description
Clean	Nontraumatic, surgical wound; no break in aseptic technique; no involvement of the respiratory, alimentary, or genitourinary tracts
Clean-contaminated	Minor break in aseptic technique OR minimal involvement of the respiratory, alimentary, or genitourinary tracts without significant spillage or infection
Contaminated	Major break in aseptic technique OR gross spillage from a hollow organ or infected tract OR a traumatic open wound less than 6 hours old
Dirty	A traumatic wound more than 6 hours old OR transection of "clean" tissues to gain access to an abscess; acute bacterial infection usually encountered

d. Accurate and complete hemostasis decreases the incidence of blood clots and minimizes bacterial growth.
    (1) Judicious use of electrocautery and ligatures is important to decrease the incidence of ischemic tissue within the wound.
    (2) Careful suture selection is necessary to leave the least possible amount of foreign material within the wound and to minimize tissue reaction to suture material.
        (a) Multifilament sutures, particularly nonabsorbables, generally increase the infection rate and should be avoided.
        (b) Monofilament, synthetic sutures (e.g., **nylon** or **polypropylene**) are preferred when it is necessary to bury sutures in tissue because these materials are inert and of a consistent strength.
        (c) Monofilament absorbable sutures (e.g., **polyglyconate** or **polydioxanone**) are acceptable sutures for all tissues except dermis.

II. SURGICAL ASEPSIS

A. Definitions

1. Asepsis refers to the maintenance of a pathogen-free environment on or within living tissue.

2. Sterilization is the elimination of all organisms from animate or inanimate surfaces.

B. Surgical site preparation. Surgical site preparation entails hair removal, skin antisepsis, and proper surgical draping.

1. Hair removal at the surgical site is necessary to enhance the removal of pathogens, increase visibility during skin incision, improve skin apposition during closure, and decrease foreign body deposition within the surgical wound.
    a. Timing. Hair should be removed immediately before surgery, because the incidence of postsurgical wound infections increases as the interval between hair removal and surgery increases. Initial hair removal is performed outside the operating room.
    b. Methods. All current methods of hair removal cause minor trauma to the skin and skin inflammation, followed by bacterial colonization of the skin.
        (1) Clipping, which causes the least skin trauma, is the currently recommended technique of hair removal. Skin trauma can be minimized by using clean, sharp, intact blades.
        (2) Shaving is not recommended because it results in multiple small lacerations and has been associated with increased postoperative wound infection rates.
        (3) Depilatories are not routinely used in veterinary medicine because of their expense and poor action on the coarse hair of animals.
    c. Technique
        (1) The surgical area should be liberally clipped to allow for extension of the incision during surgery. Extension of the incision is occasionally necessary to facilitate the surgical procedure or achieve cosmetic skin closure.
        (2) In preparation for a major orthopedic procedure to be performed on a limb, **the entire limb should be clipped to the dorsal body midline,** and potential graft sites should be prepared simultaneously.
        (3) The areas surrounding open wounds should be covered with saline-moistened gauze sponges or water-soluble gels **to minimize wound contamination with loose hair or debris.**

2. Skin antisepsis
    a. Definitions
        (1) Antiseptics are chemical agents that kill or inhibit the growth of microorganisms in or on living tissue. They are used during preoperative patient prepa-

ration to decrease the overall burden of skin bacteria and eliminate potential pathogens.

   (2) Disinfectants are chemical agents that kill microorganisms on inanimate objects.

   b. **Antiseptic agents** (Table 3–2). The ideal skin antiseptic is a broad-spectrum bactericidal agent that is also effective against spores, viruses, and fungi. ***Staphylococcus, Micrococcus, Streptococcus, Acinetobacter, Clostridium,*** and **gram-negative rods** commonly reside on feline and canine hair and skin surfaces and within dermal and subcutaneous glands.

   (1) Povidone-iodophor compounds (e.g., **povidone-iodine**) are water-soluble complexes of polyvinylpyrrolidone and iodine that allow slow release of the active iodine component. Iodine acts by binding to bacterial cell walls, forming reactive ions and protein complexes.

TABLE 3–2. Antiseptic Agents

Agent	Activity	Residual Activity	Adverse Effects
Povidone-iodine	Bactericidal (kills 99% of bacteria within 30 seconds of application) Sporicidal (with contact times greater than 15 minutes) Fungicidal Effective against viruses and protozoa	Minimal; effectiveness reduced by the presence of organic material (e.g., blood, necrotic debris); inactivated by alcohol	Contact dermatitis; hyperthyroidism; residual staining
Chlorhexidine	Bactericidal (kills 99% of bacteria within 30 seconds of application) Not effective against some *Pseudomonas* species Minimal activity against viruses and spores	Excellent; remains effective in the presence of organic material, alcohol, soaps	Prolonged use may cause photosensitivity or dermatitis (rare)
Aliphatic alcohols	Bactericidal Variable activity against fungi and viruses No activity against spores	Minimal	Repeated use causes skin irritation; application to open wounds causes necrosis
Quaternary ammonium compounds	Slow bactericidal action	Inactivated in the presence of organic material	Neurotoxicity
Hexachlorophene	Bacteriostatic for gram-positive bacteria No activity against gram-negative bacteria and spores; repeated use may favor overgrowth of gram-negative bacteria	Inactivated by organic material and alcohol	Skin ulcerations

(2) Chlorhexidine is a bisdiguanide compound that alters bacterial cell wall permeability and causes precipitation of intracellular contents.

(3) Aliphatic alcohols. Isopropyl alcohol is more effective than **ethyl alcohol,** but isopropyl alcohol is more irritating to the skin. Used alone, alcohols are slightly less effective than chlorhexidine or povidone-iodine, but combinations with either increase the efficacy of alcohol. Alcohols destroy bacterial cell membranes and precipitate intracellular proteins.

(4) Quaternary ammonium compounds (e.g., **benzalkonium chloride**) are cationic surface agents used in the past in antiseptic and disinfectant solutions.

   (a) Nosocomial infection outbreaks have been reported with the sole use of quaternary ammonium compounds.

   (b) Use of these agents is **limited to the cleaning of nonsterile areas.**

   (c) These compounds alter bacterial cell membrane permeability.

(5) Hexachlorophene is a chlorinated phenol derivative. The other antiseptics are more effective; hexachlorophene is **not recommended for use as a preoperative skin antiseptic.** It inhibits bacterial membrane enzyme systems.

c. Technique

(1) Antibacterial detergents are applied using wet gauze sponges.

   (a) Scrubbing is performed in a circular motion, beginning at the incision site and working outward in enlarging concentric circles, ending at the outer margins of the clipped areas. The sponge is replaced with a clean one and the process repeated until visible dirt is absent on discarded sponges.

     (i) If a limb is being prepared, the limb should be suspended (**hanging limb preparation**) so access to the entire circumference is possible without contacting unclipped areas.

     (ii) Gentle pressure is preferable to vigorous scrubbing. Vigorous scrubbing dislodges bacteria from the hair follicles and carries it to the skin surface, where it may colonize abrasions introduced by aggressive scrubbing.

(2) Contamination of the prepared area is avoided while the patient is moved to the operating room. If contamination occurs during transport or positioning, the entire site preparation is repeated.

(3) The surgical scrub is repeated in the operating room. The surgical site is wiped with a **non-detergent antiseptic solution** to complete the preparation.

3. Draping isolates and protects the surgical site from bacteria and debris for the duration of the surgery.

a. Materials. The draping material must remain impermeable and securely fastened to the skin despite moisture or manipulation.

(1) Both **reusable and disposable drapes** are used in veterinary surgery. If reusable drapes are used, they should be well maintained and carefully laundered to avoid enlarging pore size and increasing permeability.

(2) Polyethylene adhesive incise drapes may be useful in surgical procedures where extensive lavage or drainage often moistens drape material. Contrary to early reports, bacterial buildup does not occur beneath the drape during surgery.

(3) Orthopedic stockinettes. Animal paws have a high resident bacterial population; therefore, if access to the paw is not required, it should be covered by impermeable material.

   (a) An orthopedic stockinette is useful to prevent gross contamination of the surgical site, but its barrier properties are often compromised by wetting and manipulation.

   (b) Not using an orthopedic stockinette has not been accompanied by increased risk of surgical infection.

b. Technique. Contamination during surgery decreases with increasing intervening layers of drape material; a minimum of two layers should be used.

(1) The **first layer** isolates a central area containing the proposed incision site. Drapes should be placed at the boundary between clipped and non-clipped skin areas.

(2) The **second layer** is often a single sheet that completely covers the animal and table. An opening in the sheet slightly larger than the anticipated surgical incision should be made to allow access directly to the surgical site.

C. **Equipment preparation**

1. **Sterilization.** All surgical equipment and materials that will come in contact with tissue should be sterilized in suitable fashion, either through **steam** or **chemical** (i.e., **ethylene oxide**) **sterilization.**

2. **Storage**
   a. Sterilized surgical packs should be kept in closed cabinets or shelves to increase shelf life.
      (1) **Muslin packs**
         (a) **Single-wrapped muslin packs** (i.e., two layers of muslin) will keep for 2 days on open shelves, or 1 week in closed cabinets.
         (b) **Double-wrapped muslin packs** (i.e., four layers of muslin) will keep for 3 weeks on open shelves, or 7 weeks in closed cabinets.
      (2) **Crepe paper-wrapped packs** may be kept for 3 weeks on open shelves, or 8 weeks in closed cabinets.
   b. Sterilized surgical packs should be dated and periodically resterilized if unused.

III. **ANTIMICROBIAL PROPHYLAXIS.** Prophylactic antibiotic use during surgical procedures in the absence of existing infection is widely accepted as an important means of reducing the incidence of surgical infection.

A. **Indications** (Table 3–3)

1. **Procedures that carry a high (i.e., greater than 5%) risk of infection.** Risk of infection approximately doubles for each hour the incision is open, so most procedures longer than 2 hours in duration fall under this category.

2. **Procedures where infection would seriously endanger a patient or render the operation unsuccessful**

B. **Selection of antibiotics.** As with all antimicrobial therapy, the choice of antibiotic is dictated by the most likely causative organism. Coagulase-positive *Staphylococcus* and *Escherichia coli* are the bacteria most frequently cultured from wounds in small animal surgical patients; therefore, **cefazolin**, with 99% in vitro activity against *Staphylococcus* and 90% activity against *E. coli,* is the antibiotic of choice for antimicrobial prophylaxis in small animals.

C. **Administration of antibiotics**

1. Prophylactic antibiotics should be administered in a **single dose** to minimize side effects, toxicity, and the development of antimicrobial resistance, and to maximize economic benefits.

TABLE 3–3. Surgical Procedures Requiring Antimicrobial Prophylaxis

High Risk of Infection	Potential for Disastrous Outcome
Comminuted fracture repairs	Total hip prosthesis
Perineal hernia repair	Pacemaker implantation
Esophageal resection	Neurosurgical procedures
Biliary surgery	Hernia repair with nonabsorbable mesh
Rectal or anal surgery	Cortical bone grafts
Colon resection	

2. Prophylactic antibiotics **must attain effective concentrations at the surgical site.**
   a. This requirement necessitates careful agent selection to provide adequate levels of antibiotics in cerebrospinal fluid, the prostate gland, or the urinary bladder.
   b. Intravenous administration provides quick plasma and tissue fluid concentrations of the drug, whereas intramuscular or subcutaneous injection produces sustained levels of the drug.

3. Timing. Antibiotics should be present at the surgical site when the risk of contamination is highest.
   a. Antibiotics do not affect bacteria present in the tissue more than 3 hours before the antibiotic is administered.
   b. There is no evidence that continuing antibiotic therapy for long periods following surgery decreases the incidence of wound infection.
   c. Most frequently, cefazolin (22 mg/kg) is given intravenously at the onset of surgery and repeated intravenously every 2 hours during the operation. Alternatively, oxacillin (22 mg/kg) is used for prophylaxis.

TREATMENT OF WOUND INFECTIONS

A. **Detection of wound infections.** Wound infection should be suspected if any of the following are observed:

1. Redness, swelling, heat, pain, or **discharge** at or during palpation of a surgical incision

2. Decreased appetite, alertness, or **activity**

3. Increased systemic temperature (more than 24 hours postsurgery)

4. Increased white blood cell count

5. Increased serum fibrinogen level

B. **Treatment**

1. Débridement. During and following débridement, infected surgical incisions should be opened to allow access to the wound depth.
   a. All foreign material and necrotic debris should be removed from the wound, until clean, healthy tissue margins are reached.
   b. Infected wounds should not be closed for primary healing, but should be left open to heal by secondary healing, or prepared for delayed closure and second intention healing (see Chapter 4).

2. Lavage. Following removal of necrotic debris, the wound should be copiously irrigated with a sterile, isotonic fluid (e.g., lactated Ringer's solution, normal saline).
   a. **Addition of antiseptics or antibiotics** is unnecessary when an adequate volume of fluid is used. Incorrect concentrations of antiseptics or antibiotics may be detrimental to the wound healing process.
   b. **Volume.** The volume of lavage fluid depends on the degree of contamination and the size of the wound.
      (1) Volumes ranging from 0.5–1.0 L are usually appropriate.
      (2) Gross discoloration and edema of tissues should be avoided.

3. Surgical drains should be placed in wounds that cannot be left open because of position or temperament of the animal. Surgical drains should be used to reduce dead space, hematomas, seromas, or purulence, and the fewest drains possible should be used.
   a. **Selection.** Increasing the number of drain lumina increases the volume of effluent.
   b. **Placement.** The drain should be **placed away from anastomotic sites and major vessels**.
   c. **Exit site.** The drain should **exit through a separate stab incision,** away from the surgical incision.

(1) The drain exit site should be **prepared in an aseptic manner.**
(2) The drain exit should be **covered by sterile bandages** to prevent **premature removal or loss** of the drain and to provide a means of evaluating the nature of the effluent.

d. **Removal.** The drain should be removed **as soon as drainage decreases** or **the character of the effluent changes** from a purulent to a serous discharge.

4. **Antimicrobial therapy**
   a. **Selection of antimicrobial agent**
      (1) **Culture.** Aerobic and anaerobic culture of the wound is the preferred means of selecting a proper antimicrobial agent. Ideally, the wound is cultured both before and after wound débridement and lavage.
         (a) If fungal or unusual organisms are suspected, as in nosocomial infections, special culture procedures (e.g., incubation in broth, dilution in blood culture media) may be required.
         (b) Tissue biopsy may be necessary to isolate the responsible organism. Joint culture, for example, is best accomplished by inoculation of broth media with homogenized synovial tissue.
      (2) **Empirical antimicrobial selection** (Table 3–4) is indicated in **life-threatening infections** that exist or develop while awaiting culture and sensitivity results, and in **minor infections** that do not economically warrant culture and sensitivity testing.
   b. In most instances, animals with existing wound infections are treated initially with **intravenous medication and hospitalization.**
   c. **Duration of therapy** is based on clinical and laboratory parameters.
      (1) A normal temperature for 72 hours, a normal white blood cell count, and absence of drainage from infected sites are indications that therapy can be terminated.
      (2) Most veterinary surgical patients with wound infections are treated for 10–14 days.

5. **Bandaging.** Infected wounds should be maintained during healing under a **sterile bandage** to prevent colonization of the wound by opportunistic or resistant hospital organisms, and to prevent contamination of the environment with the infective agent. The wound should remain bandaged until it is completely covered by epithelium.

TABLE 3–4. Empirical Antibiotic Therapy

Source of Infection	Probable Organism	Effective Antibiotics
Urogenital tract, oral cavity	*Streptococcus*	Penicillins
Skin, urogenital tract, osteomyelitis, discospondylitis	*Staphylococcus*	Amoxicillin–clavulanate, cephalosporins, gentamicin, clindamycin, oxacillin, trimethoprim–sulfamethoxazole
Traumatic wounds, alimentary or urogenital tracts	*Escherichia coli*	Amoxicillin–clavulanate, cefazolin, gentamicin, enrofloxacin, amikacin
Soft-tissue infection in cats, respiratory tract	*Pasteurella*	Amoxicillin, ampicillin, cefazolin, chloramphenicol
Urinary tract, burns	*Pseudomonas*	Ticarcillin, ciprofloxacin
Abscesses, respiratory tract	*Bacteroides fragilis*	Amoxicillin–clavulanate
Urogenital tract	*Proteus*	Amikacin, amoxicillin–clavulanate, cefazolin
Nosocomial, respiratory or alimentary tracts	*Klebsiella*	Amikacin, enrofloxacin, cefazolin

V. **NOSOCOMIAL INFECTIONS** are infections, not present or incubating at the time of admittance, that develop during hospitalization (e.g., all primary surgical wound infections, secondary remote infections caused by the same organism as a surgical wound infection).

A. **Epidemiology**

1. **Pathogens.** Nosocomial pathogens are commonly endogenous patient microflora that cause disease by entering sterile tissue through anatomic, physiologic, or biochemical defects in the host defenses. Bacteria (e.g., *Chlamydia, Mycoplasma, Salmonella, Klebsiella, Serratia marcescens, Clostridium perfringens, Pseudomonas aeruginosa, Pasteurella multocida, E. coli, Enterobacter cloacae, Staphylococcus, Streptococcus*) remain the most common nosocomial pathogens, but other common pathogens include viruses and fungi.

2. **Common veterinary nosocomial infections** include urinary tract infections, respiratory infections, surgical wound infections, and bacteremia associated with intravenous catheters.

3. **Transmission** of nosocomial pathogens occurs through contact between animals, between hospital staff and animals, or through contaminated vehicles.
   a. Contaminated vehicles are unlikely sources of nosocomial pathogen transmission unless there is a disruption of aseptic technique or disinfection or sterilization procedures.
   b. The general environment of a hospitalized animal is probably the least likely cause of nosocomial infection if a clean environment is maintained. Routine cleaning of operating room surfaces reduces bacterial contamination by 60%.

B. **Factors leading to increased risk of nosocomial infection**

1. **Hospital factors** include the duration of the hospital stay and the number of personnel in contact with the animal.

2. **Individual factors** include age extremes (i.e., neonate or geriatric animals), severe chronic illness, immunosuppressive or antimicrobial therapy, and the presence of remote infections.

3. **Invasive procedures and devices** (e.g., **drains, catheters, tubes**) increase susceptibility to infection by transgressing natural host defenses.

C. **Control** of nosocomial infections consists of eliminating the source of infection, interrupting contact spread, and modifying risk factors.

1. **Proper handwashing before and after contact with each animal** is considered the most important measure to prevent nosocomial infections.

2. **Animals with nosocomial infections, immunocompromised animals, or animals that are reservoirs of potential nosocomial organisms** should be isolated.

3. **Surveillance routines** should be established in each facility to recognize infection and identify the agent and infection reservoir. A complete surveillance program provides for recognition of an atypical infectious disease problem, timely identification of the agent, prompt reporting of nosocomial infections, and determination of the endemic level in hospitalized animals.
   a. **Microbial sampling**
      (1) **Periodic microbial sampling** of the hospital environment to monitor the level of contamination is **not cost-effective** and is not recommended.
      (2) **Random microbial sampling** should be limited to investigation of epidemics caused by a single organism.
   b. **Hospital equipment.** For purposes of surveillance, hospital equipment is divided into critical, semicritical, and noncritical categories to determine necessary disinfection levels.
      (1) **Critical items** (i.e., those that are introduced directly into the body) should be

sterilized. Closed system drainage should be used for surgical drains and urinary catheters to prevent luminal contamination by environmental organisms.

   (2) Semicritical items contact mucous membranes and include thermometers, oral and vaginal specula, endotracheal tubes, and stethoscopes.

      (a) Semicritical items should be disinfected in a manner to kill all live organisms.

      (b) Glutaraldehyde, povidone-iodine, and chlorhexidine are acceptable disinfectants for semicritical equipment if fresh solutions are used for disinfection and immediately discarded.

   (3) Noncritical items (e.g., environmental surfaces, clippers) require only routine cleaning.

4. **Proper surgical technique** that includes minimal tissue devitalization, minimal intraoperative time, and avoidance of surgical implants or foreign bodies when possible aids in the control of nosocomial surgical infections.

SELECTED READINGS

Berg J: Sterilization. In *Textbook of Small Animal Surgery*, 2nd ed. Edited by Slatter D. Philadelphia, WB Saunders, 1993, pp 124–129.

Fries CL: Assessment and preparation of the surgical patient. In *Textbook of Small Animal Surgery*, 2nd ed. Edited by Slatter D. Philadelphia, WB Saunders, 1993, pp 137–147.

Harari J: Perioperative antibiotic therapy. In *Surgical Complications and Wound Healing in the Small Animal Practice.* Edited by Harari J. Philadelphia, WB Saunders, 1993, pp 279–305.

Hirsh DC, Jang SS: Antimicrobial susceptibility of selected infectious bacterial agents obtained from dogs. *J Am Anim Hosp* 30:487–494, 1994.

Knecht CD, Allen AR, Williams DJ, Johnson JHP: *Fundamental Techniques in Veterinary Surgery.* Philadelphia, WB Saunders, 1981, pp 74–103.

McCurnin DM, Jones RL: Principles of surgical asepsis. In *Textbook of Small Animal Surgery*, 2nd ed. Edited by Slatter D. Philadelphia, WB Saunders, 1993, pp 114–123.

Riviere JE, Vaden SL: Antimicrobial prophylaxis. In *Disease Mechanisms in Small Animal Surgery*, 2nd ed. Edited by Bojrab JM, Bloomberg MS, Smeak DD. Philadelphia, Lea & Febiger, 1993, pp 66–69.

Rosin E, Dow SW, Daly WR, Petersen SW, Penwick RC: Surgical wound infection and use of antibiotics. In *Textbook of Small Animal Surgery*, 2nd ed. Edited by Slatter D. Philadelphia, WB Saunders, 1993, pp 84–95.

Roush JK: Use and misuse of drains in surgical practice. In *Problems in Veterinary Medicine: Reconstructive Surgery.* Edited by Lindsay WA. Philadelphia, JB Lippincott, 1990, pp 482–493.

Roush JK: Nosocomial infections. In *Surgical Complications and Wound Healing in the Small Animal Practice.* Edited by Harari J. Philadelphia, WB Saunders, 1993, pp 279–292.

Waldron DR: Detection of sepsis in the postoperative patient. In *Surgical Complications and Wound Healing in the Small Animal Practice.* Edited by Harari J. Philadelphia, WB Saunders, 1993, pp 307–318.

Wendelburg K: Surgical wound infection. In *Disease Mechanisms in Small Animal Surgery*, 2nd ed. Edited by Bojrab MJ, Bloomberg MS, Smeak DD. Philadelphia, Lea & Febiger, 1993, pp 54–65.

Chapter 4

Wound Healing

Joseph Harari

I. **INTRODUCTION.** A wound is a disruption of the normal anatomic continuity of an organ.

A. **Wounding is the immediate phase** of injury prior to stimulation of healing processes.

B. **Causes of wounding** include:

   1. Trauma (e.g., vehicular, firearm, animal fight injuries)

   2. Surgery

   3. Noxious physical agents, including:
      a. Excessive heat or cold
      b. Chemicals
      c. Irradiation
      d. Infection
      e. Neoplasia

II. **WOUND HEALING** is the biological restoration of organ structure and function. It is characterized by cellular and metabolic processes that occur in a sequence that is relatively constant. Healing can occur via several pathways.

A. **First intention,** or **primary wound healing,** is closure of the wound by sutures, staples, or tape.

   1. Delayed primary closure is closure of a previously contaminated open wound 3–5 days following injury (before granulation tissue has formed).

   2. During the time interval prior to delayed closure, the wound is kept clean. Lavage solutions and dressings are used to reduce infection and wound dehiscence.

B. **Second intention** wound healing occurs when large cutaneous defects granulate and are allowed to close by epithelialization and contraction without tissue approximation by sutures (Figure 4–1).

   1. Granulation
      a. Granulation tissue develops 4–6 days following injury. It is bright red and granular, and is composed of capillaries, lymph vessels, fibroblasts, and macrophages (see III B).
      b. Granulation tissue serves as a barrier to infection, a bed for epithelialization, and a source of tissue for wound contraction and support.

   2. Epithelialization is the proliferation and migration of epidermal cells across a developing granulation bed.
      a. Epithelialization begins 4–5 days following wounding and may be incomplete or weak (thin) in large wounds.
      b. Invading epithelial cells move under a scab and secrete collagenase, causing the scab to shed.
      c. Epithelialization provides a barrier to wound infection and fluid loss.

   3. Contraction is the reduction of the wound by centripetal movement of the whole thickness of skin.

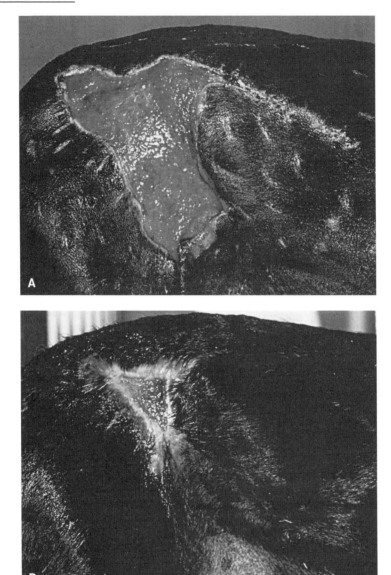

FIGURE 4–1. *(A)* Open wound with a healthy bed of granulation tissue and peripheral reepithelialization. *(B)* Wound contraction 1 month later with reduced exposure of granulation tissue. (Reprinted with permission from Harari J (ed): *Surgical Complications and Wound Healing in the Small Animal Practice.* Philadelphia, WB Saunders, 1993, p 5.)

    a. Contraction begins 5–10 days following wounding and proceeds along lines of skin tension.
    b. Myofibroblasts mediate contraction. These cells have extensive intercellular connections that attach to each other and surrounding tissues.
    c. Large defects may heal with excessive contraction, producing a tight skin that limits limb or body movements.

C. **Third intention** wound healing is secondary wound closure, using sutures or staples, of a healthy granulating wound that is at least 5–6 days old.

    1. In this procedure, the granulation tissue is excised and closure performed; alternatively, the epithelial margins can be freshened and sutured over the granulation tissue.

2. These wounds may heal more rapidly and gain tensile strength faster than primary-closed wounds because of the immediate reparative response characterized by tissue proliferation and collagen synthesis (see III B). The inflammation stage has already occurred before third intention wound healing begins.

III. PHASES OF WOUND HEALING

A. **Inflammation** occurs within minutes of wounding and is termed the **lag phase,** or **substrate phase.** It lasts for 1–3 days in uninfected wounds.

1. Classic signs include the following:
  a. Redness **(rubor)**
  b. Swelling **(tumor)**
  c. Pain **(dolor)**
  d. Heat **(calor)**
  e. Loss of function **(functio laesa)**

2. Process
  a. Initial vasoconstriction is followed by vasodilation and subsequent vascular fluid leakage. This is initiated by the release of chemical mediators (histamine, serotonin, prostaglandins) by mast cells and platelets.
  b. Neutrophils and monocytes migrate into the wound for phagocytosis and enzymatic destruction of tissue debris.
  c. Macrophages release chemotactic substances responsible for fibroplasia, angiogenesis, and collagen synthesis.

3. Wound strength during inflammation is minimal and dehiscence is prevented by sutures or staples.

B. The **repair phase,** or **proliferative phase,** begins on the third or fourth day following wounding and lasts 1–3 weeks. It is characterized by fibroblast proliferation, capillary infiltration, and reepithelialization.

1. Fibroblasts originate from undifferentiated mesenchymal cells in surrounding connective tissue and migrate into the wound along fibrin clot fibers and ingrowing capillaries.
  a. Fibroblasts produce the wound's amorphous ground substance and collagen, which is responsible for wound tensile strength.
  b. Cellular activity and collagen synthesis diminish at the end of the reparative phase, as wound maturation and remodeling begin.

2. Capillary infiltration and branching occur secondary to reduced oxygen tension in the wound and are necessary for fibroblastic activity.

3. Epithelial proliferation and migration begin at the wound margins. These processes are affected by inhibition resulting from cell-to-cell contact, oxygenation, temperature, and contact with dressings.

C. The **maturation phase,** or **remodeling phase,** develops 3 weeks following injury and lasts months to years.

1. This phase is characterized by a stable wound collagen content. Wound strength increases because of cross-linking of collagen fibers and a change in the physical weave of the fibers. They become less densely packed as the wound matures, and there is a loose basket-weave arrangement with fibers deposited along lines of stress.

2. The scar tissue that develops lacks the strength of surrounding normal tissue. It con-

sists of fewer cells than are present in earlier stages of repair, vessels and elastic fibers, and a dense collagen network.

IV. FACTORS AFFECTING WOUND HEALING

A. Local factors

1. **Vascularity** provides tissue oxygenation and nutrients that augment wound healing
   by promoting local cellular metabolism and collagen cross-linking.

2. **Foreign material,** such as soil, debris, or nonabsorbable braided suture material, delays healing by exacerbating the inflammatory response and inciting infection.

3. **Dead space and fluid accumulation** delay healing by limiting migration of reparative
   cells and increasing the risk of infection.

4. Exposure to **ionizing radiation** within 2 weeks of surgery retards wound healing by
   decreasing fibroblast formation, collagen synthesis, and capillary regeneration.

5. **Bacterial wound infection** may impede healing owing to persistence of inflammation, tissue necrosis, and accumulation of fluids. Bacterial infection also delays reparative processes, especially fibroplasia and collagen synthesis (see Chapter 3).

6. **Topical medications and dressings** can promote wound healing by reducing bacterial
   infection and protecting healing tissues.
   a. Lavage with sterile isotonic solutions (saline, lactated Ringer's) aids healing by me-
      chanically reducing contamination and bacterial infection.
   b. Lavage with dilute antimicrobial solutions (0.05% chlorhexidine, 0.1% povidone-
      iodine) promotes healing by reducing bacterial contamination.
   c. Nonadherent, moist dressings promote epithelialization. Adherent gauze dressings
      are useful for mechanical débridement of contaminated wounds.
   d. Antibacterial ointments (e.g., bacitracin-neomycin-polymixin, silver sulfadiazine,
      chlorhexidine, nitrofurazone) may be useful in reducing the bacterial content of
      contaminated wounds.

7. **Surgical technique** can directly promote wound healing if **Halsted's principles** are followed:
   a. Gentle tissue handling
   b. Accurate hemostasis and preservation of blood supply to tissues
   c. Aseptic surgical technique
   d. Careful tissue approximation without tension and with obliteration of dead space
   e. Removal of necrotic tissue

B. Systemic factors

1. **Hypoproteinemia** caused by protein loss, malnutrition, or fluid overload slows healing by delaying fibroplasia, decreasing wound tensile strength, and producing
   edema.

2. **Uremia** depresses granulation tissue formation, epithelial proliferation, and wound
   strength.

3. **Long-term, high doses of corticosteroids** inhibit the inflammatory phase and decrease collagen synthesis.

4. **Chemotherapeutic agents** may delay wound healing.
   a. They act directly by inhibiting cell division (reparative phase) or collagen synthe-
      sis (maturation phase).
   b. They can delay healing indirectly by depressing immune function, epithelializa-
      tion and contraction, and by causing anorexia.

5. **Vitamin and mineral imbalances** affect wound healing.

    a. High doses of **vitamin A** reverse corticosteroid inhibition of wound healing and stimulate fibroplasia and collagen synthesis.

    b. Excessive doses of **vitamin E** impair wound healing and collagen production.

    c. **Vitamin C** is needed for hydroxylation of the lysine and proline moieties of collagen; a deficiency delays wound healing and reduces wound strength.

    d. **Zinc** deficiency may impair granulation tissue formation and delay healing by inhibiting epithelial and fibroblastic cellular proliferation.

6. **Advanced age** slows healing. In experimental cases, epithelialization rates and wound strength decreased in old animals as compared to young animals.

7. A **malignancy** elsewhere in the body impairs wound healing by producing cachexia, altering metabolism, and reducing inflammatory cell function.

8. In people, **uncontrolled diabetes** delays healing. Hyperglycemia impairs collagen synthesis, vascular ingrowth, and granulocyte cell functions. These effects may occur in animals, as well.

V. ABNORMAL WOUND HEALING

A. **Wound dehiscence** is the splitting and separation of previously closed wound layers. **Evisceration** is protrusion of viscera through the wound. **Eventration** is protrusion of the bowels from the abdomen.

1. **Causes** include improper surgical technique, and the local and systemic factors described in IV A–B.

2. **Signs** include incisional swelling, discoloration, necrosis, and a serosanguineous discharge. Dehiscence usually occurs 3–5 days after surgery, before collagen deposition increases wound tensile strength.

3. **Treatment** depends on the severity and cause of the lesion.
    a. **Wound closure**
        (1) Wound closure can be primary if infection is controlled.
        (2) Second intention healing takes place in small dehiscences that close on their own with no complications.
        (3) Third intention healing is necessary for large defects that need skin coverage over pressure points, or to avoid excessive contraction.
        (4) In contaminated (open) wounds, nonreactive, absorbable or nonabsorbable monofilament sutures should be used to maintain wound strength and reduce infection.
    b. **Wound management** includes lavage to reduce contamination and sterile dressings or bandages for protection and support.
    c. **Wound drainage** is performed using Penrose drains, plastic or rubber tubes, or open drainage with bandage support. The goal is to reduce fluid accumulation and dead space.

B. **Treatment of delayed or nonhealing wounds** requires accurate identification of the predisposing causes, and appropriate local or systemic therapies.

1. These wounds may require **tension-relieving incisions** and, in lesions with an adequate granulation tissue bed, **second or third intention healing.**

2. **Promotion of a viable granulation bed** is performed by reducing infection, removing necrotic tissue, draining excessive tissue fluid, and protecting healing tissues.

3. **Skin grafts** are useful in promoting healing of delayed or nonhealing wounds.
    a. **Pedicle grafts** are skin flaps with subcutaneous tissue and an intact vascular supply that are transferred either to a neighboring region or to an extremity far from the donor site.
    b. **Free skin grafts** are full or split thicknesses of skin transferred to another body

site. These grafts can be pinch, strip, stamp mesh, or sheet grafts, depending on the shape of the donor tissue.

4. Wound healing stimulators such as transforming growth factor-β (TGF-β), platelet-derived growth factor (PDGF), and epidermal growth factor (EGF) have been used successfully in experimental trials. They may be useful for clinical patients in the future.

SELECTED READINGS

Cohen IK, Diegelmann RF, Lindblad WJ (eds): *Wound Healing. Biochemical and Clinical Aspects.* Philadelphia, WB Saunders, 1992.

Dernell WS, Wheaton LG: Surgical management of radiation injury. *Comp Cont Educ Pract Vet* 17:181–187, 1995.

Fitch RB, Swaim SF: The role of epitheliazation in wound healing. *Comp Cont Educ Pract Vet* 17:167–177, 1995.

Harari J (ed): *Surgical Complications and Wound Healing in the Small Animal Practice.* Philadelphia, WB Saunders, 1993, pp 1–32, 125–142.

Hosgood G: Wound healing. The role of platelet-derived growth factor and transforming growth factor beta. *Vet Surg* 22:490–495, 1993.

Pavletic MM: *Atlas of Small Animal Reconstructive Surgery.* Philadelphia, JB Lippincott, 1993.

Pope ER (ed): Wound healing. *Semin Vet Med* 4:255–320, 1989.

Probst CW: Wound healing and specific tissue regeneration. In *Textbook of Small Animal Surgery,* 2nd ed. Edited by Slatter D. Philadelphia, WB Saunders, 1993, pp 53–62.

Swaim SF, Henderson RA: *Small Animal Wound Management.* Philadelphia, Lea & Febiger, 1990.

Chapter 5

Nutritional Support of Surgical Patients

Candace E. Layton

I. **INTRODUCTION.** Malnutrition is a significant problem in the surgical patient. Although the exact prevalence of malnutrition in veterinary patients is not known, in people the incidence of malnutrition has been reported to be as high as 50% of hospitalized patients.

A. **Patient assessment**

1. **Goals of assessment**
   a. Identification of animals that are malnourished or are likely to become malnourished
   b. Evaluation of the response to nutritional support

2. **Methods of assessment.** Because of the complex relationship between the nutritive state and disease, no single parameter or test can reliably evaluate nutritional status or response to nutritional support.
   a. **Patient history and physical examination** are the most valid means of assessing nutritional status (Table 5–1).
   b. The **animal's attitude** and **appetite** and **normalization of systemic signs** are good indicators of response to a nutritional protocol. Body weight gain is an insensitive indicator.

B. **Consequences of malnutrition**

1. **General systemic effects**
   a. **Cardiac function.** Protein-calorie malnutrition decreases contractility. With adaptation to food deprivation, there is a decrease in the use of lactic acid as an energy source.
   b. **Pulmonary function.** The response to hypoxia decreases and changes in acid–base status occur, decreasing pulmonary function.
   c. **Gastrointestinal function.** Blunting of the intestinal villi reduces the gastrointestinal mass, leading to malabsorption, diarrhea, and bacterial translocation.
   d. **Renal function.** Renal mass usually does not decrease, but response to acid–base abnormalities is impaired.
   e. **Muscle strength** rapidly diminishes because of increased muscle catabolism and decreased synthesis of muscle protein.

2. **Effects of malnutrition in surgical patients**
   a. **Wound healing** is impaired. In malnourished animals, wound tensile strength is decreased, and postoperative wound infection and wound dehiscence rates are increased.
      (1) **Protein** needed for the **inflammatory response and wound healing** is utilized instead for energy. **Callus production and fracture healing** are decreased with limited protein-calorie intake.
      (2) **Energy** is required by fibroblasts and epithelial cells for migration to the wound and for ribonucleic acid (RNA), deoxyribonucleic acid (DNA), and protein synthesis.
      (3) **Amino acids and carbohydrates** are required for collagen and ground substance production.
   b. **Immunity.** The relationship between nutrition and immunity is complex. Because the immune system is composed of a large population of metabolically active cells with an increased rate of cell division and synthesis, it is in continuous demand of energy and protein.

Table 5–1. Guidelines for Nutritional Assessment

Historical evidence
  Vomiting
  Diarrhea
  Chronic draining wounds
  Catabolic drugs (e.g., steroids, chemotherapeutic drugs)
  Anorexia
    > 1–2 days in young animals
    > 4–5 days in adult animals
  Anticipated causes (e.g., surgical resection, neurologic problems, postoperative infections, or ileus)
Physical examination
  Depression
  Lack of body fat
  Muscle wasting
  Dull, dry haircoat
  Structural impediments (e.g., fractured jaw)
  Weight loss
    > 10% in adult animals
    > 5% in young animals
Laboratory parameters
  Lymphopenia
    < 1000/μl in dogs
    < 1500/μl in cats
  Hypoalbuminemia, < 2.5 mg/dl

Reprinted with permission from Layton CE: Nutritional support of the surgical patient. In *Surgical Complications and Wound Healing in the Small Animal Practice.* Edited by Harari J. Philadelphia, WB Saunders, 1993, p 96.

(1) Effects of nutrients on immunity. Compromise of the immune system persists for a period of time after the nutritional imbalance has been corrected.
  (a) Protein deficiencies produce immunodeficiencies.
    (i) Immunoglobulins, lymphokines, and **bacterial enzymes** are composed of protein.
    (ii) Cell-mediated and **humoral immune responses** are blunted. Amino acid imbalances can depress cellular and humoral immune responses.
  (b) Fatty acid imbalances affect the immune system.
    (i) Omega-6 fatty acids (long-chain fatty acids) have been shown to be immunosuppressive.
    (ii) Omega-3 fatty acids (found in fish oils or derived from linolenic acid) are less immunosuppressive.
(2) Effects of body weight on immunity
  (a) Caloric restriction has variable effects on immunity.
    (i) Mild caloric restriction may be beneficial in preventing disease. However, in patients undergoing significant stress (e.g., disease, trauma, or surgery), nutritional support is needed to improve the immune state.
    (ii) Moderate caloric restriction may improve life span and delay the normal aging of the immune system.
    (iii) Extreme caloric restriction. Immune response seems to be preserved until the animal's weight decreases **below 60% of the ideal weight.** Decreased complement proteins, decreased immunoglobulins, and delayed hypersensitivity response occur in extremely underweight animals.
  (b) Obese animals have decreased cutaneous-delayed hypersensitivity reac-

tions, decreased neutrophil bactericidal capacity, and impaired cell-mediated immunity.

II. METABOLIC CHANGES ASSOCIATED WITH STARVATION

A. **"Simple" starvation.** The overall effect of simple starvation (i.e., starvation without the stress of disease or surgery) is reduction of the basal metabolic rate, conservation of reproductive capability, and utilization of fats and protein as an energy source.

1. **Visceral protein** (e.g., albumin, transthyretin, retinol-binding protein) **is conserved** and lipolysis takes place; most tissues convert to using ketones as an energy source.

2. **Plasma insulin decreases.**

B. **Starvation complicated by the stress of disease or surgery** contributes to a **hypermetabolic state.**

1. **General metabolic changes**
   a. **Glycogen stores are depleted** in 24–48 hours.
   b. **Insulin resistance** and **glucose intolerance** develop.
   c. **Plasma levels** of insulin, growth hormones, catecholamines, glucocorticoids, glucagon, antidiuretic hormone, and aldosterone increase. These hormones contribute to an increase in the metabolic rate, stress diabetes mellitus, and a negative nitrogen balance.
   d. Energy needs, protein losses (e.g., via exudates, enteropathy, nephropathy), decreased protein production, and requirements for wound healing and the inflammatory reaction **increase the body's demand for protein.**
      (1) **Visceral protein is rapidly depleted.**
      (2) **Catabolism of skeletal muscle and skin proteins** increases to supply amino acids for gluconeogenesis.
         (a) Fat stores are not mobilized and used effectively for energy in sepsis and other hypermetabolic states.
         (b) Muscle-derived gluconeogenesis continues in animals or people with sepsis or severe trauma, even with supplementation of exogenous protein and calories.

2. **Metabolic changes associated with cancer.** Cancer causes metabolic derangements of fats, carbohydrates, and proteins.
   a. **Carbohydrate metabolism.** Tumor cells metabolize carbohydrates (instead of fat or proteins) via anaerobic pathways that are inefficient, produce lactic acid, and operate at an energy deficit for the patient.
      (1) The lactate is transported to the liver and converted to glucose via the Cori cycle.
      (2) Instead of producing approximately 38 millimoles of adenosine triphosphate (ATP) as with normal glycolysis, the Cori cycle produces only 2 millimoles of ATP. Conversion of lactic acid to glucose requires additional energy from the host.
      (3) In cancer and cachexia, glucose tolerance tests reveal insulin resistance, which affects carbohydrate metabolism.
   b. **Protein metabolism** may be impaired, leading to altered protein synthesis and catabolism and changes in whole body protein turnover rates, plasma amino acids, and liver protein metabolism.
   c. Nutritional support in cancer patients raises the concern about increasing the rate of tumor growth or metastasis, although there is **no clear evidence that nutritional support positively affects tumor growth.** In general, nutritional support benefits cancer patients by improving the quality of life, permitting completion of therapeutic protocols, and decreasing the duration of hospitalization.

III. DIETARY REQUIREMENTS

A. **Energy requirements** are not directly related to body weight—they may be affected by body temperature, status of reproduction and growth, state of health, or even breed. It is important to monitor the animal's response to the protocol and make adjustments based on clinical evaluations.

1. The **resting energy requirement (RER)** is the energy required by a dog or cat, in a postabsorptive phase, resting quietly in a thermoneutral environment. The term is often used interchangeably with "basal energy requirement" and "basal metabolic rate;" however, there are subtle differences. The RER of a healthy animal is approximately 60–80 kcal/kg/day; controversy exists as to which formula, linear or allometric, more accurately predicts the energy requirements for dogs and cats.

   a. **Allometric formula:** $RER = 70 \times (BW^{0.75})$, where

   $$RER = \text{resting energy requirement (in kcal/day)}$$

   $$BW = \text{body weight (in kg)}$$

   b. **Linear formula:** $RER = 30 \times BW + 70$. This formula may only be used for dogs weighing between 2 and 45 kg.

2. The **maintenance energy requirement (MER)** is the energy required by a dog or cat performing a normal level of activity in a thermoneutral environment. MER requirements are increased in growing or lactating animals.
   a. **Dogs.** In dogs, the **MER = 2 × RER.** Active work dogs may have requirements 2–3 times greater than average.
   b. **Cats.** In cats, the **MER = 1.4 × RER.** Because of the uniform size of most cats, a standard formula of 80 kcal/kg body weight (for an active cat) or 70 kcal/kg body weight (for an inactive cat) can also be used.

3. The **illness energy requirement (IER)** is the energy required by an animal with a disease or injury. The IER equals the RER multiplied by a mathematical factor that represents a subjective assessment of the severity of the disease or injury.
   a. These factors generally range from 1.25–2 (Table 5–2).
   b. Because of the degree of inactivity imposed by hospitalization and disease, it is rare for the IER to exceed the MER. Only with problems such as severe burn, sepsis, or head trauma do energy requirements increase to almost twice the RER.

4. **Food dose**
   a. The food dose is calculated by dividing the caloric requirement of the patient (in kcal/day) by the energy density of the food (in kcal/ml). The volume of food is then divided by the number of feedings to get the volume per feeding.
   b. With animals that have been anorectic, feeding is started at one quarter to one

Table 5–2. Illness Energy Requirement Factors for Dogs and Cats

Status	Mathematical Factor
Cage rest	1.25
Postsurgery	1.25–1.35
Trauma	1.35–1.5
Cancer	1.35–1.5
Sepsis	1.5–1.7
Major burn	1.7–2.0

Adapted with permission from Layton CE: Nutritional support of the surgical patient. In *Surgical Complications and Wound Healing in the Small Animal Practice.* Edited by Harari J. Philadelphia, WB Saunders, 1993, p 114.

third of the total calories and gradually increased over 3–5 days to the total amount.

B. **Water requirements** are often met because food contains a high percentage of water. Additional fluids can be given intravenously if necessary.

C. **Protein requirements.** The exact protein requirement in critically ill dogs and cats is not known but is influenced by the disease, trauma, the type of condition (chronic or acute), and situations of increased loss (e.g., burns, sepsis, fever) or increased use (e.g., wound healing, fracture repair). Most critical care diets have high levels of protein.

1. **Minimum protein requirements**
   a. **Dogs.** The minimum protein requirement in dogs is 4 g/100 kcal of metabolizable energy (i.e., approximately 16% of the energy requirement).
      (1) Protein intake should be **increased in critically ill dogs** to 6–8 g/100 kcal metabolizable energy.
      (2) Protein intake should be **decreased in dogs with hepatic or renal failure** to 2–3 g/100 kcal metabolizable energy.
   b. **Cats.** The minimum protein requirement in cats is 6 g/100 kcal metabolizable energy (i.e., approximately 24% of the energy requirement). Cats require more protein than dogs because they use protein as an energy source.
      (1) Protein should be **increased in critically ill cats** to 9 g/100 kcal metabolizable energy.
      (2) Protein should be **decreased in cats with hepatic or renal failure** to 4 g/100 kcal metabolizable energy.

2. **Protein supplementation** may be needed in some dogs or cats with severe protein loss or excessive protein needs, especially if the diet is a human-based product.

3. **Amino acid supplementation.** Critical care patients may need specific amino acids.
   a. **Glutamine**
      (1) Glutamine is the preferred fuel for enterocytes and colonocytes during catabolic illness.
      (2) It is an energy source for immunologically active cells and other rapidly proliferating tissues such as fibroblasts.
      (3) It is important in renal acid–base homeostasis because it acts as an ammonia donor for the excretion of hydrogen ions.
   b. **Arginine** is an essential amino acid in dogs and cats.
      (1) Supplementation may augment wound healing, enhance immune function, and increase nitrogen retention.
      (2) Arginine is a secretagogue for growth hormone, prolactin, insulin, and glucagon.
      (3) Arginine is a major source of nitrous and nitric oxides, which play a role in electron transport in hepatic mitochondria, hepatic protein synthesis, and vascular dilation.
   c. **Leucine, isoleucine,** and **valine** (branched-chain amino acids) are preferentially utilized by critically ill patients; supplementation may improve nitrogen retention.
   d. **Taurine** is an essential amino acid in cats and supplementation is necessary, especially if diets formulated for humans are being used for extended periods of time (i.e., longer than 1 week).

D. **Lipid requirements.** Critically ill animals have an increased need for fat. The recommended fat content of diets for critically ill animals ranges from 35%–50% of the energy requirement.

1. **Composition.** Dietary fat (lipid) is composed of triglyceride subunits with sterols and phospholipids. **Medium-chain triglycerides** are the most easily digested. In addition, they are absorbed relatively independently of the influence of pancreatic lipase, bile salts, and enterocyte transformation.

2. **Functions**
   a. Fats **provide concentrated energy** (2.25 times the kilocalories on a dry matter

basis as protein or carbohydrate). Increasing the fat content increases the calorie density of the diet.

    b. Fats are a **source of essential fatty acids** (linoleic acid in dogs, and both linoleic and arachidonic acid in cats). These fatty acids are precursors for prostaglandins and leukotrienes, and they preserve the functional integrity of cell membranes.

E. **Dietary fiber requirements.** Dietary fiber may play an important role in the management of critical care patients.

    1. Source
        a. **Insoluble fiber** (e.g., cellulose, hemicellulose, pectin, lignin) usually comes from plant cell walls.
        b. **Soluble fiber** (e.g., gums, mucilages) comes from intracellular polysaccharides.

    2. Function. Fiber helps normalize intestinal motility and may improve the normal bacterial colonization of the colon.

F. **Carbohydrate requirements.** Carbohydrate levels for critically ill dogs and cats are minimal; the majority of the calories are supplied as proteins and fats.

    1. Sources
        a. Carbohydrates are **polysaccharides** (starch, cellulose), **disaccharides** (lactose, sucrose), and **monosaccharides** (glucose, fructose).
        b. **Gluconeogenesis** takes place in the liver, utilizing lactate and alanine as substrates.

    2. Function. Glucose is an essential energy source for the central nervous system (CNS), red and white blood cells, and the renal medulla. During starvation, some adaptation occurs for utilization of ketones as an energy source.

IV. ENTERIC FEEDING

A. **Introduction.** Generally the simplest, least invasive route or technique is tried first. If possible, the digestive tract should be used because it is physiologic for the patient. Even patients with vomiting and diarrhea can benefit from appropriately administered enteric feedings.

    1. Advantages
        a. **Enteric** feeding is **safer, easier, less expensive,** and **more physiologic** than parenteral feeding (see V).
        b. Experimentally, enteral feeding has **improved wound healing** and **tensile strength of intestinal anastomoses.**

    2. Contraindications for enteral feeding are **intractable vomiting** and **intestinal obstruction.** Diarrhea, even that resulting from malabsorption, is not necessarily a contraindication.
        a. **Continuous infusion or frequent, small, bolus feedings** may allow enteral feeding even in animals with vomiting or diarrhea.
        b. **Partial parenteral nutrition** can be used as a supplement if enteral feeding does not meet all of the animal's nutritional needs.

B. **Methods**

    1. Stimulation of appetite. Merely getting an animal to start eating may be all that is required to overcome its anorexia.
        a. **Force feeding** or **orogastric intubation** requires a docile animal. These techniques can only be used effectively for a few feedings.
        b. **Drugs** used to stimulate appetite in dogs and cats include the following.
            (1) **Benzodiazepine derivatives** (e.g., diazepam, oxazepam) affect the appetite

center in the hypothalamus by increasing levels of the neurotransmitter γ-aminobutyric acid (GABA), which blocks serotonin.

   (a) Intravenous administration is more effective than oral or intramuscular administration. This effectiveness tends to decrease with repeated administration.

   (b) Appetite stimulation following intravenous administration occurs within minutes and lasts for a variable amount of time; therefore, it is important to feed a protein- and calorie-dense diet because only small volumes of food are consumed.

  (2) Corticosteroids are often prescribed to stimulate appetite, although their action is variable. Negative effects of corticosteroids include increased catabolism and breakdown of protein and fats, and depression of the immune and inflammatory response.

  (3) Anabolic steroids (e.g., stanozolol) may be beneficial in reversing some of the catabolic effects of disease, surgery, or trauma. The improvement in nitrogen balance results from an increase in appetite, rather than an altered metabolism.

  (4) B vitamins have been given empirically to improve appetite, especially in cats.

2. Nasoesophageal feeding tube. This method of feeding involves placement of a small-bore tube through the nasal passage, terminating at the caudal aspect of the esophagus to prevent gastroesophageal reflux and esophagitis.

  a. Advantages

   (1) Tube placement does not require general anesthesia of the patient.

   (2) Nasoesophageal feeding tubes are generally well tolerated and can be used for outpatients because intubation is not an invasive surgical procedure.

  b. Disadvantages

   (1) The technique limits the animal to a liquid diet and is only appropriate for short-term nutritional support (i.e., support lasting less than 1 week).

   (2) Complications associated with nasoesophageal tubes include rhinitis, regurgitation, vomiting, and nutrient pneumonia caused by aspiration or incorrect tube placement.

  c. Contraindications. A nasoesophageal feeding tube cannot be used in comatose animals or animals with a depressed gag reflex.

  d. Technique

   (1) Sizes of tubes range from $3\frac{1}{2}$- to 8-French; small, flexible tubes are best tolerated.

   (2) The distance from the tip of the nose to the eleventh rib (in dogs) or the seventh rib (in cats) is measured to determine the length of the tube.

   (3) Several drops of a local anesthetic (e.g., 2% lidocaine) are placed into the animal's nose.

   (4) With the patient's head in a neutral position, the lubricated tube is directed into the nose in a caudoventral and medial manner.

    (a) Some animals will salivate, sneeze, or violently shake their heads during tube insertion. **Gentle, slow advancement** can help eliminate these problems.

    (b) Tubes are available with stylets that make placement easier. Alternatively, angiography guidewires may be used. Use of a stylet or guidewire may increase the chances of nasal trauma or inadvertent intratracheal placement.

   (5) The tube is secured to the animal's nose using sutures or glue, and an Elizabethan collar is placed on the patient to prevent self-trauma.

   (6) Verification of tube location (using radiography or saline injection) is imperative, because it is relatively easy to pass small-bore tubes into the trachea with little objection from some animals.

  e. Feeding. Commercial liquid diets are usually used instead of blenderized pet foods because of the small bore size of the tube.

   (1) The preparation is administered by slow bolus several times a day or by continuous infusion.

(2) Flushing of the feeding tube before and after use is necessary to avoid obstruction of the tube by dried food.

3. Pharyngostomy feeding tube. This method of feeding is characterized by the percutaneous placement of a feeding tube through the pharyngeal wall. The tube is then directed over the glottis and into the esophagus.
   a. Advantages
   (1) A large-bone tube can be used, so that blenderized pet foods or gruels may be fed to the animal.
   (2) The tube can be left in place for 2–3 weeks and managed as an outpatient condition.
   b. Disadvantages
   (1) General anesthesia and surgical placement of the tube are required.
   (2) **Complications** such as **cellulitis** or **aspiration pneumonia** resulting from improper placement of the tube can occur; for this reason, some surgeons prefer other techniques, such as gastrostomy or esophagostomy. Other complications include **esophagitis** and **regurgitation.**

4. Esophagostomy feeding tube. This method of feeding involves the percutaneous placement of a feeding tube (either surgically or with a needle catheter) through the cranial cervical area directly into the esophagus. The tube, like the nasoesophageal tube, ends in the caudal esophagus.
   a. Advantages
   (1) If surgical placement is used, tubes with a relatively larger bore than those used for nasoesophageal feeding can be used.
   (2) The technique bypasses the pharynx and glottis; therefore, it lessens the risk of aspiration and airway obstruction disorders.
   (3) An esophageal feeding tube can be used for 1–4 weeks on an outpatient basis.
   b. Disadvantages
   (1) Placement of the tube requires heavy sedation or general anesthesia.
   (2) The needle catheter technique is less traumatic than the surgical technique, but the small size of the catheter limits feeding to liquid diets; kinking and obstruction of the catheter are common.
   (3) **Complications** include esophageal stricture, esophagitis, and local infection.
   c. Technique
   (1) The cranial cervical area is clipped and surgically prepared. A large-bore needle (10- to 14-gauge) is used as a guide for the smaller feeding catheter. Alternatively, a surgical cutdown can be made directly over the tip of a small, curved forceps, allowing placement of a larger feeding tube.
   (2) After passing the needle through the cervical skin, through the subcutaneous tissue, and into the cranial esophagus, the premeasured catheter is threaded into the caudal aspect of the esophagus.
   (3) The tube is capped and bandaged, and the stoma is cleaned to prevent infection.
   (4) When the tube is no longer needed, it is removed and the stoma is allowed to heal by second intention.

5. Gastrostomy feeding tubes are placed into the stomach surgically, endoscopically, or blindly. Gastrostomy tubes can be used in animals with esophageal disease, regurgitation, a depressed gag reflex, or occasional vomiting; however, there may be more potential for aspiration in these animals.
   a. Advantages
   (1) Gastrostomy feeding tubes permit long-term treatment (e.g., for several months).
   (2) The large tube is well tolerated by patients.
   b. Disadvantages include the need for general anesthesia, a risk of leakage around the tube and subsequent peritonitis, and if a flange is used to secure the tube to the stomach and abdominal wall, necrosis around the tube with subsequent tube dislodgment.

c. Techniques
   (1) Surgical gastrostomy is done during abdominal exploratory surgery, or as a separate surgical procedure.
      (a) A purse-string suture is placed in the fundus (body) of the stomach.
         (i) The feeding tube (a Foley or Pezzer urologic catheter) is passed into the stomach through the abdominal wall and through a stab incision centered in the purse-string suture.
         (ii) Tightening the purse-string suture everts the layer of tissue around the tube, forming a "tunnel" that minimizes leakage.
      (b) The gastrostomy site is secured to the body wall with sutures. Leakage around the tube can be further limited by placing omentum around the tube.
      (c) The feeding tube is secured to the skin and the exit site bandaged.
   (2) Endoscopic percutaneous gastrostomy uses an endoscope and biopsy forceps to position a mushroom-tipped feeding catheter.
      (a) An endoscope is passed into the stomach and the stomach is inflated with gas. A suture leader is passed through a catheter placed percutaneously into the stomach, and biopsy forceps are used to grasp the end of the suture leader and draw it through the mouth.
      (b) Next, the leader is attached to the distal end of a mushroom-tipped catheter. The free end of the suture leader is pulled back to pull the feeding tube through the mouth, into the stomach, and out through the abdominal wall.
   (3) Blind percutaneous gastrostomy involves passage of a large orogastric tube to a level where the end can be palpated through the abdominal wall.
      (a) A needle or catheter guide is used to puncture the abdominal wall and enter the lumen of the orogastric tube. A guidewire (with suture attached) is passed into the orogastric tube until the wire passes out of the mouth.
      (b) The guidewire is withdrawn until the suture is visible. The end of a mushroom-tipped catheter is tied to the suture (as with the endoscopic technique) and the suture is retracted, drawing the catheter into the stomach and through the abdominal wall.

6. Enterostomy feeding tubes are small-bore feeding tubes placed surgically into the duodenum or jejunum. A variety of tubes can be used, including commercial human enterostomy tubes, red rubber urinary catheters, polyurethane urinary or feeding tubes, and intravenous jugular catheters.
   a. Advantages. Enterostomy is indicated for animals with obstruction or dysfunction at any point along the gastrointestinal tract, up to and including the stomach.
      (1) Enterostomy feeding tubes are well tolerated by animals with a depressed gag reflex, esophageal motility disorders, or those who are comatose or recumbent.
      (2) The small bowel generally retains normal peristalsis postoperatively while the stomach is hypoperistaltic.
      (3) Enterostomy feeding can be initiated immediately after surgery, which may help normalize bowel motility and maintain a positive nitrogen balance.
   b. Disadvantages
      (1) The small bore size of the tube mandates a liquid diet.
      (2) Kinking or obstruction of the tube is common, especially if a jugular catheter is used.
      (3) Constant infusion using a gravity or infusion pump is required, because this method is more physiologic and less problematic than slow hourly bolus feeding. Constant infusion helps to minimize diarrhea, which can also be caused by the osmolarity of the diet.
      (4) Complications include peritonitis secondary to catheter displacement and bowel perforation.
         (a) The catheter should be passed a sufficient distance (20–30 cm) aborally to limit catheter displacement when the animal moves.
         (b) A flexible catheter should be used to avoid bowel erosion.

C. Enteric diet formulations

1. **Meal replacement (polymeric) diets** contain nutrients (polysaccharides and polypeptides) that require digestion.
   a. **Preparations.** These diets may be meat-based, milk-based, or vegetable- and casein-based, and they tend to be isotonic or slightly hyperosmolar. Generally, **meat-based diets are preferred** in animals.
      (1) **Commercial formulations, blended pet food,** or **homemade diets** (e.g., baby food, eggs, and corn syrup) may be used. Some commercial diets are specifically formulated for the management of catabolic animals with malnutrition (i.e., they contain high levels of protein and fat in an energy-dense form).
      (2) **Human diets** often contain more carbohydrate than is required for dogs and cats, which can cause diarrhea. Diluting the food may help, but the resultant food is less energy-dense.
   b. **Indications.** Polymeric diets can be used with nasoesophageal, esophageal, gastrostomy, and jejunostomy feeding tubes, although liquid diets work better than blended diets with smaller bore tubes.

2. **Elemental (monomeric) diets** contain nutrients that do not require additional digestion, such as monosaccharides, amino acids, dipeptides, and tripeptides.
   a. Elemental diets are usually hyperosmolar and may be diluted initially to allow the bowel time to adapt.
   b. Elemental diets may be preferred for patients with hypoproteinemia, because they are absorbed more effectively. In addition, they are indicated with jejunostomy feeding, or for animals with inflammatory bowel disease, lymphangiectasia, or other diseases that interfere with digestive function.
   c. **Modular diets** are concentrated forms of single nutrients (e.g., protein, carbohydrates, fats). These diets are used either as a supplement or combined with each other to form specific diets.

V. PARENTERAL NUTRITION

A. Introduction

1. **Total parenteral nutrition (TPN)** is the administration of all essential nutrients (proteins, carbohydrates, fats, vitamins, minerals, and water) directly into the systemic vascular system. **Partial parenteral nutrition** involves the administration of nutrients by infusion in addition to enteral feeding.
   a. The **nutritional components are given in their basic form.** For example, fats are given as medium- or long-chain fatty acids; glucose supplies carbohydrates for energy and amino acids to be used as an energy source or for protein.
   b. **Parenteral infusions tend to be hyperosmolar and extremely irritating to veins.** Increasing the lipid content tends to decrease the osmolarity of the solution.
      (1) In TPN, the solution is generally administered directly into large central veins (e.g., the cranial vena cava) through dedicated catheters.
      (2) Partial parenteral nutrition with an isosmolar solution can sometimes be administered through catheters placed in peripheral veins. Because of the volume and hyperosmolarity of the nutrient solution, it is difficult to give the total protein-calorie requirement through a peripheral catheter.

2. **Indications for TPN**
   a. **Malnourished or anorectic animals** that cannot absorb nutrients given enterally are candidates for TPN.
   b. **Pancreatitis** may also be an indication for TPN. By infusing nutrients intravenously, adverse stimulation of pancreatic digestive enzymes may be avoided.

3. **Advantages of TPN**
   a. **General anesthesia is not required** to place the intravenous catheters, as it is for placement of some of the enteral feeding tubes.
   b. **Animals with vomiting or diarrhea receive their total calorie requirement.**

4. Disadvantages of TPN

a. **Sepsis and bacteremia** are common and possibly life-threatening complications, especially in malnourished animals (see V D 2).

b. **Metabolic complications** (e.g., hyperglycemia, hyperlipidemia, electrolyte and blood–gas abnormalities) are common (see V D 1).

c. **Catheter-related problems** can range from mild complications (e.g., occlusion, phlebitis) to severe complications (e.g., thromboembolism).

d. **Gastrointestinal atrophy** occurs and may be associated with bacterial translocation from the gut to the systemic circulation.

e. **Secretory immunoglobulin A (S-IgA) production or function may be impaired** with TPN; S-IgA has an important role in the immune surveillance associated with the intestinal tract.

B. TPN solution

1. Calculation of protein and energy requirements

a. Worksheets have been developed that are helpful in the basic formulation of TPN (Figure 5–1). In general, the calculation of individual patient requirements for protein and energy is based on the same assumptions described for the calculation of enteral feeding requirements (see III).

b. Some controversy exists as to whether to include the calories supplied as protein.

(1) This may be a more important consideration for cats, because overfeeding can result in complications such as glucose intolerance and excessive hepatic glycogen storage.

(2) Because protein continues to be used as a fuel source, current recommendations are to supply sufficient protein and to include the calories supplied as protein in the total calories needed (4 kcal/g of protein).

2. Basic TPN solution is composed of dextrose, amino acids, and lipids.

a. **Dextrose solutions** are available in a wide range of concentrations; the 50% concentration is used most often. Hyperglycemia and hyperosmolarity are problems associated with the dextrose solution. Dilution of the formulation or a slower rate of administration to allow for adaptation can minimize these problems.

b. **Crystalline amino acid solutions,** which may contain electrolytes, supply protein. These solutions contain all essential amino acids for dogs and cats, except for taurine. Taurine should be added for cats receiving TPN for more than 1 week.

c. **Lipid solutions,** which serve as a source of essential fatty acids and energy, contain soybean or safflower oil, egg yolk phospholipids, and glycerol.

3. Supplements to the basic TPN solution

a. **Electrolytes.** Some patients with excessive loss may require specific electrolyte supplementation.

b. **Vitamins,** with the exception of fat-soluble vitamin K (which is given by subcutaneous injection), are added to the TPN solution.

c. **Trace elements or minerals** are not usually added unless TPN administration lasts longer than 1 week.

4. Mixing of the parenteral ingredients should be done under strict aseptic conditions.

a. Three-in-one compounding bags simplify mixing and maintain sterility.

b. To prevent disruption of the lipid emulsion, compounding should always be done in the following order: dextrose, amino acids, lipids.

C. Catheterization

1. Placement of the catheter must be performed under strict aseptic conditions because the catheter is left in place for several days and the TPN solution supports bacterial growth.

2. Percutaneous catheter placement is preferred, but a surgical cutdown may be needed in some animals.

3. Catheters require sterile bandaging that must be changed daily. The catheter site should be inspected for redness, swelling, or discharge.

Parenteral Feeding Worksheet

1. Calculate resting energy requirement (RER)

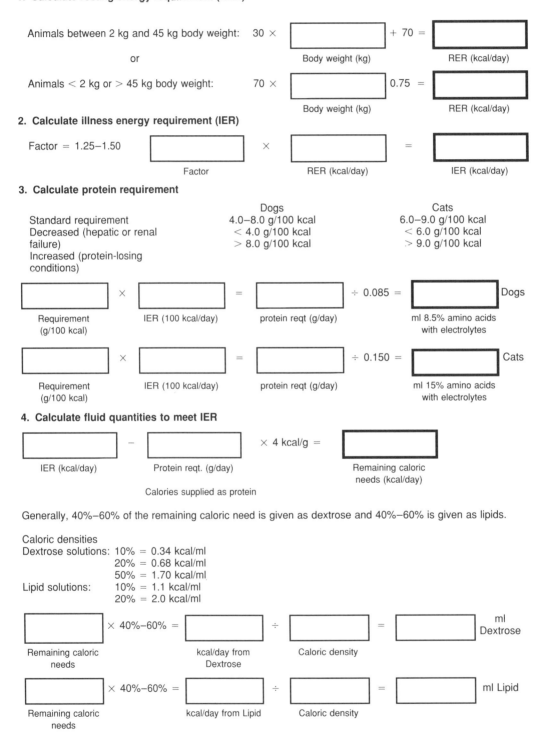

Animals between 2 kg and 45 kg body weight: $30 \times$ [Body weight (kg)] $+ 70 =$ [RER (kcal/day)]

or

Animals < 2 kg or > 45 kg body weight: $70 \times$ [Body weight (kg)] $0.75 =$ [RER (kcal/day)]

2. Calculate illness energy requirement (IER)

Factor = 1.25–1.50 [Factor] $\times$ [RER (kcal/day)] $=$ [IER (kcal/day)]

3. Calculate protein requirement

	Dogs	Cats
Standard requirement	4.0–8.0 g/100 kcal	6.0–9.0 g/100 kcal
Decreased (hepatic or renal failure)	< 4.0 g/100 kcal	< 6.0 g/100 kcal
Increased (protein-losing conditions)	> 8.0 g/100 kcal	> 9.0 g/100 kcal

[Requirement (g/100 kcal)] $\times$ [IER (100 kcal/day)] $=$ [protein reqt (g/day)] $\div 0.085 =$ [ ]Dogs
ml 8.5% amino acids with electrolytes

[Requirement (g/100 kcal)] $\times$ [IER (100 kcal/day)] $=$ [protein reqt (g/day)] $\div 0.150 =$ [ ]Cats
ml 15% amino acids with electrolytes

4. Calculate fluid quantities to meet IER

[IER (kcal/day)] $-$ [Protein reqt. (g/day)] $\times$ 4 kcal/g $=$ [Remaining caloric needs (kcal/day)]

Calories supplied as protein

Generally, 40%–60% of the remaining caloric need is given as dextrose and 40%–60% is given as lipids.

Caloric densities
Dextrose solutions: 10% = 0.34 kcal/ml
20% = 0.68 kcal/ml
50% = 1.70 kcal/ml
Lipid solutions: 10% = 1.1 kcal/ml
20% = 2.0 kcal/ml

[Remaining caloric needs] $\times$ 40%–60% = [kcal/day from Dextrose] $\div$ [Caloric density] $=$ [ ] ml Dextrose

[Remaining caloric needs] $\times$ 40%–60% = [kcal/day from Lipid] $\div$ [Caloric density] $=$ [ ] ml Lipid

FIGURE 5–1. Example of the parenteral nutritional support worksheet that was designed by Mark Morris Associates and is currently in use at Kansas State University. (Mark Morris Associates, Science and Technology Center, P.O. Box 1493, Topeka, KS 66601.)

Parenteral Feeding Worksheet *(continued)*

5. Calculate total daily volume and delivery rate

Volume dextrose = [   ] ml

Volume lipid = [   ] ml

Volume amino acids with electrolytes = [   ] ml

Volume balanced multielectrolyte solution* = [   ] ml

Vitamin B complex = [1–2] ml

Total daily volume = [   ] ml ÷ 24 hours = [   ]

ml/hour

* Calculate based on animal's fluid and electrolyte requirements.

FIGURE 5–1. *(continued)*.

D. **Monitoring for complications**

1. **Metabolic abnormalities** can be limited by careful monitoring of the patient.
   a. **Hyperglycemia** is seen most often in cats.
      (1) If significant hyperglycemia occurs (> 500 mg/dl), the calculated calories contributed by glucose should be decreased by half.
      (2) If significant hyperglycemia continues, insulin may be added to the TPN solution or given by subcutaneous injection.
   b. **Hypokalemia** is one of the most common electrolyte abnormalities and can usually be corrected by the addition of potassium to the TPN solution.
   c. **Lipemia** may be observed, especially the first few days after TPN is initiated. If the serum triglyceride level is greater than 300 mg/dl after 3 or 4 days, the calories provided by lipid should be decreased and the concentration of glucose should be increased.
   d. **Cholestasis** may also be associated with TPN.
      (1) Cholestasis may occur in cats because they require taurine to conjugate bile acids. Lack of taurine may result in secretion of abnormal bile acid.
      (2) Cholestasis may also result from a change in the intestinal flora caused by a lack of enteral nutrients or usage of broad-spectrum antibiotics. The change in intestinal flora causes absorption of hepatic endotoxins and bile acids.
      (3) Metronidazole may alleviate signs of cholestasis.

2. **Sepsis** may result from contamination of the catheter or the solution.
   a. **Signs of sepsis** include fever, hypoglycemia, depression, leukocytosis with a left shift, degenerative left shift, and hypotension. Leukocytosis or fever that cannot be attributed to another septic process indicates that a blood culture should be performed.
      (1) Ideally, the catheter is removed if the blood culture taken at the catheter tip is positive.
      (2) In many animals, TPN can be reinitiated 24–36 hours following removal of the catheter, after the fever has subsided.
   b. **Signs of infection** at the catheter site that could lead to sepsis include swelling, redness, heat, or discharge. The catheter should be removed, the catheter tip cultured, and appropriate antibiotics used.

SELECTED READINGS

Armstrong PJ: Enteral feeding of critically ill pets: The choices and techniques. *Vet Med* 87: 900–909, 1992.

Bright RM, Okrasinski EB, Pardo AD, et al: Percutaneous tube gastrostomy for enteral alimentation in small animals. *Comp Cont Educ Pract Vet* 13:15–23, 1991.

Burkholder WJ, Swecker WS, Jr.: Nutritional influences on immunity. *Semin Vet Med and Surg* 5:154–166, 1990.

Crowe DT: Clinical use of an indwelling nasogastric tube for enteral nutrition and fluid therapy in the dog and cat. *J Am Anim Hosp Assoc* 22:677–682, 1986.

Crowe DT: Nutritional support for the hospitalized patient: An introduction to tube feeding. *Comp Cont Educ Pract Vet* 12:1711–1721, 1990.

Labato, MA: Nutritional management of the critical care patient. In *Current Veterinary Therapy XI.* Edited by Kirk RW, Bonagura JD. Philadelphia, WB Saunders, 1992, pp 117–125.

Layton CE: Nutritional support of the surgical patient. In *Surgical Complications and Wound Healing in the Small Animal Practice.* Edited by Harari J. Philadelphia, WB Saunders, 1993, pp 89–124.

Mauterer JV, Abood SK, Buffington CA, et al: New technique and management guidelines for percutaneous nonendoscopic tube gastrostomy. *J Am Vet Med Assoc* 205:574–579, 1994.

McCrackin MA, DeNovo RC, Bright RM, et al: Endoscopic placement of a percutaneous gastrostomy feeding tube in dogs. *J Am Vet Med Assoc* 203:792–797, 1993.

Ogilvie GK, Vail DM: Nutrition and cancer: recent developments. *Vet Clin North Am* 20: 969–985, 1990.

Rawlings CA: Percutaneous placement of a midcervical esophagotomy tube: new technique and representative cases. *J Am Anim Hosp Assoc* 29:526–530, 1993.

Ray PA, Thatcher CD, Swecker WS: Nutritional management of dogs and cats with cancer. *Vet Med* 87:1185–1194, 1992.

Remillard RL, Martin RA: Nutritional support in the surgical patient. *Semin Vet Med and Surg* 5:197–207, 1990.

Chapter 6
Bandages and Physical Therapy
Joseph Harari

BANDAGES

  Applications. Bandages serve to **protect open wounds and incisions,** as well as **support body parts.**

1. **Wound healing.** Bandages enhance wound healing by:
   a. Promoting wound débridement
   b. Preserving wound homeostasis to ensure healing
   c. Providing for the application of topical medications (especially antimicrobial agents)
   d. Reducing pain secondary to wounding
   e. Providing pressure to reduce hemorrhage, edema, or dead space (i.e., the abnormal space between tissues created by trauma where blood or serum can accumulate)

2. **Immobilization of limbs.** Bandages immobilize limbs and provide support following orthopedic and soft tissue injuries or surgery.

  Layers. Bandages are composed of **three functional layers.**

1. The **primary (contact) layer** is in direct contact with the wound or incision and may be adherent or nonadherent. Prior to bandaging, open wounds require débridement of necrotic tissue, removal of foreign debris, and lavage with isotonic fluids or 0.05% chlorhexidine solution. Irrigation should be performed using a 60-cc syringe and 18-gauge needle with a volume dependent on the nature and character of the wound.
   a. **Adherent dressings** utilize gauze (either wet or dry) to mechanically débride necrotic tissues in the early phases of wound healing.
      (1) A **wet-to-dry dressing** [i.e., a wet contact layer covered by an absorbent secondary (intermediate) layer] helps dilute and evacuate viscous wound exudate. Sterile saline or dilute 0.05% chlorhexidine solution may be used as wetting agents.
      (2) A **dry-to-dry** dressing absorbs fluid and debris from the wound.
   b. **Nonadherent dressings** are used in the early reparative stages of wound healing (e.g., the granulation tissue, serosanguineous discharge, and epithelialization stages). Nonadherent dressings may be occlusive or semiocclusive.
      (1) **Semiocclusive dressings** utilize sterile petrolatum-impregnated gauze or commercially available products (e.g., Telfa pads) to prevent tissue dehydration and protect re-epithelialization. Topical antimicrobial ointments (e.g., gentamicin, bacitracin–polymyxin B–neomycin, silver sulfadiazine, nitrofurazone, chlorhexidine) may be used with these dressings to reduce wound infection.
      (2) **Occlusive dressings,** which enhance epithelialization and collagen synthesis more than semiocclusive dressings, are impermeable to wound fluids.
         (a) Materials used for occlusive dressings include films, foams, hydrocolloids, and hydrogels.
         (b) Occlusive dressings require less frequent changes and permit more visualization of the wound than semiocclusive dressings; however, they are more expensive and more difficult to secure.

2. The **secondary (intermediate) layer** absorbs wound exudate, secures the primary layer to the wound, and provides support. Materials used for this layer include cast padding, combine roll, cotton roll, or disposable diapers.

3. The **tertiary (outer) layer** provides support, pressure, and protection for the other

bandage layers. This layer is composed of surgical tape, which may be porous or waterproof, adhesive or nonadhesive, or elastic or inelastic.

   a. Porous tape permits evaporation; however, the porous nature of the tape necessitates daily changing of the dressing to prevent external contamination of heavily exudative wounds.

   b. Elastic adhesive tape provides continuous pressure to control hemorrhage and edema, and, because it is self-adherent, requires less tape than nonadherent material.

C. **Bandaging techniques.** Bandages are applied to various regions of the body to facilitate recovery following injury or surgery. In general, bandages should be applied **evenly and without excessive tightness** to avoid circulatory impairment and edema distal to the bandage.

1. **Head bandages** are useful for protecting incisions and tissues following surgery of the ear. Cast padding covered by elastic gauze and adhesive elastic tape are used to cover the skull and often the pinna as well.

2. **Paw bandages** are routinely used on a temporary basis (i.e., for 24 hours) following declawing to control hemorrhage and provide support. Nonadherent dressings covered by gauze and adhesive tape also prevent excessive self-trauma.

3. **Limb bandages**
   a. The **Schanz padded limb bandage** (sometimes referred to as a modified Robert-Jones bandage) is the most frequently used bandage for support and protection of limb tissues in animals.
      (1) **Description.** Adhesive tape stirrups are used to secure cast padding, elastic gauze, and elastic tape to the leg. The bandage may extend from the digits to the axillary or inguinal regions, leaving the middle toes exposed so that the limb may be evaluated for circulatory compromise.
      (2) **Modifications and applications**
         (a) The padded limb bandage may be circumferentially covered by **casting material** to increase support of damaged osseous structures (e.g., incomplete or minimally displaced radial or tibial fractures in young animals, carpal arthrodesis), if the joints above and below the affected tissues are included in the cast.
         (b) Application of **plastic or aluminum spoon splints** to the palmar or plantar aspect of the bandage is useful for treatment of fractures or luxations distal to the carpal or tarsal joint (Figure 6–1).
         (c) Application of a lateral splint (i.e., casting material and an aluminum rod along the lateral aspect of the limb) over a padded bandage is useful for external support following reconstructive surgery involving ligaments or tendons.

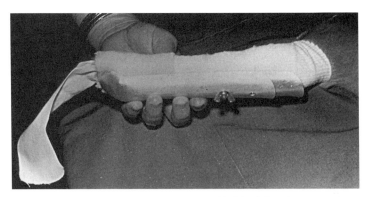

FIGURE 6–1. An aluminum spoon splint applied over a padded limb bandage provides support for metacarpal or carpal injuries.

(d) Application of a **Spica splint** (i.e., a lateral splint that reaches from the digits to over the shoulder or hip joint and adjacent vertebrae) is useful for temporary support of femoral or humeral fractures.

(e) Application of a padded limb bandage to a flexed forelimb held in close apposition to the thorax (i.e., a **Velpeau sling**) is used for treatment of shoulder luxations or scapular fractures.

(f) Application of a padded bandage to the distal aspect of the forelimb while the carpus is flexed (i.e., a **carpal flexion bandage**) is used to prevent weight-bearing following repair of flexor tendon or forelimb orthopedic injuries.

b. A **Robert-Jones bandage** is a bulky compressive support wrap that provides excellent temporary stabilization for severe orthopedic and soft tissue injuries below the elbow or stifle joint. Following placement of adhesive stirrups, cotton roll (1 lb cotton/20 lb body weight) is applied and securely covered by conforming gauze and elastic adhesive tape (Figure 6–2).

c. An **Ehmer sling** is often applied to the pelvic limb to internally rotate and abduct the limb following repair of coxofemoral luxation or femoral head and neck fractures. Application of adhesive tape around the stifle and hock joints and the caudal aspect of the abdomen prevents weight-bearing on the limb.

d. A **pelvic (Robinson) limb sling** prevents hindlimb weight-bearing following repair of bone or joint injuries while permitting joint movement to prevent tissue contracture and fibrosis. Elastic gauze and adhesive tape are applied around the trunk to form a bellyband. Strips of tape from around the tibia and metatarsal bones are then attached to the bellyband to form the sling.

e. The **Schroeder-Thomas splint,** which is used for minimally displaced fractures below the elbow or stifle joint, is a traction device composed of aluminum rods secured to cotton padding or combine roll.

(1) This splint requires meticulous care in application and maintenance to avoid soft tissue complications (e.g., necrosis, edema) and orthopedic complications (e.g., malunion, muscle contracture, and fibrosis).

(2) Misuse of the device for femoral or humeral fractures puts the limb in traction, leading to fibrosis or contracture of the muscles, tendons, ligaments, and joint tissue. The limb is rendered nonfunctional, in effect, becoming a "peg leg."

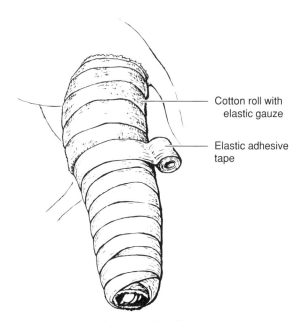

Cotton roll with
elastic gauze

Elastic adhesive
tape

FIGURE 6–2. A Robert-Jones bandage applied to the hindlimb for stabilization of a comminuted tibial fracture.

4. **Trunk bandages** may be applied to protect and stabilize thoracolumbar vertebral injuries, fractured ribs, soft tissue injuries of the thoracic or abdominal wall, and externally directed drains. These soft, padded bandages use nonadherent dressings to protect incisions. In addition, cast padding, elastic gauze, and tape are often applied circumferentially. For stabilization of rib or vertebral fractures or luxations, aluminum rods, casting, or wooden material may be incorporated into the bandage.

II. **PHYSICAL THERAPY** is the treatment of injured tissues by physical or mechanical agents to reduce morbidity and promote rapid return to normal function.

A. Applications

1. **General applications.** Physical therapy is useful for reducing inflammation, stimulating blood and lymph flows, improving muscle and joint function, and promoting the psychological well-being of the animal and client.

2. **Common injuries** in which physical therapy is useful include:
   a. Femoral fractures associated with quadriceps fibrosis in young dogs
   b. Intra-articular elbow joint fractures and luxations associated with joint stiffness
   c. Tarsal bone fractures in racing greyhounds
   d. Disk disease or trauma to the spine
   e. Pseudarthrosis formation following femoral head ostectomy

B. **Regimens.** The selection of an appropriate physical therapy regimen is based on evaluation of the type of patient (size, demeanor, overall health), type of injury or surgery (musculoskeletal, neurologic, soft tissue), owner compliance, and available facilities or equipment (pads, blankets, whirlpools, ultrasound units).

1. **Physical agents** used for therapy include the application of cold, heat, sound, and electricity.
   a. **Hypothermia.** Local hypothermia is useful in the early post-injury period. It causes vasoconstriction (which reduces inflammation) and decreases cutaneous nerve conduction (which produces analgesia and muscle relaxation).
      (1) Local hypothermia is accomplished by applying cold bags or ice packs in short sessions lasting approximately 10 minutes, 3–4 times a day.
      (2) Gentle pressure wraps are applied after treatment to prevent reflex vasodilation and edema.
   b. **Hyperthermia** is useful 48–72 hours after injury to produce vasodilation and interstitial fluid resorption, reduce muscle spasms, provide relief from pain, and enhance tissue metabolism.
      (1) **Local hyperthermia** [40°C–45°C (104°F–113°F)] is accomplished by applying warm packs, towels, or circulating water blankets to the affected area. Use of insulated heat sources and continuous monitoring protects the animal from burns.
      (2) **Superficial hyperthermia** is applied in sessions lasting 10–20 minutes. When used prior to massage and exercise, superficial hyperthermia enhances the effects of these treatments.
      (3) **Deep hyperthermia.** Ultrasonography and short-wave diathermy produce deep hyperthermia using sound waves and electrical currents.
         (a) **Ultrasonography** produces heat at muscles, the bone–tissue interface, ligaments, and tendons to reduce spasms and contracture. Proper and extensive technical expertise and equipment are required to prevent complications associated with ultrasonography (e.g., tissue burns, nerve damage, and gaseous cavitation of tissues).
         (b) **Short-wave diathermy** uses high-frequency currents to create tissue energy and heat. Diathermy application requires technical expertise and avoidance of metal in or around the patient to prevent burns.

2. **Mechanical agents** used in physical therapy include massage and exercise.
   a. **Massage** improves local circulation to promote nutrient delivery and removal of waste products, reduces adhesions to stimulate muscular function, and relaxes uncomfortable animals. Massage is often an integral part of combination therapy programs (see II B 3).
      (1) **Types of massage**
         (a) **Stroking** *(effleurage)* **massage** is superficial and light, and proceeds toward the heart.
         (b) **Kneading** *(petrissage)* **massage** involves picking up and manipulating skin and muscle to produce tissue motion.
      (2) **Massage sessions** should last 10–20 minutes every 24–48 hours and should not be performed if tissue infection is present.
   b. **Exercise** involves active or passive motion and is used to improve circulation, promote sensory awareness and voluntary movement, increase muscular strength and coordination, and prevent muscle atrophy and joint stiffness.
      (1) **Passive exercise** is accomplished by directed movement of joints and limbs at a rate of 10–20 cycles per minute for 5 minutes, 2–3 times a day by an owner or therapist.
      (2) **Active exercise** is performed voluntarily by the animal in assisted or resisted sessions of short duration several times a day.
         (a) **Assisted exercise** involves weight support using towels, slings, harnesses, or water.
         (b) **Resisted exercise** improves muscle strength by applying external manual resistance during movement of the limb or joint.

3. **Combination therapy programs** use superficial hyperthermia, massage, and passive or active exercise to provide multiple benefits in severely affected patients. **Whirlpools** are extremely useful for providing these therapies in one unit. In addition, they contribute to the maintenance of animal cleanliness.
   a. Manual therapy during immersion of the animal in water enhances the massage action of circulating water.
   b. **Important considerations** involved with hydrotherapy include patient compliance and the status of wounds or incisions. Disinfection of the water is critical.

C. Adjuncts to physical therapy
1. **Analgesic drugs or sedatives** may be useful in permitting manipulation of painful and injured limbs.
   a. Injectable compounds such as **acepromazine maleate** alone or in combination with **butorphanol, oxymorphone,** or **buprenorphine** should be considered.
   b. Oral medication of patients with **aspirin** may also help alleviate postoperative discomfort and aid in physical rehabilitation.

2. **Established treatment protocols** and **adequate documentation** (e.g., gait analysis, muscle circumference measurement, goniometer measurements) should be used to produce desirable and repeatable results. Furthermore, encouragement of the owner by the veterinarian is critical for successful therapy at home.

SELECTED READINGS

Bartels KE: Orthopedic bandaging: principles and application. In *Current Techniques in Small Animal Surgery,* 3rd ed. Edited by Bojrab JM. Philadelphia, Lea & Febiger, 1990, pp 911–929.

DeCamp CE: External coaptation. In *Textbook of Small Animal Surgery,* 2nd ed. Edited by Slatter D. Philadelphia, WB Saunders, 1993, pp 1661–1667.

Hodges CC, Palmer RH: Postoperative physical therapy. In *Surgical Complications and Wound Healing in the Small Animal Practice.* Edited by Harari J. Philadelphia, WB Saunders, 1993, pp 389–405.

Knecht CD: *Fundamental Techniques in Veterinary Surgery,* 3rd ed. Philadelphia, WB Saunders, 1987, pp 106–149.

Lozier SL: Topical wound therapy. In *Surgical Complications and Wound Healing in the Small Animal Practice.* Edited by Harari J. Philadelphia, WB Saunders, 1993, pp 63–88.

Swaim SF, Henderson RA: *Small Animal Wound Management.* Philadelphia, Lea & Febiger, 1990, pp 34–51.

Tangner CH: Physical therapy in small animal patients: basic principles and application. *Compend Contin Educ Pract Vet* 6:933–936, 1984.

Taylor RL: Postsurgical physical therapy; the missing link. *Compend Contin Educ Pract Vet* 14: 1583–1593, 1992.

PART II

SOFT TISSUE SURGERY

Chapter 7

Respiratory System

Giselle Hosgood

I. **ANATOMY.** The respiratory tract is divided at the cricotracheal junction into the upper and lower tracts.

A. **Upper respiratory tract**

1. **Nose.** The nose comprises the **planum nasale** and **nasal chambers**. The **nasolacrimal duct** opens on the floor of the **nasal vestibule**, just inside the nostril opening.

2. **Nostrils (nares).** The nostrils are comma-shaped openings in the planum nasale that impede airflow into the nasal chambers.

3. **Nasal cavity**
   a. The **nasal septum** divides the nasal cavity into **left** and **right fossae.**
   b. **Conchae** are scroll-like structures of soft bone or cartilage that fill the nasal cavity.
      (1) The conchae are **covered by a vascular, glandular mucosa.**
      (2) **Conchae of the caudal nasal cavity** are referred to as **turbinates.**
   c. **Blood supply.** The **sphenopalatine** and **major palatine arteries** and **their branches** vascularize the nasal cavity and nose. Both the sphenopalatine and major palatine arteries are branches of the **maxillary artery**, a branch of the carotid artery.

4. **Paranasal sinuses**
   a. **Frontal sinus** (Figure 7–1) **and maxillary recess.** Frontal sinuses are the largest sinuses. The right and left frontal sinuses, separated by a median septum, contain lateral, medial, and rostral compartments in the dog, but not in the cat.
   b. **Sphenoidal sinus.** Cats have a sphenoidal sinus in addition to the frontal sinus and maxillary recess.

5. **Pharynx.** The pharynx comprises the **nasopharynx** and the **soft palate.**
   a. **Nasopharynx.** The lateral walls of the nasopharynx contain the **slit-like openings of the auditory tubes.** A flat **pharyngeal tonsil** is present on either side of the nasopharyngeal roof.
   b. **Soft palate.** The soft palate forms the floor of the nasopharynx. Nerves from the pharyngeal plexus (**cranial nerves IX and X**) supply the soft palate.

6. **Larynx**
   a. **Cartilage**
      (1) **Major.** The larynx is composed of five major cartilages: the **paired arytenoid cartilages**, and the **unpaired thyroid, cricoid,** and **epiglottis cartilages.**
      (2) **Minor.** Two very small cartilages, the **sesamoid** and **interarytenoid cartilages**, are also present.
   b. **Vocal ligaments** and **muscles** arise from the **vocal process** (i.e., the ventral portion) of both arytenoid cartilages and meet at the internal midline on the thyroid cartilage.
   c. **Muscles**
      (1) **Extrinsic.** The **hyopharyngeal, thyropharyngeal,** and **cricopharyngeal** muscles elevate, depress, and retract the larynx.
      (2) **Intrinsic**
         (a) The **lateral cricoarytenoid** and **thyroarytenoid muscles** adduct the arytenoid cartilages.
         (b) The **dorsal cricoarytenoid muscle** is the only muscle to abduct the arytenoid cartilages.
         (c) The **cricothyroid muscle** constricts the laryngeal lumen.
   d. **Innervation**

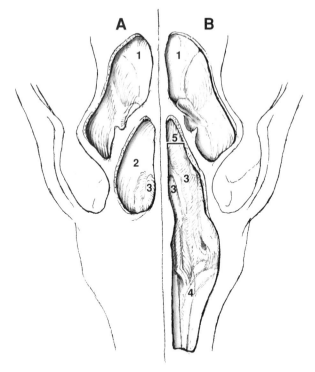

FIGURE 7–1. Dorsal view of the sinuses of the dog. On the right-hand side, the floor of the rostral compartment has been removed to expose the medial compartment. (*1*) Lateral and (*2*) rostral compartments of the frontal sinus. (*3*) Turbinates. (*4*) Nasal concha. (*5*) Medial compartment of frontal sinus.

    (1) The **caudal laryngeal nerve**, an extension of the recurrent laryngeal branch of the vagal nerve, **supplies all intrinsic muscles of the larynx except the cricothyroid.**

    (2) The **cranial laryngeal nerve**, also a branch of the vagus nerve, innervates the **cricothyroid muscle.**

  e. Blood supply. The larynx receives blood primarily from the **cranial laryngeal artery**, a branch of the external carotid artery.

B. **Lower respiratory tract**

  1. Trachea. The trachea is composed of 35–40 C-shaped cartilages that are approximately 4 mm wide.

    a. The **cartilage ends** are joined dorsally by the **trachealis muscle.** The **cartilage rings** are joined ventrally and laterally by **fibroelastic annular ligaments,** which give the trachea its flexibility.

    b. Blood supply

      (1) Arterial. Branches of the **cranial thyroid, caudal thyroid,** and **bronchoesophageal arteries** penetrate the annular ligaments of the trachea.

      (2) Venous. Drainage is through the **thyroid, internal jugular,** and **bronchoesophageal veins.**

    c. Innervation. The innervation of the trachea is **autonomic.**

      (1) Sympathetic stimulation (from the **middle cervical ganglion** and **sympathetic trunk**) **inhibits** tracheal muscle contraction and glandular secretions.

      (2) Parasympathetic stimulation (from the **vagal** or **recurrent laryngeal nerves**) **induces** tracheal muscle contraction and glandular secretions.

2. **Bronchi.** The trachea bifurcates into the **two main-stem (principal) bronchi** at the level of the fourth or fifth thoracic vertebrae.
    a. The left and right main-stem bronchi divide into **lobar** and **segmental bronchi**, which divide into several generations of smaller bronchi.
    b. The smaller bronchi branch into **bronchioles**, which are less than 1 mm in diameter and have no cartilage support.
    c. **Terminal bronchioles** branch into **respiratory bronchioles,** which are surrounded by alveoli.

3. **Lungs.** The right lung is larger than the left in the dog and cat.
    a. **Lobes.** Both lungs are divided into cranial and caudal lung lobes; the right lung also has middle and accessory lobes.
    b. **Blood supply**
        (1) **Pulmonary arteries and veins** accompany the bronchi to form bronchovascular bundles. Radiographically, the pulmonary arteries course laterally and the pulmonary veins course medially to most airways.
        (2) **Pulmonary lymphatics** drain into the tracheobronchial lymph nodes located at the tracheal bifurcation.

II. PREOPERATIVE CONSIDERATIONS

A. Evaluation of animals with respiratory disease

1. **Physical examination**
    a. **Evaluating the breathing pattern** can help the clinician distinguish between restrictive and obstructive disorders.
    b. **Auscultation** is useful for detecting abnormal lung sounds.
    c. **Percussion of the thorax**
        (1) Dullness on percussion suggests thoracic masses, pleural fluid, or atelectasis.
        (2) Increased resonance suggests pneumothorax.

2. **Survey radiography** is suitable for evaluation of the upper and lower respiratory tracts.
    a. **Nasal cavity.** Radiographic examination of the nasal cavity requires general anesthesia to facilitate positioning.
        (1) The **open-mouth ventrodorsal view** using a detail rare-earth intensifying screen is recommended to avoid superimposition of structures over the nasal cavity.
        (2) Alternatively, an **occlusal dorsoventral view** using nonscreen film can be performed.
    b. **Pharynx, larynx, and trachea.** Lateral radiographs of these structures are useful, although computed tomography may provide more accurate visualization of masses in the region of the larynx and pharynx.
    c. **Thorax.** Radiographs of the thorax should be made during inspiration.
        (1) **Visualization of lesions.** When checking for small masses or focal lesions, both left and right lateral radiographic projections, in addition to a ventrodorsal projection, should be made. Pleural fluid should be removed to facilitate observation.
        (2) **Visualization of pulmonary arteries** in the caudal lung lobes requires a **dorsoventral**, rather than a ventrodorsal, **projection.**

3. **Computed tomography** is superior to radiographs for evaluation of the caudal nasal cavity, particularly to determine tumor extent.

4. **Arterial blood gas analysis** provides information regarding ventilation, gas exchange, and perfusion mismatching.

5. **Endoscopy** of the nasal passages (**rhinoscopy**), larynx (**laryngoscopy**), and trachea and bronchi (**tracheobronchoscopy**) is performed while the animal is anesthetized.

B. **Anesthetic considerations**

1. **All animals with respiratory conditions**
   a. Prior to anesthesia, the animal must be kept calm to avoid accentuating respiratory distress. Hyperoxygenating the animal during the immediate preanesthetic period is beneficial.
   b. An induction protocol that allows rapid induction of anesthesia and endotracheal intubation is essential. If airway control cannot be gained by endotracheal intubation, emergency tracheostomy is performed.
   c. Perioperative systemic corticosteroid administration may minimize airway obstruction secondary to swelling.

2. **Brachycephalic breeds**
   a. **All brachycephalic dogs are high-risk anesthetic patients.** Preoxygenation, rapid induction of anesthesia, immediate intubation, assisted intraoperative ventilation, and postoperative administration of oxygen are required.
   b. In brachycephalic breeds with upper airway disease, vagal tone is frequently high; therefore, preanesthetic administration of an anticholinergic drug (e.g., atropine, glycopyrrolate) is indicated.

III. UPPER RESPIRATORY TRACT CONDITIONS TREATED BY SURGERY

A. **Brachycephalic syndrome** affects brachycephalic breeds of dogs and other short-nosed dogs or cats, including cocker spaniels, Sharpeis, and Persian and Himalayan cats. Anatomic changes in the skulls of these animals distort the nasopharynx.

1. **Pathogenesis. Stenotic nares** and an **elongated soft palate** increase resistance to airflow. The resultant increased inspiratory effort generates an increased negative pressure during each respiratory cycle, which leads to **eversion of the laryngeal saccules,** edema, thickening of the laryngeal and pharyngeal mucosae, and collapse of the cuneiform and corniculate processes of the arytenoid cartilages.
   a. Noncardiogenic pulmonary edema may also develop.
   b. Tracheal hypoplasia is often present concurrently.

2. **Clinical signs** include respiratory distress, stridor, mouth breathing, gagging, cyanosis, and collapse; signs are exacerbated by exercise, excitement, or high ambient temperatures.

3. **Diagnosis** is based on history, signalment, clinical signs, physical examination, endoscopy, and radiography.

4. **Treatment.** The stenotic nares are corrected surgically, usually in conjunction with resection of the elongated palate and everted laryngeal saccules. To avoid severe postoperative edema, perioperative corticosteroids should be administered.
   a. **Surgical correction of stenotic nares** requires resection of a wedge from the wing of the nostril and suturing the cut tissue edges.
   b. **Resection of the elongated soft palate (staphylectomy).** The excessive length is resected, and the oral and nasal mucosae are sutured over the cut edge.
      (1) **Electrosurgical** or **laser resection** is possible.
      (2) **Postoperative complications** include edema, hemorrhage, and nasal regurgitation if excessive palatal tissue is removed.
   c. **Resection of everted laryngeal saccules.** The everted tissue is grasped with forceps and cut with scissors or biopsy forceps. The resection sites heal by second intention. **Postoperative complications** include hemorrhage and edema.
   d. If laryngeal collapse has occurred, **arytenoid cartilage lateralization** may be necessary (see III F 4 a).
   e. In severe cases, **permanent tracheostomy** may be indicated.

5. **Prognosis** depends on the age of the animal and the severity of the disease.

B. **Trauma and neoplasia**

1. **Trauma to the planum nasale** results in hemorrhage. Lacerations usually heal without complication if **cleansed, débrided,** and **left to heal by primary, secondary,** or **third intention,** depending on the severity of the injury.

2. **Squamous cell carcinoma** is the most common tumor of the planum nasale in dogs and cats. White-nosed cats are particularly susceptible.
   a. **Etiology**
      (1) In **dogs,** squamous cell carcinoma of the planum nasale usually originates within the medial wall of the nasal vestibule.
      (2) In **cats,** squamous cell carcinoma typically begins as a bleeding ulcer on the external surface. Tumor growth may be stimulated by exposure to ultraviolet light; carcinoma of the pinna may also be seen in the same cat [see Chapter 14 III A 2 c (1)].
   b. **Treatment. Radiation, surgical excision** with complete resection of the planum nasale, and **cryosurgery** are treatment alternatives.

C. **Chronic rhinitis**

1. **Etiology.** Chronic rhinitis can result from inhalation of foreign bodies, periodontal disease, bacterial or mycotic infections, or neoplasia.
   a. **Foreign bodies** (e.g., grass awns) are inhaled through the nares into the anterior nasal cavity. Foreign bodies may also gain access to the nasal cavity through palatine defects. Occasionally, bones or sticks gain access to the posterior nasal cavity from the nasopharynx.
      (1) **Clinical signs** include violent sneezing (possibly associated with epistaxis), head-shaking, and nose-pawing.
         (a) Sneezing may dislodge the foreign body; however, a mild rhinitis may persist for 2–3 days.
         (b) A retained foreign body will cause persistent sneezing and a mucopurulent nasal discharge resulting from a secondary bacterial or fungal infection.
      (2) **Diagnosis.** Radiography of the skull may only reveal inorganic foreign bodies, whereas rhinoscopy may identify foreign bodies in the ventral or dorsal meatus.
      (3) **Treatment. Exploratory rhinotomy** (see II C 2) may be necessary to remove the foreign body and treat secondary bacterial or fungal rhinitis.
      (4) **Prognosis.** The prognosis is good if the foreign body can be removed and there are minimal inflammatory changes in the sinuses.
   b. **Periodontal disease,** especially that involving the canine teeth, is a common cause of chronic rhinitis. Treatment requires removal of the tooth, curettage of the alveolus, and creation of a buccal or mucoperiosteal flap to close the oronasal fistula that remains (see III E 4 b).
   c. **Infection**
      (1) **Chronic bacterial rhinitis** occurs as a result of inflammatory change or damage to the nasal cavity.
         (a) **Etiology.** *Bordetella bronchiseptica, Pasteurella multocida, Staphylococcus aureus,* and gram-negative bacteria (e.g., *Pseudomonas aeruginosa, Escherichia coli*) are often encountered.
         (b) **Treatment.** Chronic, initially untreated bacterial rhinitis is often responsive to **antibiotic therapy**, but recurrence is likely and **turbinectomy via a rhinotomy may be necessary.**
      (2) **Chronic fungal rhinitis** is much more common in dogs than in cats.
         (a) **Etiology**
            (i) **Dogs.** *Aspergillus fumigatus* is the most common cause of canine rhinomycosis; *Penicillium* species and *Cryptococcus neoformans* are implicated less frequently. *Rhinosporidium seeberi,* which causes growth of granulomatous masses in the anterior nasal cavity, occasionally causes disease in dogs.

       (ii) Cats. *Cryptococcus neoformans* is the most common fungal pathogen in cats; *Aspergillus* and *Penicillium* are rarely isolated.

    (b) Treatment is **systemic or topical antifungal therapy.** At this time, enilconazole applied topically is considered the most effective treatment for dogs. In cats, oral administration of ketoconazole is the treatment of choice.

       (i) Rhinotomy is **only indicated when** a diagnosis cannot be obtained from assessment of the nasal discharge and antibody titer, or it is necessary to establish drainage.

       (ii) Turbinectomy is **not indicated.**

  d. Neoplasia

    (1) Etiology

      (a) Dogs. Adenocarcinoma is the most common neoplasia of the nasal cavity in dogs, but **fibrosarcoma, osteosarcoma,** and **squamous cell carcinoma** have all been reported.

      (b) Cats. Lymphosarcoma is the most common neoplasia of the nasal cavity in cats.

    (2) Clinical signs of nasal tumors in dogs and cats include:

      (a) Mucopurulent nasal discharge that is initially unilateral but becomes bilateral with transeptal spread

      (b) Epistaxis (either spontaneous or associated with **violent sneezing**)

      (c) Retching or coughing associated with posterior drainage from the nasal cavity

      (d) Ocular discharge resulting from erosion of the nasolacrimal duct

      (e) Facial deformity, which denotes local invasion but does not affect prognosis

    (3) Diagnosis

      (a) A definitive diagnosis is based on **cytology or histopathology of aspirates or tissue** biopsied from the nasal cavity.

      (b) Radiographs of the nasal cavity are evaluated for evidence of increased soft tissue density, distortion or loss of turbinate structure, and asymmetry between the left and right nasal cavities. Bony proliferation may also occur.

      (c) Computed tomography is necessary to determine the extent of disease and evaluate the integrity of the cribriform plate.

    (4) Treatment

      (a) Surgery alone is not effective but may temporarily ameliorate symptoms.

      (b) Radiation—either megavoltage alone, orthovoltage in combination with surgical debulking, or brachytherapy—**is the treatment of choice for nasal tumors.**

       (i) Megavoltage therapy. Surgery in combination with megavoltage radiation therapy has no advantage over megavoltage therapy alone.

         □ Median survival times with megavoltage alone range from 8.1–12 months.

         □ One-year survival rates of over 50% are reported, with two-year survival rates decreasing by 28%.

       (ii) Orthovoltage therapy. Because orthovoltage has minimal penetration (i.e., 3–4 cm), surgery to reduce tumor bulk is required. Orthovoltage therapy is more effective than megavoltage therapy.

         □ Median survival times with orthovoltage and cytoreduction surgery range from 8.1–23 months.

         □ One-year survival rates of over 50% are reported, with two-year survival rates decreasing by 10%.

       (iii) Brachytherapy involves placement of radioactive implants within the nasal cavity after surgical removal of the primary neoplasm. Iridium[192] is most commonly used. Variable results have been reported; complications include local bone and soft tissue necrosis.

(c) **Chemotherapy alone is unsuccessful** for the treatment of nasal neoplasia.

2. **Diagnosis and treatment. Rhinotomy** for the diagnosis and treatment of various sinus disorders can be performed via a dorsal, ventral, or lateral approach.

  a. **Dorsal rhinotomy** (Figure 7–2) exposes the rostral nasal cavity.

    (1) Technique

      (a) Exposure of the nasal cavity. A bone flap (which is later secured in place with a large gauge suture) is created, or the dorsal nasal bone is removed. Removal of the bone is associated with minimal postoperative deformity.

      (b) Curettage and lavage. The nasal cavity is curetted and lavaged.

      (c) Hemorrhage control

        (i) Temporary ligation of both carotids can be used to reduce hemorrhage during intranasal surgery.

        (ii) Use of chilled lavage fluid may help decrease hemorrhage.

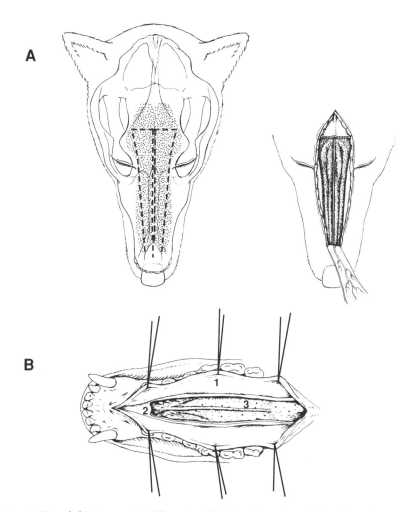

A

B

FIGURE 7–2. (*A*) Dorsal rhinotomy. A midline dorsal incision is made and the skin, subcutaneous tissue, and periosteum are reflected to expose the nasal cavities and frontal sinuses (*shaded*). The incision in the bone is indicated by the *broken line*. The bone is hinged at its cartilaginous junction. (*B*) Ventral rhinotomy. A midline incision is made, and the mucoperiosteum (*1*) is reflected. The central portion of the hard palate (*2*) is removed and the ventral nasal passages (*3*) are exposed.

          (iii) Packing the nasal cavity with gauze that is removed over the course of 2–3 days helps reduce hemorrhage.

      (d) Drainage and postoperative care. A temporary rhinostomy can be created at the sinus end of the rhinotomy to allow postoperative flushing and medication of the frontal sinuses and nasal passages, and to prevent postoperative subcutaneous emphysema. Alternatively, fenestrated drains can be placed in each nasal cavity, entering dorsally and exiting through the nostril.

    (2) Postoperative complications include hemorrhage, sneezing, and subcutaneous emphysema, which resolve with time.

      (a) Packing over the incision may help to reduce subcutaneous emphysema.

      (b) Sedation reduces sneezing and hemorrhage.

  b. Ventral rhinotomy (see Figure 7–2). The ventral approach to the nasal cavity provides access to the region rostral to the major palatine artery foramen (through the hard palate) or the caudal region (through the hard and soft palate).

    (1) Technique. After reflection of the mucoperiosteum, a section of hard palate is removed and discarded.

      (a) This approach may damage the vomer bone in growing dogs, resulting in muzzle shortening.

      (b) A two-layer closure of the mucoperiosteum over the bony defect is performed.

    (2) Postoperative complications are similar to those of dorsal rhinotomy. In addition, **oronasal fistula formation** may occur.

  c. Lateral rhinotomy. The lateral approach exposes the nasal vestibule.

    (1) An excision extending caudally from the wing of the nostril through the cutaneous junction is made.

    (2) The wing of the nostril and alar cartilage are reflected dorsally to expose the vestibule.

    (3) The tissue layers are closed in three layers.

D. **Chronic sinusitis**

  1. Etiology and pathogenesis. Chronic sinusitis occurs infrequently in dogs but is **common in cats, most often secondary to feline viral rhinotracheitis or calicivirus.**

    a. **Severe turbinate damage** allows **secondary bacterial infection** (e.g., by *Streptococci, Staphylococci, Pasteurella,* or coliforms).

    b. **Normal drainage of the frontal sinus is impeded** as a result of thickening of the mucosa around the sinus ostium.

  2. Clinical signs are similar to those of rhinitis, because sinusitis is usually an extension of rhinitis. Erosion of the frontal bones and subcutaneous mucocele formation cause facial deformity.

  3. Diagnosis

    a. Radiography. An anteroposterior radiographic projection of the skull highlights the frontal sinus, revealing the soft tissue density of the sinus, asymmetry, and frontal bone erosion consistent with sinusitis.

    b. Cytology of aspirate obtained from the frontal sinus through the frontal bone may be useful for detecting organisms, inflammatory cells, and possibly, neoplastic cells.

    c. Surgical exploration of the sinuses may be necessary if aspirates are nondiagnostic.

  4. Treatment entails medical and surgical therapies.

    a. Flushing. The sinus can be flushed with a dilute antiseptic solution (e.g., 0.1% povidone-iodine or 0.5% chlorhexidine) and drained through a trephine hole in the frontal region.

    b. Surgical exploration and drainage

      (1) The bone overlying the sinus is removed with rongeurs or a burr.

      (2) The sinus is curettaged, the septum between the sinuses is resected to establish drainage, and the nasosinus ostium is enlarged.

(3) Drains, passed into the sinus and through the ostium into the nasal cavity, are sutured in place to allow postoperative irrigation of the sinuses.

   c. **Sinus obliteration** is indicated in cats with sinusitis that is unresponsive to medical therapy.

      (1) A temporal fascial graft is placed over each ostium and the cavities are filled with autogenous fat (from the ventral abdomen) or bone chips. The sinuses heal and become occluded within 6–12 months.

      (2) Recurrence may be a problem unless all sinus mucosa is removed.

   d. **Systemic antibiotic therapy,** based on bacterial culture and antibiotic sensitivity testing, is used in conjunction with surgical procedures.

5. **Prognosis.** The prognosis for chronic sinusitis, without surgical treatment, is poor. Surgical intervention may improve the prognosis.

E. **Cleft palates and oronasal fistulae** are abnormal communications between the oral and nasal cavities.

   1. **Etiology**
      a. **Cleft palates** are **usually congenital. Congenital cleft palates are rare in cats.**
         (1) **Primary cleft palates (harelips)** are anterior to the incisive foramen and involve the lip.
            (a) Isolated cleft of the primary plate is rare. Male animals and brachycephalic breeds are at greatest risk.
            (b) The left side appears to be affected more often than the right side.
         (2) **Secondary cleft palates** are posterior to the incisive foramen and involve the hard and soft palates. Clefts of the secondary palate, alone or in combination with primary cleft palate, occur more frequently than isolated primary lesions.
      b. **Oronasal fistulae** are **acquired.**
         (1) They may be **secondary to trauma, surgical resection of maxillary lesions,** or **dental lesions.** Acquired oronasal fistulas secondary to **head trauma** and **maxillary fracture** are fairly common in cats.
         (2) In dogs, oronasal fistulae commonly occur **secondary to severe periodontal disease with maxillary bone resorption.**
         (3) **Failure of previous surgical repair of congenital cleft palates** may also result in secondary oronasal fistulae.

   2. **Clinical signs**
      a. **Nasal discharge,** which may be **purulent or hemorrhagic,** is the predominant clinical sign of cleft palates and oronasal fistulae. Discharge may be **unilateral or bilateral.**
      b. **Nasal regurgitation of fluid or food** may be evident in animals with **cleft palates.**

   3. **Diagnosis** is by **visual examination of the oral cavity.** Thorough examination may require sedation or anesthesia, especially to detect small fistulae secondary to periodontal disease.

   4. **Treatment. Surgical correction** is the treatment of choice for all types of oronasal fistulae and cleft palates. Correction of cleft palate is possible once the animal has attained a suitable size for anesthesia and surgery, usually at 6–8 weeks of age.
      a. **Preoperative considerations**
         (1) **Preoperative radiographs of the maxilla** are recommended for animals with cleft palates and oronasal fistulae secondary to neoplasia, infection, or trauma, so that the extent of bone deformity or destruction can be ascertained.
         (2) **Preoperative radiographs of the thorax** are also indicated to rule out the presence of aspiration pneumonia.
      b. **General technique.** Repair of cleft palates and oronasal fistulae is based on the creation of a mucoperiosteal or a gingival/buccal mucosal flap, or both, to cover the defect.
         (1) **Principles**
            (a) The flap must be larger than the defect.

   (b) The apposed edges must be cleanly incised because a flap sutured to an intact epithelial surface will not heal.
   (c) Suture lines should be placed over connective tissue, rather than the defect itself, whenever possible.
   (d) Tension on suture lines should be minimized by adequately mobilizing the flaps and using large bites of tissue when placing sutures.
   (e) Care should be taken to preserve the major palatine artery when elevating mucoperiosteal flaps near the point of its emergence from the palatine bone (approximately 1 cm medial to the carnassial tooth).
   (2) Wound closure
   (a) Absorbable or nonabsorbable sutures (except stainless steel) are used in an **appositional suture pattern** (e.g., simple interrupted).
      (i) If possible, a **two-layer closure is advised** to minimize tension on the epithelial suture line.
      (ii) Nonabsorbable sutures have to be removed, often requiring sedation or anesthesia of the animal; however, this provides an opportunity to examine the suture line.
   (b) Electrocautery should be avoided to prevent tissue damage, avoid delayed wound healing, and decrease the likelihood of wound dehiscence.
   (c) Use of perioperative antibiotics. In healthy wounds, perioperative antibiotics are unnecessary. If there is moderate to severe periodontal disease, perioperative antibiotics should be used.
c. Repair of primary cleft palate. The floor of the nasal orifice is closed so it is confluent with the mucosal side of the lip closure, and then the nasal and cutaneous lip clefts are closed.
d. Repair of secondary cleft palate. The two most frequently used procedures for treatment of secondary cleft palates involve creation of sliding bipedicle flaps and overlapping flaps.
   (1) Sliding bipedicle flaps are created on either side of the cleft along the length of the defect by making bilateral incisions in the mucoperiosteum along the dental arcade.
      (a) The mucoperiosteal layer is elevated from the incisions to the defect on both sides and the edges of the defect are incised and sutured in two layers (i.e., nasal and oral mucosae).
      (b) This procedure places the suture line over the defect.
   (2) Overlapping flaps are created when a mucoperiosteal pedicle at the margin of the defect is reflected and overlapped by the opposite incised edge of the defect. This procedure avoids placing the suture line over the defect and is usually associated with less tension on the suture line than the bipedicle procedure.
   (3) Combinations or modifications of these two procedures are feasible. Defects that extend into the soft palate can be closed by incising the margins of the defect, undermining the oral and nasal mucosa, and apposing the nasal mucosa and oral mucosa in separate layers.
e. Repair of oronasal fistulae secondary to trauma or severe periodontal disease requires careful débridement and excision of devitalized and infected tissue.
   (1) For **mild periodontal oronasal fistulae,** the tooth can be removed and the alveolar bone débrided with rongeurs.
   (2) For **severe periodontal oronasal fistulae,** *en bloc* removal of the tooth and surrounding bone by partial maxillectomy may be necessary. Closure of an oronasal fistula may be performed with a gingival/buccal mucosal flap, a mucoperiosteal flap elevated from the hard palate, or a combination of both in a double reposition flap procedure (Figure 7–3).
      (a) The **gingival/buccal mucosal flap** is an advancement flap created in the buccal mucosae at the edge of the fistula. The flap is elevated and advanced until it will cover the defect without tension. The flap is positioned over the defect and sutured (in two layers if possible) to the edges of the defect.

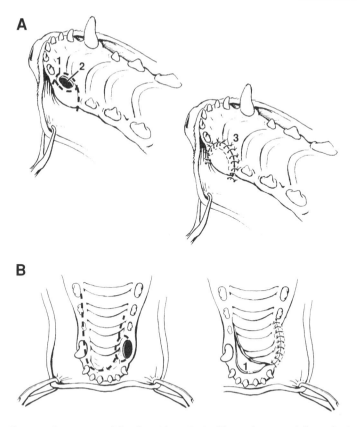

FIGURE 7–3. (*A*) Closure of an oronasal fistula with a gingival/buccal mucosal flap. The incision (*1*) around the fistula (*2*) extends into the buccal gingiva. The flap is advanced over the defect and sutured to the mucoperiosteum of the hard palate (*3*), using a two-layer closure. (*B*) Closure of an oronasal fistula with a mucoperiosteal flap. An incision (*broken line*) in the mucoperiosteum is made. The flap is elevated, advanced over the defect, and sutured to the buccal margin of the defect. Note the secondary defect (*1*) created with this procedure.

      (i) This procedure is suitable for oronasal fistulae positioned close to the gingival margin.

      (ii) Nasal epithelium covers the exposed submucosal tissue facing the nasal cavity within 30 days.

(b) Mucoperiosteal flaps elevated from the hard palate may be hinged, advanced, or rotated over the defect, depending on the location of the fistula and the availability of nearby tissue.

      (i) Mucoperiosteal flaps are usually used for oronasal fistulae located toward the center of the hard palate, or in combination with gingival/buccal mucosal flaps.

      (ii) A secondary defect is often created, but the exposed bone of the hard palate is covered by epithelium within 3–4 weeks.

(c) Double reposition flap. A hinged mucoperiosteal flap, based at the medial edge of the defect, is elevated and reflected over the defect. This flap and the exposed palatine bone are then covered by a gingival/buccal mucosal advancement flap.

      (i) A double reposition flap is used to repair large oronasal fistulae that require several flaps to cover the defect, or for repair of failed closures of oronasal fistula near the gingival margin.

      (ii) Advantages include a strong double-layer closure and a bacteria-resistant epithelial surface in both the nasal and oral cavities.

5. Postoperative considerations
  a. Dehiscence, the most common complication of oronasal fistula repair, is often the result of technical difficulties and poor tissue integrity. **Prevention of self-mutilation** is extremely important; an Elizabethan collar should be placed on the animal immediately after recovery from anesthesia.
  b. Enteral feeding. Some form of enteral feeding that bypasses the oral cavity may be required to prevent impaction of food and irritation of the suture line. Definitive evidence of any beneficial effect on healing by doing this is, however, lacking.
    (1) Pharyngostomy and **gastrostomy** (percutaneous if possible) are suitable methods (see Chapter 5 IV B 3, 5).
    (2) The **duration** of enteral feeding **is arbitrary** but should probably cover at least the first 7 days.
  c. Inspection of the surgical site daily is important to monitor healing.
    (1) Nonabsorbable sutures can be removed in 14 days.
    (2) Open palatine defects usually require 3–4 weeks to become completely covered with epithelium. Unless the area is obviously infected (e.g., necrotic stomatitis), postoperative antibiotics are unnecessary.

F. Laryngeal paralysis

1. Etiology
  a. Idiopathic laryngeal paralysis is the result of **neurogenic atrophy of the intrinsic laryngeal muscles.** Older, large and giant breed dogs (e.g., St. Bernard, Labrador retriever, golden retriever, Siberian husky) are most often affected. A heritable form has been described in Siberian huskies and Bouvier des Flandres, and may occur in younger animals of these breeds.
  b. Other causes of laryngeal paralysis include trauma to the recurrent laryngeal or vagal nerves, mass lesions of the cervical or cranial mediastinal regions, iatrogenic damage to the nerves during cervical surgery, and polyneuropathy.

2. Clinical signs. Early clinical signs of laryngeal paralysis include **dysphonia** and **postprandial gagging** and **coughing. Exercise intolerance, stridor, severe dyspnea, cyanosis,** and **collapse** become apparent as the disease progresses.

3. Diagnosis. Visual examination of the larynx while the animal is sedated reveals the inability of the arytenoid cartilages and vocal folds to abduct during inspiration.
  a. The **arytenoid processes lie in a more medial position,** reducing the size of the laryngeal lumen.
  b. Idiopathic laryngeal paralysis, which is most common, results in **bilateral** paralysis. Other causes usually result in **unilateral** paralysis.

4. Treatment is surgical and may involve arytenoid cartilage lateralization, vocal cordectomy alone or with partial arytenoidectomy, modified castellated laryngofissure, reinnervation of laryngeal muscles, or permanent tracheostomy. A temporary tracheostomy may facilitate anesthetization and visualization for laryngectomy and castellated laryngofissure procedures.
  a. Arytenoid cartilage lateralization (Figure 7–4) involves placement of a nonabsorbable, monofilament suture from the muscular process of the arytenoid cartilage (the insertion of the dorsal cricoarytenoid muscle) to the caudodorsal midline of the cricoid cartilage.
    (1) Technique. Incision of the interarytenoid ligament can be performed but is not essential. Disarticulation of the cricoarytenoid articulation allows better visualization of the muscular process of the arytenoid cartilage for suture placement.
    (2) Unilateral or bilateral procedures can be performed. Bilateral lateralization increases the chance of postoperative aspiration pneumonia, although this is also a potential complication of unilateral lateralization.
    (3) A **lateral or ventral approach** can be taken.
  b. Vocal cordectomy and partial arytenoidectomy
    (1) Oral approach (Figure 7–5)

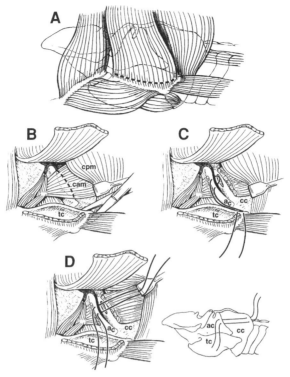

FIGURE 7–4. Arytenoid cartilage lateralization. (*A*) The larynx and adjacent musculature. The thyropharyngeal muscle is transected (*broken line*) to expose the thyroid cartilage. (*B*) The cricothyroid articulation is severed to allow reflection of the thyroid cartilage (*tc*) ventrally. The cricopharyngeal muscle (*cpm*) is retracted caudally, exposing the dorsal cricoarytenoid muscle (*cam*). The dorsal cricoarytenoid muscle is transected over the cricoarytenoid articulation and the cricoarytenoid articulation is severed. The junction between the corniculate processes (sesamoid band) is severed to completely mobilize the arytenoid cartilage. (*C*) A suture is placed between the muscular process of the arytenoid cartilage (*ac*) and the caudodorsal edge of the thyroid cartilage (*tc*). Cricoid cartilage (*cc*) is visible. (*D*) Alternatively, the suture may be placed between the muscular process of the arytenoid cartilage (*ac*) and the cricoid cartilage (*cc*) in the region of the now-exposed cricothyroid articular surface (*tc*).

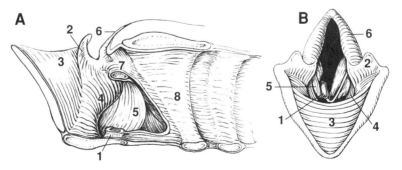

FIGURE 7–5. Vocal cordectomy (oral approach). (*A*) Medial view after vocal cordectomy, showing the ventral remnant of the vocal cord and muscle (*1*), the cuneiform process (*2*), the epiglottis (*3*), the false vocal cord (*4*), the mucosa lateral to the excised vocal cord and muscle (*5*), the corniculate process (*6*), the arytenoid cartilage (*7*), and the cricoid cartilage (*8*). (*B*) Rostral view of the larynx after vocal cordectomy.

(a) **Vocal cordectomy.** The vocal folds are resected using a long-handled instrument or equine uterine biopsy forceps.
(i) **Bilateral resection** is performed if only the vocal folds are excised.
(ii) **Unilateral resection** is done in conjunction with partial arytenoidectomy.
(b) **Partial arytenoidectomy.** Unilateral resection of the corniculate process of the arytenoid cartilage is performed, while the interarytenoid groove, ventral commissure, and ventral vocal fold tissues are preserved.
(c) **Resection of the cuneiform process, muscular process,** and **aryepiglottic fold** can be performed if necessary.
(d) **Healing.** The operative wounds are left open to heal by second intention.
(e) **Postoperative complications** include contraction and formation of an obstructive web across the laryngeal lumen, and development of excessive granulation tissue. Excessive scarring may require additional tissue resection and the creation of mucosal flaps to attain primary healing.
(2) **Ventral approach.** Vocal cordectomy and partial arytenoidectomy can be performed more accurately through a ventral laryngotomy incision in the thyroid cartilage. This approach allows incision of the mucosa over the arytenoid, which facilitates the removal of cartilage and vocal folds and allows suturing of the mucosa to reduce granulation tissue formation.
c. **Modified castellated laryngofissure** is performed via a ventral laryngotomy through the thyroid cartilage (Figure 7–6).
d. **Reinnervation of the laryngeal muscles** may be possible using nerve anastomosis or neuromuscular pedicle graft techniques.
(1) Anastomosis of the recurrent laryngeal nerve may be possible in traumatic cases.
(2) Alternately, ventral motor branches of the first cervical nerve (and the sternothyroid muscle) or a portion of the phrenic nerve may be used.
e. **Permanent tracheostomy** is discussed in IV B 2.

G. **Laryngeal collapse** is characterized by medial and rostral collapse of the arytenoid cartilages and aryepiglottic folds.

1. **Etiology.** Trauma or conditions that diminish cartilage support (e.g., **brachycephalic syndrome**) lead to laryngeal collapse.

2. **Pathogenesis.** Laryngeal collapse occurs in stages characterized by laryngeal saccule eversion (stage 1), medial collapse of the cuneiform process (stage 2), and medial collapse of the corniculate process (stage 3).

3. **Clinical signs** are similar to those of laryngeal paralysis.

4. **Treatment.** Conservative treatment (i.e., medication and rest) may help some animals, although surgery can provide more reliable relief of clinical signs.
a. In brachycephalic breeds, resection of nares, the elongated soft palate, and everted saccules is performed. A permanent tracheostomy may be indicated in severe disease.
b. In other breeds, a permanent tracheostomy is indicated.

H. **Laryngeal neoplasia** comprises benign polyps, granulation or scar tissue, and malignant disease.

1. **Inflammatory polyps** are rare but may be removed by simple excision, via an oral or ventral laryngotomy approach.

2. **Granulation or scar tissue** secondary to partial laryngectomy procedures is removed following a ventral laryngotomy. Mucosal apposition is necessary to prevent recurrence.

3. **Malignant disease** is rare but adenocarcinoma, osteosarcoma, chondrosarcoma, mast cell tumors, and leiomyomas have been reported and will cause obstructive dyspnea. Local excision through a ventral laryngotomy may be palliative, but total laryngec-

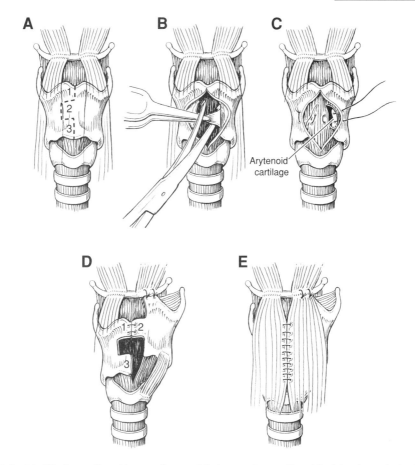

FIGURE 7–6. Modified castellated laryngofissure. (*A*) A ventral, castellated incision is made in the thyroid cartilage. (*B*) The vocal folds are resected. (*C*) Intraglottic arytenoid lateralization is performed by placing a single horizontal mattress suture through the vocal process of the arytenoid cartilage and the lamina of the thyroid cartilage, traversing the recess of the lateral ventricle. Nonabsorbable, monofilament suture material is used. (*D*) The castellated incision is closed. One side of the "stepped" thyroid cartilage is advanced cranially. The apposed edge of the flap and the opposite cut edge of the thyroid cartilage are sutured. (*E*) The defects remaining between the cut edges are covered by apposed sternohyoid muscles. (Modified with permission from Gourley IM, Gregory CR: *Atlas of Small Animal Surgery.* New York, Gower, 1992, p 5.7.)

tomy in conjunction with a permanent tracheostomy may be indicated to achieve adequate margins and relieve the obstruction.

 LOWER RESPIRATORY TRACT CONDITIONS TREATED BY SURGERY

A. **Tracheal collapse** typically occurs in middle-aged to older toy and miniature-breed dogs (e.g., pomeranians, toy and miniature poodles, Yorkshire terriers, pugs, chihuahuas).

1. **Etiology.** The specific cause of the condition is unknown.

2. **Pathogenesis.** Affected tracheal cartilage progressively degenerates and cannot maintain its shape during respiration.

    a. **Grade I collapse** is characterized by a 25% reduction in lumen diameter. The trachealis muscle is slightly pendulous and the cartilage is still somewhat circular in shape.

    b. Grade II collapse is characterized by a 50% reduction in lumen diameter. The trachealis muscle is stretched and pendulous and the cartilage is somewhat flattened.

    c. Grade III collapse is characterized by a 75% reduction in lumen diameter. The trachealis muscle is stretched and pendulous and the cartilage is nearly completely flattened.

    d. Grade IV collapse. The lumen is essentially obliterated and the trachealis muscle is in contact with cartilage.

3. Clinical signs. A history of mild to moderate **productive coughing** and **mild exercise intolerance** is common. The cough progresses to a typical **"goose-honk"** and excitement often precipitates coughing and dyspnea.

4. Diagnosis is based on history, clinical signs, possible palpation of flattened cervical tracheal rings, and radiography and endoscopy findings.

    a. Thoracic radiographs may reveal **cardiomegaly. Inspiratory and expiratory thoracic radiographs** reveal a **collapsed trachea** in approximately 60% of dogs with severe (grade II or more) collapse.

        (1) The cervical trachea collapses on inspiration, while the thoracic trachea collapses on expiration.

        (2) Fluoroscopy may facilitate diagnosis.

    b. Endoscopy is performed with the animal under light anesthesia to determine the grade of collapse. Tracheal inflammation and infection are often present; therefore, bronchotracheal washing samples should be collected for bacterial culture and sensitivity testing and cytology studies.

        (1) Laryngeal paresis or paralysis has been reported in approximately 30% of dogs with tracheal collapse.

        (2) Fifty percent of dogs with tracheal collapse have some degree of bronchial collapse, worsening the prognosis.

5. Treatment

    a. Weight reduction and medical therapy (i.e., antitussives, bronchodilators, antibiotics, corticosteroids, sedatives) may alleviate symptoms in some dogs.

    b. Surgical treatment is indicated for dogs with 50% or more reduction in tracheal lumen diameter. **Plastic prosthetic rings** (Figure 7–7) or **a spiral** is placed around the trachea. Although using a prosthetic spiral instead of individual rings has produced favorable results, placement of the spiral requires extensive dissection, which may compromise the tracheal blood supply and cause necrosis.

        (1) Preparation of rings. The rings are fashioned from 3-cc polypropylene syringe cases, have five or six predrilled holes, and are autoclaved prior to surgery.

        (2) Support of the cervical trachea. The rings are placed around the cervical trachea through a ventral cervical approach and sutured in place. At least one suture should be through the trachealis muscle.

        (3) Support of the thoracic trachea. The portion of the trachea at the thoracic inlet and the intrathoracic tracheal portion are exposed by cranial traction on the cervical trachea. Five or six rings are usually placed.

            (a) If intrathoracic exposure is required, the trachea can be approached by

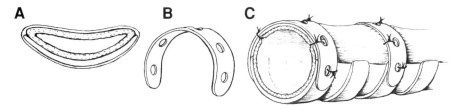

FIGURE 7–7. (*A*) Grade III tracheal collapse. (*B*) Plastic ring prosthesis. (*C*) The plastic ring is sutured to the trachea and dorsal membrane (tracheal muscle).

extension of the cervical incision to a median sternotomy or through a right lateral thoracotomy at the third to fifth intercostal space.

(b) The morbidity rate substantially increases with intrathoracic exposure.

(4) **Postoperative complications** include respiratory distress resulting from inflammation and edema of the tracheal mucosa. Corticosteroids, supplemental oxygen, cough suppressants, and sedatives may be indicated. **Early postoperative results** may not be improved over preoperative status because of tracheitis and suture irritation. By 4 weeks, coughing and dyspnea should improve.

B. **Upper airway obstruction. Tracheostomy** is used to bypass upper airway obstruction. It can be **temporary** or **permanent.** Tracheostomy may be an **elective** procedure (preoperative temporary tube tracheostomy, permanent tracheostomy) or an **emergency** procedure.

1. **Temporary (tube) tracheostomy** is performed aseptically through a ventral midline incision over the trachea.

   a. **Tracheal incision.** A transverse incision is made between the third and fourth or fourth and fifth tracheal rings. Other incisions (e.g., vertical, elliptical, "U," window-type) have also been described.

   b. **Tracheostomy tubes** may be metal or plastic, cuffed or noncuffed, and cannulated or noncannulated. In order to prevent total obstruction should the tube become occluded, the diameter of the tube should be approximately one half the diameter of the trachea.

   c. **Postoperative care**
      (1) Initially, intense postoperative care is required. The tube may need cleaning as often as every 15 minutes using a sterile suction cannula inserted into the tube lumen. Sterile saline can be infused into the trachea immediately before suctioning to loosen secretions.
      (2) The tracheostomy tube is removed when an adequate airway is established. Alternatively, smaller tubes can replace larger ones until adequate ventilation is resumed.
      (3) After tube removal, the incision is allowed to heal by second intention.

   d. **Complications** include gagging, vomiting, tube obstruction, tube dislodgment, emphysema, tracheal stenosis, tracheocutaneous or tracheoesophageal fistula formation, and tracheal malacia.

2. **Permanent tracheostomy** provides relief of upper airway obstruction that is not responsive to other methods of treatment. It is performed at the level of the third to sixth tracheal rings, via a ventral approach (Figure 7–8).

   a. **Resection of the tracheal wall.** A ventral segment of the tracheal wall, approximately 3 to 4 tracheal rings long and one third of the tracheal circumference in width, is resected.

   b. **Creation of a tracheostoma.** An "I" or "H" incision is made in the mucosa and the edges sutured to the edges of the skin to create a tracheostoma.

   c. **Postoperative management** requires inspection of the tracheostoma every 1–3 hours.
      (1) Mucus accumulation is gently wiped from the stoma. The distal trachea can be suctioned using sterile equipment. After 1 week, cleansing can be reduced to every 4–6 hours and by the end of the first month, cleansing may only be required twice daily.
      (2) Hair is kept short around the stoma to prevent matting.
      (3) Exercise must be limited to clean areas and swimming is prohibited.

   d. **Postoperative complications** involve stomal occlusion resulting from skin folds or stenosis (e.g., due to contraction of the stoma, collapse of cartilage rings, or formation of excessive granulation tissue).

C. **Trauma, neoplasia,** or **stenosis of the trachea** requires **tracheal reconstruction.** Up to 20%–60% of the trachea (8 to 23 rings) can be removed in dogs. **Split-cartilage anasto-**

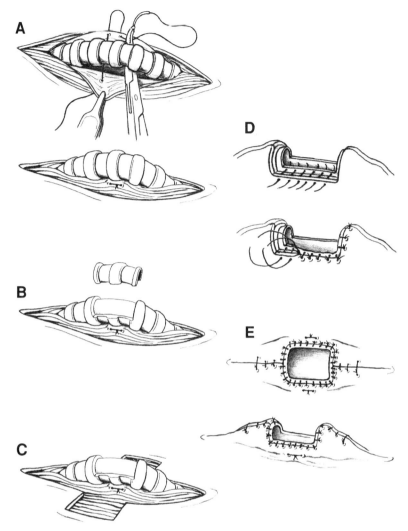

FIGURE 7–8. Permanent tracheostomy (ventral approach). (*A*) One or two horizontal mattress sutures are placed through the sternohyoid muscles to elevate the trachea. (*B*) A portion of the ventral trachea is resected. (*C*) A similarly sized section of skin is excised. (*D*) An "I"-shaped incision is made in the mucosa and the stoma is closed with simple interrupted sutures through the mucosa and skin. (*E*) Note that four large horizontal mattress sutures are preplaced through the peritracheal fascia and skin before the mucosal sutures are placed to relieve tension on the stoma closure. (Modified with permission from Hedlund CS, Tangner CH: Tracheal surgery in the dog, part II. *Comp Cont Ed* 5:738–751, 1983, p 746.)

mosis is the preferred method, because it preserves lumen size and results in more precise anatomic alignment than other techniques involving apposition of intact rings, suturing of the annular ligaments, or overlapping the rings.

1. **Technique.** The affected segment is removed by incising halfway through a cartilage ring on either end of the segment. These cartilages are reapposed and sutured together with simple interrupted absorbable or nonabsorbable sutures placed around the cartilage rings. **Preservation of blood supply is essential; only the affected segment must be freed from the surrounding peritracheal tissue.**

2. **Postoperative considerations.** Exercise is restricted and extension of the neck is avoided. Neck braces may be required. **Complications** include dehiscence and stenosis.

D. **Lung disease**

1. **Surgical techniques**
   a. **Thoracotomy.** The lungs are typically approached via a lateral thoracotomy over the affected lung area (see Chapter 9 III; Table 9–1).
   b. **Partial lobectomy** can be used to attain biopsy samples, or to treat isolated marginal lesions. The portion to be removed is isolated and cut distal to a row of absorbable continuous horizontal mattress sutures or a row of staples.
   c. **Lobectomy** is usually performed via a **lateral (right or left) thoracotomy** at the fifth or sixth intercostal space. A **median sternotomy** provides good access to the ventricles of the heart and allows exploration of the entire thoracic cavity; however, access to the hilus of the lungs is difficult, especially in deep-chested animals.
      (1) **Blood vessel ligation and bronchial suturing** is the traditional approach.
         (a) The bronchus and blood vessels are palpated at the hilus from a craniodorsal position.
         (b) The lobar artery, located dorsolateral to the bronchus, is dissected free from the bronchus using blunt-tipped right-angle forceps.
         (c) The artery is triple-ligated; two simple ligatures of 2-0 or 3-0 monofilament absorbable suture are placed first, followed by placement of a transfixation suture distal to the most proximal ligature. The artery is severed between the transfixation suture and the distal simple ligature.
         (d) The lobar vein, located ventromedial to the bronchus, is dissected free, ligated, and divided as was the artery.
         (e) The bronchus is thus exposed, and further dissection of the peribronchial tissue should be minimal.
            (i) The bronchus is double-clamped and transected between the clamps, allowing removal of the lung and, consequently, improved exposure of the bronchial stump.
            (ii) The bronchus proximal to the remaining clamp is sutured with overlapping, simple interrupted horizontal mattress sutures, using 2-0 or 3-0 monofilament absorbable or nonabsorbable suture material.
            (iii) The clamp is removed and the crushed bronchus is trimmed, leaving approximately 2 mm of crushed tissue. The stump is oversewn in a simple continuous suture pattern.
      (2) **Stapled lobectomy** is quick, safe, and inexpensive. Because stapling substantially reduces operative time, perioperative morbidity is reduced.
         (a) Even in large-breed dogs, the 50-mm thoracoabdominal stapler (TA50) is usually sufficient to extend across the bronchial hilus.
         (b) The TA50 is placed across the hilus and fired, placing a double row of 2.5-mm staples. The hilus is transected distal to the staples before the stapler is removed.
      (3) **Combination.** Alternatively, the blood vessels may be ligated and the stapler used on the bronchus only.
         (a) This is advantageous when exposure of the hilus is difficult. Ligation and division of the blood vessels improves exposure of the hilus.
         (b) It is also advantageous in very large dogs where the large staples (e.g., 3.5-mm) required to compress the bronchus do not adequately compress the blood vessels.
      (4) **Flushing.** Following removal of the lung lobe, the thorax is filled with warm saline to check for air bubbles as evidence of leakage from the bronchus (or lung parenchyma, in partial lobectomy).
      (5) **Thoracostomy tube placement** (see IV D 1 e) is required to remove air remaining in the chest and monitor for postoperative bronchial or parenchymal leakage. One tube drains both hemithoraxes in dogs and cats because the mediastinum is incomplete.
   d. **Pneumonectomy.** The entire left lung can be removed without significant compromise; however right pneumonectomy, which causes obstruction of more than

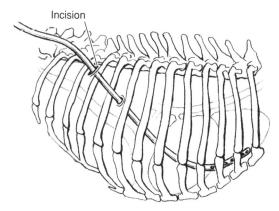

Incision

FIGURE 7–9. Placement of a thoracostomy tube (lateral view). The tube is introduced through the skin between the tenth and eleventh ribs and passed subcutaneously for three or four intercostal spaces in a cranioventral direction. Between the eighth and ninth ribs (*arrow*), the tube is threaded through the intercostal muscles and pleura to the thoracic cavity. (Redrawn with permission from Bojrab MJ: *Current Techniques in Small Animal Surgery,* 2nd ed. Philadelphia, Lea & Febiger, 1990, p 288.)

60% of pulmonary blood flow and diminishes lung capacity by more than 50%, may be fatal.

e. **Thoracostomy** (Figure 7–9). A thoracostomy tube is introduced through the skin at the level of the tenth or eleventh rib, passed subcutaneously for three or four intercostal spaces in a cranioventral direction, then introduced through the intercostal muscles and pleura using a stylet or a large hemostat. The tube is sutured to the skin and bandaged to the chest with only the end exposed, and suction is applied.

   (1) A **continuous suction system** is used for situations such as spontaneous pneumothorax or pleural effusions (chylothorax, pyothorax), using a two- or three-underwater bottle system. A one-way (Heimlich) valve is used to treat pneumothorax in medium- or large-sized dogs (i.e., those weighing more than 15 kg).

   (a) Continuous suction of 8–15 cm H_2O is effective for pneumothorax. Pressures of up to 20 cm H_2O may be needed to aspirate viscous fluid.

   (b) In the three-bottle system, the thoracostomy tube is connected to a collection bottle, which is connected to a water seal (containing 2–3 cm of water) that is connected to the suction control bottle (containing 10–20 cm water). The amount of suction is altered by raising or lowering a tube in the water in the third bottle. A vent tube in the third bottle allows air to be aspirated into the bottle as suction is applied.

   (2) **Intermittent suction** uses a three-way stopcock on the end of the thoracostomy tube.

   (a) A "C"-clamp must be used to occlude the tube between aspirations to prevent pneumothorax from developing as the result of a leaky stopcock connection.

   (b) Intermittent suction is applied every 15 minutes, lengthening the intervals as the amount of air or fluid decreases. It is imperative to completely close the stopcock and ensure that all connections are tight.

2. **Specific conditions treated by surgery**

   a. **Neoplasia**

   (1) **Primary pulmonary neoplasia** is most common in older, large-breed dogs. **Adenocarcinoma** and **alveolar carcinoma** are diagnosed most often.

   (a) **Clinical signs** may result from airway compression, regional ventilation–perfusion abnormalities, or pleural effusion.

   (i) A **persistent cough, unresponsive to antibiotics,** is a common clinical sign.

       (ii) **Exercise intolerance, respiratory distress,** and **hemoptysis** can occur.

       (iii) **Anorexia, weight loss,** and **depression** may be seen.

       (iv) Thoracic masses may cause **hypertrophic osteopathy,** a condition characterized by swollen, painful, distal limbs that show periosteal proliferation on radiographs. Regression of the clinical signs and periosteal proliferation occur with excision of the thoracic masses.

    (b) Diagnosis

       (i) **Radiography reveals a single nodule,** most commonly in the right caudal lung lobe. **Cavitation** and **calcification of the mass** may occur. **Hilar lymphadenopathy** may be evident.

       (ii) **Definitive diagnosis** is based on **cytology** or **histopathology** of pleural fluid, bronchoalveolar lavage fluid, or fine needle aspirates of the nodule.

    (c) Treatment entails either **lobectomy** or **pneumonectomy** and **biopsy of the tracheobronchial lymph nodes.**

    (d) Prognosis, based on wide excision and no evidence of metastatic disease in the lymph nodes, is good, with a median survival time of at least 1 year. Metastatic spread to the lymph nodes carries a poor prognosis with a median survival time of 2–3 months.

  (2) Secondary pulmonary neoplasia is common because the lungs are a frequent site of metastatic spread. The efficacy of surgical excision of metastatic pulmonary lesions is uncertain.

b. Lung abscesses are more common in cats than in dogs.

  (1) Etiology. Abscess formation may be secondary to foreign bodies, chronic lung infection, penetrating wounds, vascular obstruction, or neoplastic disease.

  (2) Clinical signs include pyrexia, cough, respiratory distress, exercise intolerance, anorexia, and lethargy.

  (3) Treatment is surgical excision of the affected lung lobe.

  (4) Prognosis for confined disease is very good after complete surgical excision. Disseminated disease carries a poor prognosis.

c. Lung lobe torsion is an uncommon condition, usually seen in large, deep-chested canine breeds. The right cranial and right middle lung lobe are most often affected.

  (1) Etiology. Lung lobe torsion is associated with chylothorax, trauma, neoplasia, and chronic respiratory disease.

  (2) Pathogenesis. Lung lobe torsion causes venous and bronchial obstruction, but arterial blood flow is maintained. The lung lobe consolidates and pleural effusion occurs.

  (3) Clinical signs are related to the pleural effusion and consolidated or necrotic lung lobe. **Coughing,** varying degrees of **dyspnea, anorexia,** and **weight loss** are observed. **Muffled respiratory and cardiac sounds** are noted because of the presence of pleural fluid.

  (4) Diagnosis is by **radiography** and **bronchoscopy. Exploratory thoracotomy** may be required if these methods are nondiagnostic.

    (a) The pleural fluid may be serosanguineous or chylous in nature, containing erythrocytes and leukocytes but rarely bacteria.

    (b) Radiographs reveal pleural fluid and lung consolidation. Radiographs taken after aspiration of pleural fluid may better identify the affected lung lobe; the lung lobe can be definitively identified with positive contrast bronchography or bronchoscopy.

  (5) Treatment involves **lobectomy.** To prevent endotoxin release, the affected lung lobe is not derotated.

d. Lung lacerations may be secondary to rib fractures, penetrating injury, or, occasionally, blunt trauma.

  (1) Clinical signs may be related to the type of injury.

    (a) Pain or crepitus on palpation may be associated with fractured ribs.

    (b) Respiratory distress may be associated with hemothorax or pneumothorax.

    (c) Moist lung sounds are associated with pulmonary hemorrhage or edema.

(2) Diagnosis
   (a) Radiographs may show free air and fluid within the thorax.
   (b) Bronchoscopy may be useful to locate tracheal or main-stem bronchial tears. Identification of hemorrhage within a bronchus may help to identify the affected lung lobe.
(3) Treatment. Spontaneous healing of pulmonary lacerations may occur, but surgical intervention is indicated if there is continual evidence of pneumothorax despite treatment or there is evidence of significant hemorrhage associated with the injury.
   (a) A **lateral thoracotomy** is performed over the affected lung lobe, and the laceration is first sutured using large horizontal mattress sutures.
   (b) The edges of the laceration can then be apposed with a simple continuous or a continuous Lembert suture pattern.
e. Spontaneous pneumothorax is air within the thorax caused by conditions other than trauma. This condition is considered a **closed pneumothorax** because the air originates from within the thorax (i.e., the thoracic cavity has not been penetrated).
   (1) Etiology. Causes include emphysematous bullae, cysts, or other parenchymal disease. The underlying disease may be difficult to discern radiographically. In one study of 21 animals, only 4 had radiographic evidence of underlying disease.
   (2) Treatment
      (a) Conservative therapy with **thoracostomy tubes** often results in recurrence, and early surgical intervention is indicated.
      (b) Definitive treatment involves excision of the affected lung lobe.

SELECTED READINGS

Bojrab MJ (ed): *Current Techniques in Small Animal Surgery*, 3rd ed. Philadelphia, Lea & Febiger, 1990, pp 321–366.

Ettinger SJ, Feldman EC (ed): *Textbook of Veterinary Internal Medicine*, 4th ed. Philadelphia, WB Saunders, 1995, pp 551–566, 754–811.

Gourley I, Gregory C: *Atlas of Small Animal Surgery*. New York, Gower, 1992, pp 2–2.10, 4–4.6, 5–5.6, 6–6.5.

Holt D, Harvey C: Idiopathic laryngeal paralysis: results of treatment by bilateral vocal fold reaction in 40 dogs. *J Am Anim Hosp Assoc* 30:389–395, 1994.

Holtsinger RH, Beale BS, Bellah JR, et al: Spontaneous pneumothorax in the dog: a retrospective analysis of 21 cases. *J Am Anim Hosp Assoc* 29:195–210, 1993.

Morris JS, Dunn KJ, Dobson JM, et al: Effects of radiotherapy alone and surgery and radiotherapy on survival of dogs with nasal tumours. *J Small Anim Pract* 35:567–573, 1994.

Ogilivie GK, Weigel RM, Haschek WM, et al: Prognostic factors for tumor remission and survival in dogs after surgery for primary lung tumor: 76 cases (1975–1985). *J Am Vet Med Assoc* 195:109–112, 1989.

Sharp NJH, Harvey CE, Sullivan M: Canine nasal aspergillosis and penicilliosis. *Compend Contin Educ Pract Vet* 13:41–48, 1991.

Slatter DH (ed): *Textbook of Small Animal Surgery*, 2nd ed. Philadelphia, WB Saunders, 1993, pp 692–819.

Trout NJ, Harpster NK, Berg J: Long-term results of unilateral ventriculocordectomy and partial arytenoidectomy for the treatment of laryngeal paralysis in 60 dogs. *J Am Anim Hosp Assoc* 30: 401–407, 1994.

White RAS: Unilateral arytenoid lateralization: an assessment of technique complications and long-term results in 62 dogs with laryngeal paralysis. *J Am Anim Pract* 30:543–549, 1989.

Chapter 8

Cardiovascular System

Giselle Hosgood

I. ANATOMY

A. **Orientation.** The heart and great vessels occupy the cranial thoracic cavity.

1. The heart lies obliquely, with the base directed craniodorsally and the apex directed caudoventrally.

2. The heart extends from the third to the sixth rib. The lungs cover most of its surface, except for the area of the cardiac notch over the right ventricle.

B. **Pericardium.** The heart is covered by the pericardium, which has an **outer fibrous layer** and an **inner serous layer.**

1. The **serous pericardium** is composed of two layers:
   a. The **parietal layer,** fused to the fibrous pericardium
   b. The **visceral layer,** or **epicardium,** attached to the heart

2. The **pericardial cavity,** which lies between the parietal and visceral layers of the serous pericardium, normally contains a small volume of clear fluid.

C. **Vessels.** Major vessels include the **aorta,** the **cranial and caudal venae cavae,** and the **pulmonary trunk.**

D. **Nerves.** The autonomic nervous system innervates the cardiovascular system.

1. **Parasympathetic innervation** is via the left and right vagus nerves, which pass across the left and right base of the heart, respectively.

2. **Sympathetic innervation** is through fibers originating in the thoracic spinal cord.

3. Other nerves, important because of their location within the thoracic cavity and their critical functions elsewhere in the body, are the left recurrent laryngeal nerve and the phrenic nerves.
   a. The **left recurrent laryngeal nerve** leaves the vagus at the aortic arch and loops around the aortic arch caudal to the ligamentum arteriosus.
   b. The **phrenic nerves** course across the lateral aspects of the heart, ventral to the vagus nerves.

II. CONGENITAL CARDIAC DISORDERS

A. **Epidemiology**

1. Certain dog breeds are predisposed to congenital heart defects (Table 8–1).

2. Cats have a higher incidence than dogs of multiple congenital heart defects but no breed predisposition has been found.

TABLE 8-1. Dog Breeds Predisposed to Congenital Heart Defects

Defect	Breed	
Atrial septal defect	Boxer	
	Old English sheepdog	
Patent ductus arteriosus (PDA)	Brittany spaniel	Keeshond
	Cocker spaniel	Pomeranian
	Collie	Miniature poodle
	German shepherd	Shetland sheepdog
Persistent right aortic arch (PRAA)	Doberman	
	German shepherd	
	Great Dane	
	Irish setter	
	Weimaraner	
Pulmonic stenosis	Beagle	Keeshond
	Chihuahua	Miniature schnauzer
	English bulldog	Samoyed
	German shepherd	Terriers
	Giant schnauzer	
Subaortic stenosis	Boxer	
	German shepherd	
	German short-hair pointer	
	Golden retriever	
	Newfoundland	
Tetralogy of Fallot	Keeshond	
	Miniature poodle	
	Miniature schnauzer	
	Terriers	
	Wirehaired fox terrier	
Valve dysplasia	Chihuahua	
	English bulldog	
	Great Dane	
	Weimaraner	
Ventricular septal defect	Beagle	
	English bulldog	
	German shepherd	
	Keeshond	
	Mastiff	
	Miniature poodle	
	Siberian husky	

B. **Common congenital cardiac defects** that are amenable to surgical treatment include patent ductus arteriosus (PDA), pulmonic stenosis, subaortic stenosis, and persistent right aortic arch (PRAA).

   1. **PDA** is the most common congenital cardiac defect in dogs. PDA is occasionally seen in cats.
      a. Pathogenesis
         (1) The ductus arteriosus is the normal fetal communication between the aorta and pulmonary artery. It should close within 2–3 days of birth in both dogs and cats.

    (2) Failure of the ductus arteriosus to close results in **left-to-right shunting of blood** from the aorta to the pulmonary artery.

    (3) A small number of animals with PDA develop **right-to-left shunting of blood** resulting from pulmonary hypertension. The prognosis for these animals is poor.

b. Diagnosis is by physical examination, electrocardiography, radiography, and, if necessary, echocardiography and selective angiography.

    (1) **Physical examination.** Clinical signs may not be noticeable until the pathology has progressed and the animal develops left-sided congestive heart failure and pulmonary edema.

        (a) Characteristic findings in animals with left-to-right shunting with or without clinical signs include the following:

            (i) A continuous murmur over the left heart base can be discerned, often associated with a palpable cardiac thrill.

            (ii) Femoral pulses are hyperkinetic ("water hammer"), because of rapid diastolic runoff of blood through the ductus arteriosum.

            (iii) Mucous membrane color is normal.

        (b) In animals with right-to-left shunting, caudal mucous membranes (e.g., the vulva, prepuce) are cyanotic and the animals are polycythemic. No cardiac murmur is discerned and the femoral pulse is normal.

    (2) **Electrocardiography** shows tall R waves (greater than 2.5 mV) in leads II and aVF. In leads I and aVF, deep Q waves may be present.

    (3) **Thoracic radiographs** show left atrial and ventricular enlargement, enlargement of pulmonary vessels (often described as "overcirculation" of the lungs), and dilation of the descending aorta. On the dorsoventral view, these changes represent the four "bulges" on the left side of the heart characteristic of PDA.

    (4) **Echocardiography** may confirm the cardiac changes but rarely actually identifies the shunt.

    (5) **Selective angiography,** using contrast medium injected into the ascending aorta, can be used to definitely determine the presence of PDA.

c. Treatment. Surgery should be performed as soon as possible after diagnosis. However, animals younger than 6 weeks of age or those that weigh less than 500 grams are a greater anesthetic risk. If the animal is otherwise clinically asymptomatic (apart from the murmur), delaying the surgery until this age or size is attained is desirable.

    (1) **Ligation of the left-to-right PDA** is performed through a left lateral thoracotomy at the fourth intercostal space (Figure 8–1).

        (a) Dogs with pulmonary edema should be treated with furosemide before surgery.

        (b) The PDA is bluntly dissected with right-angle forceps and double ligated with nonabsorbable suture.

            (i) Because of its limited length, the PDA is not severed.

            (ii) Care is required to isolate and retract the left vagus nerve from the PDA prior to dissection.

        (c) The PDA is ligated slowly with the arterial ligature tightened first. The heart rate may slow (Branham's sign) during ligation because of a sudden increase in arterial blood pressure.

        (d) A continuous murmur should no longer be auscultated after PDA ligation; however, a systolic murmur may be present if left ventricular dilation has caused mitral insufficiency.

    (2) **Ligation of right-to-left shunts** is contraindicated because the cardiac and pulmonary changes are irreversible, and rapid, fatal heart failure and pulmonary edema would occur.

d. Prognosis. The prognosis for long-term survival is excellent for animals with left-to-right PDA if heart failure has not occurred. Cardiac changes will reverse after ligation of the PDA.

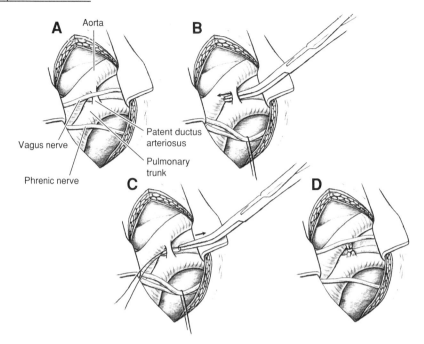

FIGURE 8–1. Ligation of patent ductus arteriosus (PDA). *(A)* A left lateral thoracotomy is performed through the fourth intercostal space, exposing the patent ductus arteriosus. Note the location of the vagus and phrenic nerves. The pericardium is incised over the ductus arteriosus and retracted, retracting the vagus nerve ventrally. *(B)* The ductus arteriosus is dissected from the caudal aspect. *(C)* A nonabsorbable, double ligature is passed around the ductus arteriosus. *(D)* Each ligature is tied separately. The ligature closest to the aorta is tied first. (Redrawn with permission from Gourley IM, Gregory CK: *Atlas of Small Animal Surgery.* New York, Gower Medical Publishing, 1992, p. 11:4.)

   2. Pulmonic stenosis may be supravalvular, valvular, or subvalvular; valvular stenosis is most common. Pulmonic stenosis is the second most common congenital cardiac defect in dogs. It is rare in cats.
   a. Pathogenesis. The increased pressure required for pulmonary outflow causes right ventricular hypertrophy. This may exacerbate the stenosis by narrowing the right ventricular outflow tract at the level of the infundibulum.
   b. Diagnosis
   (1) Physical examination. Most dogs are asymptomatic at the time of diagnosis; however, some dogs have clinical signs consistent with right-sided heart failure. A systolic murmur is auscultated over the region of the pulmonic valve (left side over base of heart).
   (2) Electrocardiographic findings indicate right ventricular enlargement and right axis deviation.
   (3) Thoracic radiographs reveal right ventricular and poststenotic pulmonary enlargement.
   (4) Echocardiography. Blood pressure gradients can be measured indirectly using Doppler echocardiography to assess the blood flow velocity in the pulmonary artery.
   (5) Cardiac catheterization can be performed to directly measure the blood pressure gradient across the pulmonic valve.
   c. Treatment
   (1) Indications for surgery. The decision to perform surgery is based on the age of the animal, clinical findings, and the blood pressure gradient across the pulmonic valve. Generally, animals with pulmonary blood pressure gradients greater than 50 mm Hg and right ventricular pressure greater than 70 mm Hg, or animals with severe right ventricular hypertrophy, are candidates for surgery.

(a) Immature or mature animals that are asymptomatic with right ventricular pressure less than 70 mm Hg can be treated conservatively.

(b) Asymptomatic or symptomatic immature animals with right ventricular pressure greater than 70 mm Hg should be treated with surgery.

(c) Symptomatic, mature animals with right ventricular pressure greater than 70 mm Hg may be poor candidates for surgery and are best treated conservatively.

(2) **Techniques** for correcting pulmonic stenosis include balloon valvuloplasty, blind valvuloplasty, valvulectomy, and patch grafting.

   (a) **Balloon valvuloplasty** is performed percutaneously.

    (i) The catheter is introduced through a jugular vein and passed into the right ventricle and across the pulmonic valve.

    (ii) The catheter is filled with contrast medium to facilitate monitoring its position fluoroscopically.

    (iii) The balloon is inflated to dilate the valve. The systolic blood pressure is monitored to evaluate the effectiveness of the dilation and the change in systolic pulmonic blood pressure gradient.

   (b) **Blind valvuloplasty (Brock procedure)** is indicated for simple valve stenosis without infundibular stenosis.

    (i) Blind valvuloplasty is performed via a lateral thoracotomy at the fourth intercostal space.

    (ii) A purse-string suture is placed at the base of the pulmonary outflow tract in the right ventricle. A valve dilator is placed through a stab incision in the middle of the purse-string suture and passed through the valve.

    (iii) The purse-string suture is tightened around the instrument to prevent hemorrhage.

    (iv) The pulmonic valve is dilated several times by opening the valve dilator. The instrument is then withdrawn and the purse-string suture tied.

   (c) **Valvulectomy** is indicated for valvular pulmonic stenosis.

    (i) Venous inflow occlusion is performed; temporary ligatures are placed around the cranial and caudal venae cavae and the azygous vein.

    (ii) The venous inflow is occluded and the heart is allowed to beat once or twice to empty the ventricles. A pulmonary arteriotomy is performed directly over the valve, and the valve leaflets are resected.

    (iii) A Satinsky clamp is placed on the arteriotomy incision to allow closure of the arteriotomy without occlusion of the pulmonary artery and to allow release of the venous inflow occlusion.

    (iv) Venous inflow occlusion should be sustained for no longer than 2 minutes. However, venous inflow can be released and re-occluded several times.

   (d) **Patch grafting** is indicated for severe valvular stenosis with infundibular hypertrophy.

    (i) A patch of pericardium or synthetic material (e.g., polytetrafluorethylene) is placed over the pulmonary outflow tract, extending from the ventricle to the supravalvular area. Some redundancy in the patch is required, especially for young, growing animals.

    (ii) Patch grafting can be performed with or without venous inflow occlusion (i.e., the grafting can be "open" or "closed," respectively).

       In **open grafting,** venous inflow occlusion is performed to allow incision into the right ventricular outflow tract and valvulectomy. The patch is then sutured to the epicardium to cover the area of the open incision.

       For **closed grafting,** a small-gauge wire is preplaced in the pulmonary outflow tract through a hole in the pulmonary artery above the pulmonic valve, emerging from a hole in the right lateral ventricular

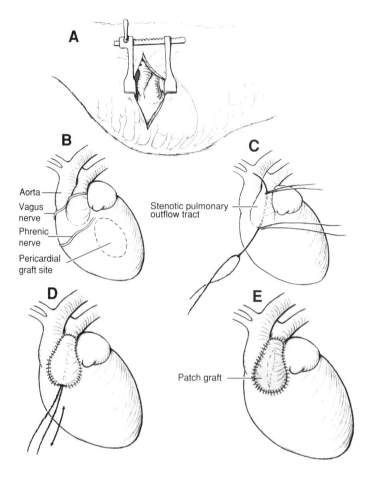

A

B

Aorta
Vagus nerve
Phrenic nerve
Pericardial graft site

C

Stenotic pulmonary outflow tract

D

E

Patch graft

FIGURE 8–2. Closed patch graft placement for pulmonic stenosis. *(A)* A left lateral thoracotomy through the fourth intercostal space (in dogs) or sixth intercostal space (in cats) is performed. *(B)* A pericardial patch is harvested. *(C)* The cutting wire is preplaced in the pulmonary artery. *(D)* The pericardial patch is sutured over the pulmonary outflow tract, leaving a small section open to allow exit of the cutting wire *(arrow)*. *(E)* The wire is removed and the patch graft completely closed. (Redrawn with permission from Caywood DO, Lipowitz AJ: *Atlas of General Small Animal Surgery.* St. Louis, CV Mosby, 1989, p 125.)

wall (Figure 8–2). The graft is sutured over the pulmonary outflow tract, leaving the last two sutures at the distal aspect of the patch open to allow for removal of the cutting wire. The wire is pulled through the lateral wall of the pulmonary outflow tract. The sutures in the graft are quickly tied once the wire is pulled free.

  d. **Prognosis.** The prognosis for dogs with pulmonic stenosis varies according to severity.

  (1) Dogs with right ventricular blood pressure less than 70 mm Hg or a pulmonic blood pressure gradient less than 50 mm Hg may be asymptomatic.

  (2) The prognosis is good for dogs that are asymptomatic until adulthood and undergo surgery for valvular or subvalvular stenosis.

  (3) The prognosis is poor for young symptomatic dogs and dogs with severe muscular hypertrophy.

3. Aortic stenosis is the third most common congenital heart defect in dogs and the most common congenital heart defect of large breed dogs. Because the most common lesion is a subvalvular ring or ridge of fibrocartilaginous tissue, the disease is often referred to as **subaortic stenosis.**

a. **Pathogenesis**
  (1) Subaortic stenosis results in pressure overload of the left ventricle, causing hypertrophy without dilation.
  (2) Tachyarrhythmias may occur, and sudden death can occur in severely affected animals.
b. **Diagnosis** is by physical examination, electrocardiography, radiography, echocardiography, and indirect pressure evaluation. Contrast angiography and direct pressure evaluation may also be required.
c. **Treatment**
  (1) **Indications for surgery.** Surgical correction is indicated in animals with **systolic aortic blood pressure gradients greater than 70 mm Hg.** Animals with gradients less than this should be reevaluated. Those developing clinical signs, progressive left ventricular hypertrophy, or increases in the gradient may require surgery.
  (2) **Techniques** for correcting aortic stenosis include blind valvuloplasty, open arteriotomy and valvulectomy, and conduit placement.
    (a) **Blind valvuloplasty** is performed through a median sternotomy. The technique is similar to the Brock procedure used for pulmonic stenosis.
      (i) A valve dilator is passed through a stab in the left ventricle into the aortic outflow tract. The instrument is passed across the aortic valve, opened to dilate the valve, and withdrawn. A suture is tied over the stab incision.
      (ii) Long-term results of this surgery are discouraging, and sustained reductions in systolic aortic blood pressure gradients are not achieved.
    (b) **Open arteriotomy** performed during extracorporeal cardiopulmonary bypass surgery appears more useful for discrete subvalvular lesions. During cardiopulmonary bypass surgery, the aorta is opened and the subvalvular lesion is excised.
    (c) Alternatively, a **prosthetic conduit** can be placed to bypass the aortic valve. The conduit passes from the left ventricle to the descending aorta.
d. **Prognosis.** The prognosis for dogs with severe subaortic stenosis is poor without surgery, and sudden death is possible. The prognosis after effective surgery is good; however, treated dogs are at risk of developing cardiomyopathy within 5–7 years as a result of underlying muscular disease.

4. **PRAA** is the most common vascular ring anomaly (and the fourth most common congenital heart defect in dogs). It is most commonly seen in German shepherds and Irish setters. Cats are less commonly affected.
a. **Pathogenesis**
  (1) PRAA is the result of the aorta developing from the right fourth aortic arch rather than the left. The persistent left ligamentum arteriosus connecting the left pulmonary artery to the descending aorta forms a ring around the esophagus. The ring is completed by the base of the heart (Figure 8–3).
  (2) Persistent left vena cava occurs with PRAA approximately 40% of the time.
  (3) The PRAA, because of the abnormal positioning of the vascular structures, causes extracardiac problems. For example, esophageal dilation proximal to the vascular ring occurs. Animals often aspirate food during regurgitation, increasing the risk of pneumonia.
b. **Diagnosis** is based on history and signalment, clinical signs, and radiography.
  (1) **Clinical signs** (e.g., postprandial regurgitation) become evident after weaning when the animal begins eating solid food. Physical examination may reveal a stunted animal in poor body condition. Murmurs are not present.
  (2) **Thoracic radiographs** reveal a dilated esophagus cranial to the heart that usually contains large amounts of food or air (see Figure 8–3B).
    (a) Evidence of pneumonia may be present, especially in the right middle lung lobe.
    (b) Positive contrast radiography using an oral barium suspension will demonstrate an **esophageal constriction at the base of the heart** with varying degrees of esophageal dilation cranial to the constriction. **The constric-**

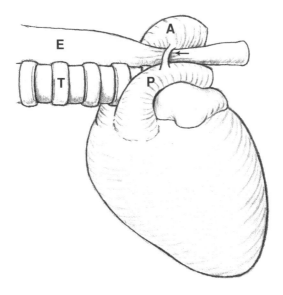

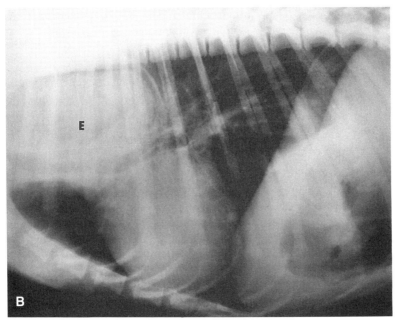

FIGURE 8–3. *(A)* Persistent right aortic arch (PRAA). The dilated esophagus *(E)* is seen anterior to the heart. The esophagus and trachea *(T)* are constricted by the ligamentum arteriosus *(arrow)*, right aorta *(A)*, pulmonary artery *(P)*, and the base of the heart. *(B)* Lateral radiographic projection of a dog with persistent right aortic arch (PRAA). Note the large dilated esophagus *(E)* filled with food cranial to the heart, with the constriction at the base of the heart.

> **tion must be in this location for a diagnosis of PRAA.** Esophagitis and idiopathic megaesophagus can cause varying degrees of esophageal dilation, but a definite stricture in the region of the base of the heart is not evident.
>
> **(3) Fluoroscopy** may confirm the constriction and evaluate the esophageal motility, which is often abnormal.

c. Treatment. Surgery is indicated to free constriction of the ligamentum arteriosus around the esophagus. The procedure is performed through a left lateral thoracotomy at the fourth intercostal space.

(1) The ligamentum arteriosus is dissected free, double ligated, and severed between the ligatures. Constricting periesophageal fibers should be dissected free. A balloon catheter passed down the esophagus intraoperatively and dilated at the site of the constriction helps to identify constricting fibers.

(2) Imbrication of the dilated esophagus is not recommended because it does not reduce postoperative regurgitation and may increase the risk of postoperative complications such as mediastinitis, pyothorax, and bronchoesophageal fistulation.

d. Prognosis. The postoperative prognosis is guarded.

(1) Esophageal motility is often abnormal, and long-term elevated feeding and diet manipulation may be required. Feeding soft food or gruels may be necessary as well.

(2) Medical management of aspiration pneumonia may be required.

(3) Surgery on very young animals carries the best prognosis.

C. **Rare congenital cardiac defects.** Tetralogy of Fallot, atrial septal defect, and ventricular septal defect are less common than the disorders already described, and they require considerable surgical expertise for correction.

1. Tetralogy of Fallot is the most common congenital heart defect that causes cyanosis.
  a. Pathogenesis
   (1) This syndrome involves four heart defects: **ventricular septal defect, pulmonic stenosis, right ventricular hypertrophy, and dextropositioning or overriding of the aorta,** allowing the aorta to accept blood from both ventricles (Figure 8–4).
   (2) Right ventricular hypertrophy is secondary to pulmonic stenosis. As blood pressure increases in the right ventricle, right-to-left shunting of blood causes mixing of blood in the aorta. Chronic hypoxia causes polycythemia.
  b. Medical treatment includes phlebotomy to maintain the packed cell volume (PCV) between 62% and 68%. Blood volume should be replaced with crystalloid fluids. Treatment with propranolol may reduce muscular contractility and muscular constriction. Use of drugs that cause systemic vasodilation should be avoided.

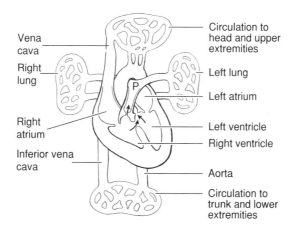

FIGURE 8–4. Tetralogy of Fallot. The obstruction at the pulmonary artery *(P)* causes increased pressure in the right ventricle and secondary muscular hypertrophy. The ventricular septal defect allows blood to exit from the high pressure right ventricle, and the overridden aorta allows diversion of low oxygen tension blood to the systemic circulation.

    c. Surgical treatment
        (1) Definitive repair of tetralogy of Fallot requires closure of the ventricular septal defect (see II C 3) and correction of the pulmonic stenosis during cardiopulmonary bypass.
        (2) Palliative procedures are designed to increase pulmonary blood flow by shunting blood from the aorta to the pulmonary artery.
            (a) A modified **Blalock-Taussig procedure** uses a harvested subclavian artery as a free graft conduit between the aorta and the pulmonary artery.
            (b) A **Pott's anastomosis** can be performed, creating a direct communication between the aorta and the pulmonary artery. However, this procedure may overload the pulmonary circulation.
    d. Prognosis. The prognosis for untreated tetralogy of Fallot is poor. Many animals may die suddenly. Surgical palliation may result in postoperative survival for up to 4 years.

2. Atrial septal defect is the rarest congenital heart defect.
    a. Pathogenesis
        (1) Atrial septal defect causes left-to-right shunting with overloading of the right ventricle and eventual right-sided congestive heart failure.
        (2) Pulmonary hypertension may occur. If right atrial pressures become elevated during heart failure, right-to-left shunting may result.
    b. Treatment involves an open heart procedure to suture or patch the defect during cardiopulmonary bypass.

3. Ventricular septal defect is more common than atrial septal defect and is the most common congenital heart defect in cats.
    a. Pathogenesis
        (1) The ventricular septal defect causes left-to-right shunting, which overloads both the left and right ventricles.
        (2) A large ventricular septal defect essentially creates a common ventricle and causes significant right ventricular dilation and hypertrophy. If pulmonary hypertension develops, right-to-left shunting can occur (Eisenmenger's syndrome).
    b. Treatment
        (1) Definitive correction of the ventricular septal defect requires open heart surgery to suture or patch the defect during cardiopulmonary bypass.
        (2) Palliative procedures include pulmonary arterial banding to decrease pulmonary blood flow. Reducing the pulmonary artery diameter by two thirds or doubling the right ventricular pressure is desired.
        (3) Surgical correction of ventricular septal defect in an animal with right-to-left shunting is contraindicated because of irreversible cardiac changes.
    c. Prognosis. The prognosis for a large, untreated ventricular septal defect is poor.

III. ACQUIRED CARDIAC DISORDERS

A. **Pericardial effusion** may be transudative, exudative, inflammatory, or, most commonly, sanguineous or serosanguineous.

1. Etiology
    a. The most common cause of pericardial effusion is **neoplasia,** including heart base tumors, right atrial hemangiosarcoma, and mesothelioma.
        (1) Pericardial effusions associated with neoplasia are generally **sanguineous** or **serosanguineous.**
        (2) Pericardial effusions associated with hemangiosarcoma are more common in large breed dogs, especially German shepherds.
    b. Idiopathic pericardial effusion is the second most common type of pericardial effusion in dogs and is more common in medium to large breed, young to middle-aged dogs. It is sanguineous or serosanguineous.

   c. Other causes of sanguineous or serosanguineous pericardial effusions include **blood dyscrasias** or **coagulopathies.**

   d. **Pericardial transudate** may occur secondary to **congestive heart failure, hypoproteinemia,** or incarceration of a liver lobe associated with a **peritoneopericardial hernia.**

   e. **Inflammatory pericardial exudate** is uncommon but may be the result of **bacterial infection,** from either hematogenous or penetrating sources. **In cats,** feline infectious peritonitis and **toxoplasmosis** may cause pericardial effusion.

2. **Clinical signs** of pericardial effusion reflect cardiac tamponade and right-sided heart failure.

   a. **Clinical signs** include **lethargy, tachypnea, cough, abdominal enlargement and ascites, weakness,** and **syncope.**

   b. The clinical signs are **usually gradual in onset,** although acute cardiac tamponade may cause sudden weakness, dyspnea, collapse, or death.

3. **Diagnosis**

   a. **Physical examination** findings depend on the amount of effusion.

      (1) Small volumes cause minimal clinical signs.

      (2) Larger volumes cause muffling of the heartbeat on both sides of the thorax, resting tachycardia, jugular distention, and diminished pulse strength.

         (a) Dysrhythmias may be present.

         (b) Signs of right-sided heart failure may be detected.

   b. **Electrocardiography** shows diminished QRS amplitudes (less than 0.1 mV).

      (1) Sinus tachycardia is usually present, although supraventricular and ventricular arrhythmias may be present.

      (2) Electrical alternans, a regular alteration in the electrical activity of the heart in the presence of a normal rhythm, is present in approximately 50% of cases. On the electrocardiogram (ECG), this manifests as variation in the height of the QRS complexes.

   c. **Radiography** shows spherical enlargement of the cardiac silhouette with loss of the normal contour of the individual chambers. Widening of the caudal vena cava and pleural effusion may be present.

   d. **Echocardiography** is very sensitive and specific for identifying the presence of pericardial fluid. It may also help to identify and localize pericardial and cardiac masses.

   e. **Pneumopericardiography** can be used to positively identify cardiac masses if echocardiography is unavailable.

      (1) Carbon dioxide or room air is injected into the pericardium after aspiration of the effusion.

      (2) Right and left lateral projections and dorsoventral and ventrodorsal projections are taken to completely evaluate the pericardial space.

   f. **Pericardiocentesis** (aspiration of fluid from the pericardial space) provides the definitive diagnosis of pericardial effusion.

      (1) Pericardiocentesis is performed using a 14- to 16-gauge over-the-needle catheter with one to three extra holes cut near the tip.

      (2) With the animal under sedation and using local anesthesia, the catheter is placed through the right fourth to sixth intercostal space.

      (3) Hemorrhagic effusions usually do not clot and have a PCV lower than that of peripheral blood.

4. **Treatment**

   a. **Pericardiocentesis** provides palliative relief for pericardial effusion.

   b. **Pericardiectomy** is often necessary to definitively treat infectious, idiopathic, or neoplastic effusions. Pericardiectomy is performed through a median sternotomy or, if right atrial hemangiosarcoma is suspected, through a right lateral thoracotomy at the fifth intercostal space (see Chapter 9 III A, C). A thoracostomy tube placed in the thorax is usually removed 5–7 days after surgery, once effusion has ceased.

(1) Total pericardiectomy requires dissection of the phrenic nerves from the parietal pericardium before excision of the entire parietal pericardium at the level of the base of the heart.

(2) Subtotal pericardiectomy is performed by excising the pericardium below the level of the phrenic nerves.

5. **Prognosis.** The prognosis after pericardiectomy is fair, depending on the cause.

B. **Constrictive pericarditis** is associated with minimal pericardial effusion.

1. **Etiology.** Constrictive pericarditis is the result of **pericardial fibrosis,** which may be caused by recurrent idiopathic hemorrhagic pericarditis, foreign bodies, bacterial or fungal infections, neoplasia, or an idiopathic disorder.

2. **Clinical signs** are similar to those in animals with pericardial effusion. The most common sign is abdominal enlargement resulting from ascites.

3. **Diagnosis** is accomplished primarily by ruling out other causes of right-sided heart failure. Echocardiography may detect pericardial effusion and help rule out other causes of right-sided heart failure. Confirmation of pericardial thickening is usually not possible.

4. **Treatment** is by parietal pericardiectomy.
   a. Total pericardiectomy is usually required, although subtotal pericardiectomy may be successful if minimal epicardial fibrosis is present.
   b. Epicardiectomy is difficult and risky, and recurrence of epicardial constriction is common.

5. The **prognosis** after parietal pericardiectomy for animals with little epicardial involvement is good, with approximately 75% of animals responding.

C. **Cardiac neoplasms** amenable to surgical excision include right atrial hemangiosarcomas, atrial wall sarcomas, chemodectomas, and other intrapericardial masses, including cysts, granulomas, and abscesses.

1. **Types of neoplasms**
   a. Sarcomas. Primary cardiac sarcomas occur infrequently in dogs. Sarcomas and carcinomas occur more commonly as metastatic disease.
      (1) Hemangiosarcoma is a highly malignant tumor of endothelial origin. It is much more common in dogs than cats.
         (a) Primary cardiac hemangiosarcoma of the right atrium is the most common primary cardiac tumor in the dog.
         (b) Primary cardiac hemangiosarcoma frequently originates at the crista terminalis, a ridge of muscle at the juncture of the right atrium and right auricle.
         (c) Hematogenous metastasis to lungs, liver, spleen, kidneys, brain, and subcutaneous tissue is common.
      (2) Lymphosarcoma is the most common metastatic cardiac tumor in cats. It may be present as discrete nodules or as a diffuse, infiltrative form within the myocardium. The pericardium, great vessels, and cardiac chambers may also be involved.
   b. Chemodectomas (e.g., aortic body tumor, heart base tumor) are tumors of the nonchromaffin paraganglia of the aortic bodies.
      (1) Chemodectomas occur more frequently in older dogs but are rare in cats.
      (2) They do not secrete hormones and clinical signs are related to their physical presence.
   c. Benign primary cardiac tumors include myxomas, fibromas, rhabdomyomas (often intraluminal), and pericardial mesotheliomas.
      (1) Myxomas, fibromas, and rhabdomyomas are often intraluminal and interfere with blood flow.
      (2) Mesotheliomas arise from the pericardial surface but may invade the adjacent myocardium.

2. **Diagnosis**
   a. **Clinical signs** associated with most cardiac neoplasia are those of right-sided heart failure secondary to development of hemorrhagic pericardial effusion. Clinical signs of cardiac sarcomas vary according to their location and the extent of tissue involvement.
      (1) **Physical examination** reveals tachycardia, dysrhythmias, muffled heart sounds, dyspnea, and possible liver and splenic enlargement.
      (2) **Hematologic studies** of animals with hemangiosarcoma reveal a microcytic hemolytic anemia with schistocytes, poikilocytes, anisocytes, and polychromasia. These animals can develop disseminated intravascular coagulation characterized by thrombocytopenia, elevated fibrin degradation products, and prolonged clotting times.
   b. **Radiography** may show enlargement of the cardiac silhouette, elevation of the trachea, caudal vena cava distention, pleural effusion, and pulmonary edema.
   c. **Electrocardiography** may reveal abnormalities consistent with pericardial effusion, such as reduced amplitude of QRS complexes and electrical alternans. Dysrhythmias may be present.
   d. **Echocardiography** is the most useful diagnostic technique for identifying the presence, location, and size of cardiac masses.
      (1) Hemangiosarcoma is typically found in the right atrium.
      (2) Aortic body tumors arise from the base of the aorta between the aorta and the pulmonary artery.
      (3) Myxomas and other benign tumors (fibromas, chondroma, rhabdomyoma) are found within the cardiac chambers.
      (4) Sarcomas and metastatic tumors are often found in the walls of the right and left ventricle and the interventricular septum.
   e. **Pericardiocentesis** is indicated if pericardial fluid is present. Cytologic diagnosis of neoplasia may be difficult, however, and biopsy is usually required.
   f. **Positive contrast angiography** may be useful in defining the extent of cardiac involvement and the possibility of resection. Direct intracardiac pressure measurement can be performed at the same time to evaluate the effect of the mass on hemodynamics.
   g. **Biopsy,** performed during exploratory thoracotomy, is usually necessary to definitively diagnose cardiac neoplasia. A lateral thoracotomy or a median sternotomy can be performed, depending on the location of the mass.

3. **Treatment**
   a. **Sarcomas** involving the right atrial wall are most amenable to surgical resection. Hemangiosarcomas of the right atrial wall or auricular appendage wall can be resected by cross-clamping the structure with a vascular clamp, excising the affected tissue, and suturing the cut edge using a continuous suture pattern.
      (1) Excision may be facilitated by the use of automatic stapling equipment.
      (2) Excision of right atrial wall tumors is facilitated by venous inflow occlusion. A prosthetic patch graft may be necessary following resection of large tumors.
   b. **Intracardiac masses of the right heart** can be removed during venous inflow occlusion. Other masses may require cardiopulmonary bypass during resection.
   c. **Aortic body tumors** are rarely resectable, but pericardiectomy may palliate clinical signs if pericardial effusion is present.

4. The **prognosis** for long-term survival of animals with cardiac tumors is guarded because most cardiac tumors are extensive at the time of presentation and often have metastasized.
   a. The prognosis for long-term survival after resection of right atrial hemangiosarcoma is poor, with a mean survival time of 4 months.
   b. Resectable benign tumors may be associated with postoperative survival of up to 2 years.

D. **Bradycardia**

1. **Etiology**
   a. **Sick sinus syndrome** is most commonly seen in miniature schnauzers and is the

result of intrinsic disease of the sinus node, characterized by intermittent, severe sinus bradycardia, sinus arrest or sinus block, supraventricular escape rhythms, and occasionally, paroxysmal supraventricular tachycardia.

b. **Persistent atrial standstill** is a heritable disease of springer spaniels and is the result of dystrophy of the cardiac atrial muscle.
   (1) It is characterized by bradycardia, absence of P waves, and a supraventricular or ventricular escape rhythm.
   (2) Normal serum potassium concentrations differentiate it from transient atrial standstill.
c. **Atrioventricular (AV) block** is the result of a delay or block of cardiac impulses through the AV node.
   (1) **First degree (primary) AV block** is often the result of exaggerated vagal tone or digitalis toxicity and causes prolongation of the P-R interval.
   (2) **Second-degree (secondary) AV block** is characterized by intermittent failure of impulse transmission through the AV node.
   (3) **Third-degree AV block** is complete failure of conduction through the AV node and is characterized by complete AV dissociation on the ECG.

2. **Surgical treatment.** Bradycardia that causes clinical signs (e.g., weakness, exercise intolerance, collapse, syncope) may be treated by **pacemaker implantation.**
   a. **Pacemaker operation.** The pacemaker paces the heart by either an endocardial or an epicardial electrode placed in the ventricle. Pulse generators can be programmed according to rate and stimulus threshold, and can be reprogrammed from outside the body. They are generally programmed at 80–100 beats per minute in dogs, and 100 beats per minute in cats.
   b. **Indications**
      (1) **Dogs.** Pacemaker implantation is generally indicated for bradycardia resulting from intrinsic causes.
         (a) Third-degree AV block is an indication for pacemaker implantation, as is second-degree AV block if clinical signs are present.
         (b) First-degree AV block is not an indication for a pacemaker.
      (2) **Cats.** Pacemaker implantation for second- and third-degree AV block has been described in cats.
   c. **Technique**
      (1) **Placement of endocardial electrodes.** Endocardial electrodes are bipolar and may be temporary or permanent. In animals that are high anesthetic risks, temporary endocardial electrodes can be placed percutaneously without anesthesia prior to implantation of a permanent pacemaker.
         (a) **Temporary.** Endocardial leads (transvenous) are introduced into the jugular vein and passed into the right ventricle. Placement of these leads does not require invasive thoracic or abdominal surgery, but the risk of dislodgment is higher. The leads are connected to an external pulse generator.
         (b) **Permanent.** The pulse generator is usually implanted within the muscles of the neck. This placement may be difficult in small dogs.
      (2) **Placement of epicardial electrodes.** Epicardial electrodes are unipolar and require invasive surgery for placement. Screw-in epicardial leads are the most common type.
         (a) A midline celiotomy and an incision in the diaphragm are made to gain access to the pericardium over the left ventricle.
         (b) The pericardium is opened and grasped to stabilize the heart as the epicardial lead is screwed into the epicardium.
         (c) The lead is usually sutured to the diaphragm to stabilize it, and the pulse generator is placed (without suturing) between the liver and the diaphragm or between the transverse abdominal and internal abdominal oblique muscles.
   d. **Complications** of pacemaker implantation include dislodgment of the leads, seroma formation around the pulse generator, rotation of the pulse generator on its long axis (twiddler's syndrome), fibrosis of the lead, and possible tumor formation

at the site of the pulse generator. Exit block may be associated with malfunction of the pulse generator.

3. The **prognosis** after pacemaker implantation is generally good. Dogs with AV block tend to do better than dogs with sick sinus syndrome or sinoatrial arrest.

E. **Caval syndrome** is an acute syndrome that occurs when a large number of adult worms lodge in the caudal vena cava and right atrium.

1. **Clinical signs** of caval syndrome include an abrupt onset of hemoglobinuria, hemoglobinemia, hemolytic anemia, dyspnea, and weakness.
   a. Liver and renal dysfunction occur.
   b. An enlarged jugular vein with a jugular pulse may be present. Jaundice may be evident.
   c. Dogs usually die 48–72 hours after onset of clinical signs if treatment is not received.

2. **Diagnosis**
   a. **Radiographs** of the thorax reveal changes associated with advanced heartworm disease, including enlarged right atrium and ventricle, enlarged pulmonary trunk, and enlarged, tortuous branches of the pulmonary artery. Abdominal radiographs may reveal hepatomegaly and splenomegaly.
   b. **Echocardiography** confirms right heart enlargement and worms in the right atrium and venae cavae.

3. **Treatment. Immediate surgical removal of worms via jugular venotomy is indicated.**
   a. General anesthesia is often unnecessary because the animals are moribund; however, analgesia should be provided.
   b. With the dog in left lateral recumbency, a local anesthetic agent (lidocaine) is infused over the right jugular vein. A skin incision is made and the jugular vein is isolated and occluded distally (away from the heart, toward the head).
   c. The vein is opened, and long alligator forceps or a spiral basket instrument is passed through the jugular into the right atrium and caudal vena cava. Fluoroscopy can be used to mark the exact location of the instruments. Worms are removed until they can no longer be grasped.
   d. The jugular vein is closed in a simple continuous suture pattern using 4-0 or 5-0 polypropylene. Alternatively, the vein can be ligated. The skin incision is closed routinely.

4. **Prognosis.** The **prognosis** for recovery is good and approximately 85% of dogs respond.

VASCULAR DISORDERS

A. **Aortic thromboembolism**

1. **Dogs.** In dogs, aortic thromboembolism occurs secondary to bacterial endocarditis, nephrotic syndrome, aberrant adult heartworms, gastric dilation or volvulus, and trauma.

2. **Cats. Feline aortic thromboembolism** is the most common vascular disorder of small animals. Approximately one-third of cats with feline cardiomyopathy develop thromboembolism of peripheral arteries.
   a. The most common site is at the trifurcation of the descending aorta into the external iliac artery, the internal iliac artery, and the median sacral artery.
   b. **Clinical signs** of feline aortic thromboembolism include **posterior paralysis** and **pain.**
      (1) Affected cats often vocalize continuously.
      (2) The rear legs are cold and cyanotic, and the toenails do not actively bleed if they are cut.

    (3) A femoral arterial pulse is absent.
  c. Diagnosis is primarily by clinical signs.
    (1) Thermography may provide conclusive evidence of poikilothermia of the hindlimbs.
    (2) The use of **radionuclide angiography** to diagnose aortic thromboembolism in dogs has been described.
  d. Treatment. Medical versus surgical treatment is controversial.
    (1) Surgical treatment. Surgical removal of the thromboembolus may be performed if presentation is within 4–6 hours. Excision of the left atrial appendage has been recommended to remove a nidus for clot formation.
      (a) Surgical removal of the thromboembolus (embolectomy) can be performed through an **aortic arteriotomy** via a ventral midline celiotomy.
      (b) Balloon catheters passed through bilateral femoral arteriotomies (performed under sedation and local analgesia) may also be used.
        (i) The balloon catheter is passed beyond the embolus with the balloon deflated.
        (ii) The balloon is then inflated and pulled distally through the femoral artery, hopefully dislodging the thromboembolus and also bringing it through the arteriotomy site.
    (2) Medical treatment. Because a delay in presentation is common, treatment is generally cage rest and supportive therapy. Improvement can be expected over 2–4 weeks.
      (a) Medical management involves **initial management of the cardiovascular crisis,** including pulmonary edema, hypothermia, and cardiogenic shock.
        (i) Identification and treatment of pre-existing cardiomyopathy are required.
        (ii) Analgesia for the pain associated with the ischemia is recommended.
      (b) The efficacy of **thrombolytic agents** is uncertain. Streptokinase and urokinase have not been clinically demonstrated to be effective in cats, although they do reduce clot size. The anticoagulant heparin does not cause clot lysis.
      (c) Vasodilating agents, such as calcium channel blockers (e.g., verapamil), may be beneficial.
      (d) For **prevention** of thromboembolism, aspirin is administered at 25 mg/kg every third day for the remainder of the cat's life.
  e. Prognosis. The **prognosis** for aortic thromboembolism is guarded.
    (1) A third of all cats with aortic thromboembolism die from acute heart failure resulting from pre-existing cardiomyopathy.
    (2) Surviving cats often have major deficits in rear limb function.

B. **Peripheral arteriovenous fistulae** are uncommon congenital or acquired defects of the vasculature in small animals.

  1. Pathogenesis. An arteriovenous fistula is an abnormal, direct communication between an artery and vein, resulting in left-to-right shunting of blood away from the capillary bed. The hemodynamic effects of an arteriovenous fistula depend on its size.

  2. Congenital arteriovenous fistulae are often multiple and extensive.
    a. The most common congenital arteriovenous fistula is a **PDA** (see II B 1).
    b. Other peripheral congenital arteriovenous fistulae most commonly involve the extremities, although they have been reported in the temporal region, eye, flank, tongue, and liver.

  3. Acquired arteriovenous fistulae are usually single and direct, although extensive collateral circulation can develop.
    a. Trauma (e.g., penetrating injury, venipuncture, extravascular injection of irritants, mass ligation of arteries and veins, aneurysm rupture) is the most common cause of peripheral arteriovenous fistulae.

    b. Neoplasia and **ischemia** induce the formation of collateral circulation, which may include arteriovenous fistulae.

    c. Surgery. Arteriovenous fistulae may be created surgically to improve venous access and reduce the time needed for blood collection.

4. Diagnosis

    a. Clinical signs of peripheral arteriovenous fistulae of the extremities include painless swelling of the extremity, bleeding from that site, hypertrophy of the limb, lameness, and possible ulceration of the distal limb. A history of trauma is not always apparent.

    b. Physical examination reveals a localized swelling at the site and distal to the arteriovenous fistula.

        (1) The area of the fistula may be hyperthermic with the distal limb hypothermic.

        (2) Dilated tortuous vessels may be apparent at the site. A continuous bruit (murmur) over the site may be auscultated, and a palpable thrill may be present.

        (3) Occlusion of the proximal artery may cause a sudden decrease in heart rate (Branham's sign) because of the sudden increase in blood pressure.

    c. Survey **radiographs** are usually unremarkable, although periosteal proliferation, limb length discrepancy in young dogs, or cortical rarefaction or thickening may be seen.

    d. Contrast angiography is the most useful diagnostic test for determining the size and location of a fistula, and local vessel changes. Ultrasonography may also demonstrate an arteriovenous fistula.

    e. Because high-output cardiac failure can develop, assessment of cardiovascular function by thoracic radiographs, electrocardiography, and echocardiography is indicated for large arteriovenous fistulae.

5. Treatment

    a. Treatment for a **single arteriovenous fistula** is most often surgery to separate the artery and the vein.

        (1) If possible, the region of the fistula is removed.

        (2) For large arteriovenous fistulae, the arterial supply should be ligated slowly to allow monitoring for bradycardia.

    b. Treatment of **multiple arteriovenous fistulae** is generally palliative (bandaging in association with partial fistula resection) because separation or resection of all the fistulae is impossible.

        (1) Arterial embolization may be attempted.

        (2) Multiple arteriovenous fistulae present in a body organ (e.g., the liver) are often totally resectable.

6. Prognosis. The prognosis for recovery of animals with either a single fistula amenable to surgery, or multiple fistulae that can be totally excised (e.g., a liver lobe) is good. The prognosis for multiple, congenital fistulae is poor if the entire region cannot be excised.

C. **Vascular repair.** Arteriotomy or venotomy and vascular anastomosis or repair are rarely performed in veterinary surgery for the treatment of vascular problems or trauma.

1. Arteriotomy or venotomy may be performed for the removal of intravascular structures (e.g., parasites, thromboemboli).

    a. If the procedure is elective, the animal is administered heparin prior to surgery.

    b. The vessel is totally or partially occluded, and the incision is made parallel to the long axis of the vessel. The incision is started with a scalpel blade and extended with sharp scissors.

    c. Loose adventitia is removed from the outer surface of the vessel and the vessel is closed with a simple continuous suture pattern using bites that penetrate the entire wall of the artery. The knots should be placed outside of the lumen.

        (1) Endothelial apposition is essential.

        (2) Polypropylene suture ranging from 4-0 to 7-0 is recommended, depending on the size of the vessel. Polypropylene is recommended for most vascular surgery because it is nonabsorbable, inert, monofilament, and the least thrombogenic of all suture materials.

   2. Vascular anastomosis can be performed as an end-to-end or an end-to-side anastomosis.

     a. For an **end-to-end anastomosis,** the vessel ends are cut slightly obliquely to maximize the anastomotic diameter.

      (1) Excess adventitia is removed from the vessel ends.

      (2) The anastomosis is divided into halves or thirds (triangulated). The anastomosis is begun at one side by tying a knot and progressing around one half of the anastomosis using a simple continuous suture pattern. The other half of the anastomosis is begun 180 degrees from the first, and progressed around the other half using simple continuous sutures. The sutures are then tied to the opposite knots.

     b. An **end-to-side anastomosis** is most often used to join a graft to a vessel.

      (1) The adventitia is removed from the graft vessel.

      (2) The graft vessel is cut at an angle and a triangular piece removed from the graft to create a "cobra head," which maximizes the diameter of the anastomosis.

      (3) An arteriotomy is made in the recipient vessel, and the anastomosis is performed as described in IV C 2 a.

      (4) Alternatively, a single double-armed suture can be used, starting at one end and progressing along the front and back side of the anastomosis with each end of the suture. The suture ends are then tied together at the opposite side of the anastomosis.

     c. The use of free, vascular skin grafts requiring vascular anastomosis is becoming a popular alternative for wound construction.

   3. Repair of traumatized vessels is difficult but should be attempted if very large vessels are involved.

     a. An end-to-end direct anastomosis should be performed if possible.

     b. The ends are débrided and the adventitia is removed from the end of the vessel.

     c. Laceration of large vessels can be repaired while the vessel is cross-clamped, to avoid the necessity for complete occlusion during the repair. Closure with a simple continuous suture is recommended. **The absence of tension on the repair is essential.**

SUGGESTED READINGS

Birchard SJ, Bonagura JD, Fingland RB: Results of ligation of patent ductus arteriosus in dogs: 201 cases (1969–1988). *J Am Vet Med Assoc* 196:2011–2013, 1990.

Bonagura JD, Darke PG: Congenital heart disease. In *Textbook of Veterinary Internal Medicine,* 4th ed. Edited by Ettinger SJ and Feldman EC. Philadelphia, WB Saunders, 1995, pp 892–943.

Bright JM, Jennings J, Toal R, et al: Percutaneous balloon valvuloplasty for treatment of pulmonic stenosis in a dog. *J Am Vet Med Assoc* 191:995–996, 1987.

Eyster GE, Gaber CE, Probst M: Cardiac disorders. In *Textbook of Small Animal Surgery,* 2nd ed. Edited by Slatter D. Philadelphia, WB Saunders, 1993, pp 856–929.

Fingland RB, Bonagura JD, Myer W: Pulmonic stenosis in the dog: 29 cases (1975–1984). *J Am Vet Med Assoc* 189:218–226, 1986.

Fox RR, Moise S, Woodfield JA, et al: Techniques and complications of pacemaker implantation in four cats. *J Am Vet Med Assoc* 12:1742–1753, 1991.

Goodwin JK, Lombard CW: Patent ductus arteriosus in adults dogs: clinical features of 14 cases. *J Am Anim Hosp Assoc* 28:350–354, 1992.

Komtebedde J, Ilkiw JE, Follette DM, et al: Resection of subvalvular aortic stenosis: surgical and perioperative management in seven dogs. *Vet Surg* 22:419–430, 1993.

Miller MW, Sisson D: Pericardial disorders. In *Textbook of Veterinary Internal Medicine,* 4th ed. Edited by Ettinger SJ and Feldman EC. Philadelphia, WB Saunders, 1995, pp 1032–1145.

Sisson D, Thomas WP, Woodfield J, et al: Permanent transvenous pacemaker implantation in forty dogs. *J Vet Int Med* 5:322–331, 1991.

Chapter 9

Thoracic Wall and Cavity

Giselle Hosgood

I. **ANATOMY.** The thoracic wall is composed of ribs, primary and secondary respiratory muscles, and other muscles.

A. **Ribs and sternebrae.** Thirteen ribs and eight sternebrae form the bony portion of the thoracic cavity in dogs and cats.

1. The **first nine ribs** are **sternal ribs** (i.e., with sternal articulation), whereas the **last four ribs** are **asternal (false) ribs** (i.e., without sternal articulation). The distal portion of each rib ends in the **costal cartilage.** The costal cartilage of ribs 10 through 12 join to form the **costal arch.**

2. The **first sternebra** is the **manubrium.** The **last sternebra** is the **xiphoid,** which gives rise to the cartilaginous **xiphoid process.**

B. **Respiratory muscles**

1. The **primary respiratory muscles** are the **internal** and **external intercostal muscles** located between each rib.

2. The **secondary respiratory muscles** include the **dorsal** and **ventral serratus, scalenus, external abdominal oblique, latissimus dorsi,** and **pectoral muscles.**

C. **Vascularization and innervation.** Intercostal vessels and nerves supply the primary respiratory muscles.

1. The **intercostal arteries** and **veins**, which run caudal to each rib, are branches of the aorta and azygous vein, respectively. They are continuous with the internal thoracic artery and vein, which run along the deep surface of the sternum.

2. The **intercostal nerves** arise from ventral branches of the thoracic nerves and course with the intercostal vessels.

II. **PRE- AND POSTOPERATIVE CONSIDERATIONS**

A. **Positive intrathoracic pressure.** The intrathoracic pressure, which is normally negative, becomes positive during thoracotomy.

1. **Effects**
   a. The tidal volume decreases, especially if the lung lobes are collapsed.
   b. The positive intrathoracic pressure reduces the effect of thoracic pumping on venous return to the heart.

2. **Assisted ventilation is required.** The ventilatory pressure should be increased to 15–20 cm H_2O (unless doing so is contraindicated by the presence of pulmonary disease) and the respiratory rate may have to be increased to 12–15 breaths per minute to avoid atelectasis and maintain adequate alveolar minute ventilation.

B. **Pain** impairs postoperative ventilation.

1. **Intercostal nerve blocks** using **bupivacaine with epinephrine** are best performed at the time of surgery.
   a. The injection is made in the region of the intercostal nerve at the proximal, caudal rib surface.

b. Blocking two or three intercostal nerves on either side of the thoracotomy incision is recommended.

2. Intrapleural administration of **bupivacaine** causes minimal adverse cardiovascular effects and provides prolonged analgesia postoperatively. Bupivacaine can be repeatedly administered through the thoracostomy tube postoperatively.

3. Intramuscular or **intravenous administration** of **opioids** provides good analgesia postoperatively, but may cause cardiorespiratory depression and prolonged postoperative hypothermia.

4. Epidural administration of **morphine** or **oxymorphone** provides good postoperative analgesia (see Chapter 2 III C 2 c).
a. Oxymorphone administered epidurally is **effective for up to 10 hours** (as opposed to 2 hours with intramuscular administration).
b. Cardiorespiratory depression will occur.

C. **Air or fluid in the thoracic cavity** impairs postoperative ventilation. Air or fluid is removed via a thoracostomy tube that is placed at the time of surgery (see Chapter 7 IV D 1 d).

III. **SURGICAL APPROACHES TO THE THORACIC CAVITY.** The approach taken depends on the structures that require exposure. A lateral thoracic radiograph may facilitate selection.

A. **Lateral (intercostal) thoracotomy** is the standard approach when the region to be exposed is defined (Table 9–1).

1. Incision of the superficial layers. The **skin** and **cutaneous trunci muscle** are incised,

TABLE 9–1. Indications for Lateral Thoracotomy in Dogs and Cats

Thoracic Structure	Intercostal Space	
	Left	Right
Heart		
Pericardium*	4, 5	4, 5
Ductus (ligamentus)		. . .
arteriosus	4, (5)	
Pulmonic valve	4	. . .
Lungs		
Cranial lobe	4–6	4–6
Middle lobe	(4), 5	(4), 5
Caudal lobe	5, (6)	5, (6)
Caudal vena cava	(6–7)	7–10
Diaphragm	7–10	7–10
Thoracic duct		
Cat	8–10	(8–10)
Dog	(8–10)	8–10
Esophagus		
Cranial intrathoracic		5
(heart base)	. . .	
Caudal intrathoracic	8–9	8–9
Trachea		
Isolated segments	. . .	3–5

Parentheses indicate an alternative approach.
* Median sternotomy may be used instead.

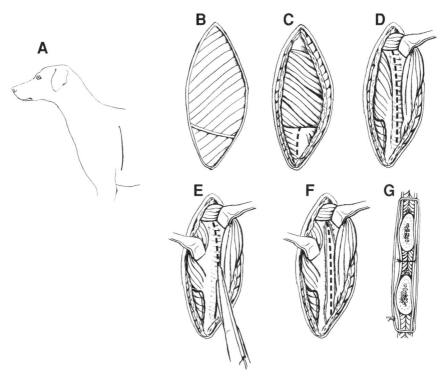

FIGURE 9–1. Lateral thoracotomy. *(A)* Incision site. *(B)* The skin and cutaneous trunci muscle are incised to expose the latissimus dorsi muscle and lateral thoracic nerve. *(C)* The latissimus dorsi muscle is incised to expose the serratus ventralis, scalenus and external abdominal oblique muscles. In caudal thoracotomies, the latissimus dorsi muscle can be reflected dorsally. *(D)* The scalenus muscle is incised and the serratus ventralis muscle is retracted. *(E)* Scissors are used to make an incision to expose the intercostal muscles. *(F)* The intercostal muscles are incised to expose the pleura. *(G)* Cross-section of the thoracic wall. Circumcostal sutures are placed to close the intercostal incision.

and the **latissimus dorsi muscle** is incised parallel to the skin incision. If a caudal approach is used, the latissimus dorsi muscle may be elevated to expose the deeper muscles (Figure 9–1).

2. **Confirmation of surgical site.** The surgical site may be confirmed by counting the intercostal spaces under the latissimus dorsi muscle. The junction of the scalenus muscle and the external abdominal oblique muscle marks the fifth intercostal space.

3. **Incision of the deeper muscles**. The **scalenus, ventral serratus,** or **external abdominal oblique muscle** is incised, depending on the area to be accessed. The muscle bellies of the ventral serratus may be separated rather than incised.

4. **Incision of the intercostal muscles.** A midline incision is made in the intercostal muscles to avoid damage to the blood vessels.

5. **Retraction of the ribs.** The ribs are spread with a Finochietto rib retractor.

6. **Closure.** The thoracotomy is closed with heavy-gauge (2-0 to 1) simple interrupted sutures.
   a. The sutures are placed circumferentially around the ribs immediately cranial and caudal to the incision.
   b. Each muscle layer is closed separately over the incision to ensure an airtight seal.

B. **Rib resection** and **rib pivot thoracotomy** permit exposure of a larger portion of the thoracic cavity.

1. **Rib resection**
   a. **Exposure.** Once the ribs are exposed, the periosteum of the rib to be resected is incised over the mid-lateral surface of the rib and elevated circumferentially from the rib.
   b. **Resection.** The rib is removed with bone cutters. The intact medial periosteum is then incised to enter the thoracic cavity.
   c. **Closure.** The thoracotomy is closed using a technique similar to that used for lateral thoracotomy.

2. **Rib pivot thoracotomy**
   a. **Exposure.** The rib is exposed and the periosteum elevated as for rib resection. While the thoracic cavity is exposed, the rib is severed with bone cutters at the costochondral junction and pivoted at the chondrovertebral articulation. The thoracic cavity is entered as for rib resection.
   b. **Closure.** The rib is reapposed using hemicerclage wires and a routine thoracotomy closure is performed.

C. **Median sternotomy** is the only thoracic approach that provides access to the entire thoracic cavity. It is primarily indicated for exploration of the thoracic cavity and for procedures that involve the base of the heart (e.g., pericardiectomy).

1. **Positioning the patient.** Median sternotomy is performed with the animal in **dorsal recumbency.** This position causes the heart to tilt downward, increasing venous pressure and reducing cardiac output.

2. **Procedure** (Figure 9–2)
   a. **Incision.** The skin and subcutaneous tissue are incised along the midline.
   b. **Exposure of the sternum.** The pectoral muscles are elevated from the midline of the sternum.
   c. **Sternotomy.** The sternum is scored with a scalpel blade, then cut with an osteotome and mallet, oscillating saw, or sternal splitter (Lebske sternal knife). To increase postoperative stability of the sternum and reduce pain, either the manubrium or the xiphoid is left intact.
   d. **Closure**

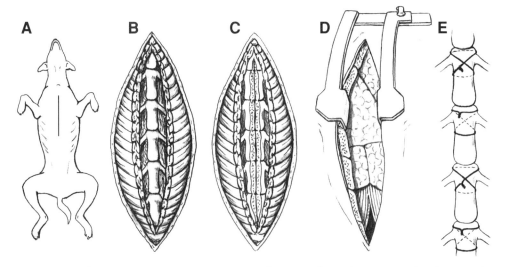

FIGURE 9–2. Median sternotomy. *(A)* Incision site. *(B)* The pectoral muscles are incised and retracted, exposing the sternum. *(C)* Sternotomy. *(D)* Retraction. The median sternotomy incision can be combined with a midline ventral celiotomy to increase exposure of the caudal thoracic cavity or diaphragm. *(E)* An alternate cruciate pattern is used to suture the sternebrae using orthopedic wire.

(1) The **sternum** is closed with cruciate (figure-of-eight) circumferential sutures passed around each costosternal junction. Heavy-gauge (2-0 to 1) suture material should be used.

(2) The **pectoral muscles, subcutaneous tissue,** and **skin** are closed in separate layers using standard technique.

3. Variations

a. Median sternotomy may be **combined with a ventral midline abdominal incision.** Incision of the diaphragm may be required to increase exposure.

b. Median sternotomy may be **combined with a lateral thoracotomy** to create a thoracic wall flap, allowing greater exposure of the thoracic cavity.

D. **Transsternal thoracotomy** increases the area exposed by a lateral thoracotomy.

1. A lateral thoracotomy incision is extended across the sternum to incorporate another lateral thoracotomy. The internal thoracic arteries must be ligated.

2. The sternal osteotomy is closed with small intramedullary pins and cerclage wire or heavy suture material.

IV. CONDITIONS OF THE THORACIC WALL TREATED BY SURGERY

A. **Congenital malformations**

1. Pectus excavatum, although uncommon, is the most frequently observed congenital malformation of the chest wall in dogs and cats. Concave, inward deformation of the caudal sternum and costal cartilages causes dorsoventral flattening of the thoracic cavity.

a. **Clinical signs** include gross deformation of the sternum, stunted growth, exercise intolerance, dyspnea, cyanosis, and vomiting. Cardiac murmurs and dysrhythmias may also occur as a result of compression of the heart and vessels.

b. **Diagnosis** can be confirmed by **radiography.** The degree of compression can be evaluated from the lateral radiographic projection and specific indices can be calculated.

c. **Treatment.** Surgical repair can be attempted if cardiopulmonary compromise is severe or for esthetic reasons.

(1) **External splints** are useful for animals less than 2 or 3 months of age. Large sutures are placed percutaneously around the sternum and tied to an external framework.

(2) **Internal fixation** with intramedullary pins or Kirschner wires may be required in older animals.

d. **Prognosis** is fair if surgical correction is performed early and the deformation is mild.

2. Rib abnormalities are fairly common and include missing ribs, fused ribs, extra ribs, and malformed ribs. Surgical treatment is usually unnecessary.

B. **Trauma**

1. Types

a. **Blunt (crushing) injury** often causes severe damage to the internal thoracic organs (e.g., **cardiac** and **pulmonary contusions**) without obviously damaging the external thoracic wall.

(1) **Fractured ribs** result from blunt trauma to the thorax.

(2) **Rupture of the intercostal muscles** may result from blunt trauma or bite wounds, possibly causing herniation of lung lobes. If the intercostal tear communicates with a skin wound, a "sucking wound" may occur, resulting in pneumothorax.

     b. Penetrating injury may cause **hemorrhage, hemothorax,** or **pneumothorax.**

  2. Etiology. Bite wounds often cause a combination of penetrating and crushing injuries. Other causes of traumatic chest wall injury include **vehicular trauma, falls,** and **abuse.**

  3. Clinical signs associated with thoracic wall trauma depend on the extent of trauma.
     a. Cardiac dysrhythmias may be associated with myocardial contusion (traumatic myocarditis) or hemothorax.
     b. Flail chest. Multiple rib fractures can result in a segment of chest wall that moves paradoxically with respiration, reducing the animal's ventilation capacity. Ruptured intercostal muscles may cause paradoxical movement of the skin that may be mistaken for flail chest.
     c. Signs of hemorrhagic shock can occur if hemorrhage is severe and acute.
     d. Respiratory distress may be associated with pneumothorax or hemothorax, flail chest, or pulmonary contusions.

  4. Diagnosis. Thoracic radiographs are important tools in the diagnosis of pneumothorax, pleural fluid accumulation (e.g., hemothorax), and rib fractures.

  5. Treatment
     a. Muscle tears and **multiple rib fractures.** Surgical repair should be delayed until the animal is stable.
       (1) Muscle tears can be sutured primarily, apposed with circumferential rib sutures, or "patched" using an omental pedicle or flaps from the latissimus dorsi or external abdominal oblique muscles.
       (2) Multiple rib fractures may necessitate primary fixation with intramedullary pins and hemicerclage wire. Alternatively, percutaneous, encircling sutures can be placed around the ribs and anchored to an external split.
     b. Isolated rib fractures can be treated conservatively with rest.
     c. Hemothorax. Treatment of hemothorax depends on the degree of respiratory impairment.
       (1) If respiratory compromise is minimal, the blood is not withdrawn from the thoracic cavity because dogs are capable of absorbing 30% of their blood volume within 90 hours. Because 70%–100% of the red blood cells are absorbed intact, pleural drainage is performed only if absolutely necessary.
       (2) If drainage of hemothorax is necessary, autotransfusion is possible, providing a readily available source of compatible blood.
     d. Continuous hemorrhage. Exploratory surgery may be required.

C. Neoplasia

  1. Benign tumors of the thoracic wall arise from the subcutaneous tissue and skin. Large lipomas are often encountered in the connective tissue between the muscles and skin.

  2. Malignant tumors. Primary osteosarcoma and **chondrosarcoma of the rib** are the most common malignant tumors of the chest wall. Other malignancies include **fibrosarcoma, mast cell tumors,** and **hemangiosarcoma.**
     a. Clinical signs are often minimal, apart from a **firm, nonpainful swelling** that is palpable over the lateral thoracic wall. Although the mass usually has a significant intrathoracic portion, clinical signs of respiratory or cardiovascular compromise are uncommon.
     b. Diagnosis is by **radiography** and **fine needle aspiration** or **incisional biopsy.** Radiographs may reveal osteolysis of the rib associated with intra- and extrathoracic soft tissue masses.
     c. Treatment is by *en bloc* **resection** of the affected portion of the thoracic wall and a margin of healthy tissue. *En bloc* resection involves removal of the pleura, ribs, muscles, fascia, and skin. The defect is repaired and a light chest bandage is applied to cover the wound and thoracostomy tube until the thoracostomy tube is removed, usually within 24 hours. **Reconstruction** involves replacement of the thoracic wall, soft tissue, and skin.

(1) Prosthetic materials (e.g., mesh) can be used to replace the thoracic wall. The prosthetic material is pulled taut over the defect. For defects of four or more ribs, paradoxical movement of the prosthesis may cause respiratory compromise. Flexible, plastic spinal plates wired to the severed ribs can be used to provide support for the prosthesis.

(2) Muscle flaps can be used on top of the mesh to replace soft tissue.
   (a) For **small thoracic soft tissue defects,** the margins of the muscle layers are elevated and closed in a centripetal, four-corner pattern.
   (b) Large thoracic soft tissue defects may require muscle flaps or an omental pedicle.
      (i) The **latissimus dorsi muscle** is used for **ventral defects.**
      (ii) The **external abdominal oblique muscle** can be elevated and reflected cranially about its craniodorsal pedicle to correct **caudal defects.**

(3) Omentum can be used as an alternative to muscle flaps to fill the soft tissue defect.
   (a) For **caudal thoracic soft tissue defects,** the omentum may be long enough to use without creating a pedicle.
   (b) For **cranial thoracic soft tissue defects,** creation of an omental pedicle through a celiotomy is required. The omental pedicle can be advanced from the abdomen through the diaphragm or subcutaneously after passing through the abdominal wall.

(4) Skin flaps. Rotation or advancement of skin flaps can be used for final coverage of the defect.
   (a) Because they include the panniculus muscle, these flaps are actually myocutaneous flaps.
   (b) Axial pattern skin flaps, based on a specific direct cutaneous artery, can also be used.

(5) Diaphragmatic advancement. For lesions caudal to the ninth rib, the thoracic wall defect can essentially be reconstructed by advancing the diaphragm cranially.
   (a) The diaphragm is removed from its normal costal attachment and sutured to the epaxial and intercostal muscles at the cranial rib margin of the defect. This converts the thoracic defect into an abdominal defect. Prosthetic materials and transpositional muscle flaps may be necessary to close the "abdominal" defect.
   (b) This procedure compromises thoracic cavity volume to some degree, but does not appear to create a problem in sedentary dogs.

d. Prognosis
   (1) The prognosis for animals with **osteosarcoma** of the rib is **guarded** because metastasis occurs early.
   (2) The prognosis for animals with **chondrosarcoma** is better because metastasis is late and long-term survival (greater than 2 years) has been reported.

V. CONDITIONS OF THE THORACIC CAVITY TREATED BY SURGERY

A. **Chylothorax** is characterized by the accumulation of chyle in the pleural space from the chylothoracic duct system. Dogs and cats are both affected; Afghan hounds are at higher risk than other dogs for developing chylothorax.

1. Etiology. The cause of chylothorax is often unknown (idiopathic), but chylothorax has been associated with trauma, dirofilariasis, blastomycosis, cardiomyopathy, lung lobe torsion, heart base tumors, thymoma, and lymphangiectasia. It is important to rule out all possible causes of chylothorax before making a diagnosis of idiopathic chylothorax.

TABLE 9–2. Characteristics of Chylous Effusion

Milky white appearance that remains after standing
Contains chylomicrons
Triglyceride concentration three times or more that of serum
Cholesterol concentration less than or equal to serum
Predominance of small lymphocytes

2. **Associated complications. Constrictive pleuritis** is a sequela to chylothorax (and other pleural effusions) reported more frequently in cats than dogs. Severe, constrictive pleural adhesions develop secondary to the irritation and inflammation associated with chyle in the thoracic cavity, causing significant respiratory compromise.

3. **Clinical signs** of chylothorax often manifest gradually and include dyspnea, tachypnea, exercise intolerance, anorexia, weight loss, and dehydration.

4. **Diagnosis**
   a. **Radiographic signs** are consistent with the presence of pleural fluid.
   b. **Evaluation of pleural fluid** (Table 9–2). Chylous effusion is characterized by a milky white appearance that remains after standing. Chyle will clear after the addition of ether; pseudochylous effusions do not clear with ether.

5. **Treatment**. An effort must be made to determine and treat the underlying cause of the chylothorax.
   a. **Medical treatment** involves drainage of the thoracic cavity and dietary manipulation to reduce the fat content of the chyle.
      (1) Percutaneous chest drainage may be performed intermittently or continuously.
      (2) Feeding a low-fat, high-protein, high-carbohydrate diet is recommended. Supplementation with fat-soluble vitamins is required.
   b. **Surgical treatment** can involve:
      (1) Transthoracic ligation of the caudal thoracic duct
      (2) Implantation of active pleurovenous shunts or pleuroperitoneal shunts (also used to palliate animals with **refractory chylothorax)**
      (3) Creation of passive pleuroperitoneal shunts by suturing fenestrated Silastic sheeting into a surgically created diaphragmatic defect, or by placing transdiaphragmatic Silastic tubes
      (4) Embolization of the thoracic duct by injecting isobutyl 2-cyanoacrylate/iophendylate through a cannulated mesenteric lymph vessel

6. **Prognosis.** Despite medical or surgical treatment, or both, the prognosis for an animal with chylothorax is poor.
   a. Approximately 50% of animals respond to treatment.
   b. If it is possible to treat the cause of the chylothorax, the prognosis may be more favorable.

B. **Pyothorax** is the accumulation of infected material and fluid within the pleural space.

1. **Etiology.** Pyothorax may be the result of systemic sepsis, spread of infection from adjacent structures, or direct introduction of organisms by penetrating trauma, foreign bodies, thoracocentesis, or surgery.

2. **Clinical signs** associated with pyothorax include fever, anorexia, weight loss, and shortness of breath.

3. **Diagnosis**
   a. **Radiographic findings**
      (1) A moderate to large pleural effusion is present. Characteristically, it is bilateral and obscures pulmonary detail and the cardiac silhouette.
      (2) Radiographs should be repeated after thoracocentesis because pulmonary in-

filtrates or consolidation may be present. The left cranial lung lobe is frequently affected in dogs and cats.
   b. **Fluid analysis** is essential to a diagnosis of pyothorax. **Thoracocentesis** through the ventral third of intercostal spaces 4 to 7 is recommended.

4. **Treatment** requires both fluid removal and the systemic administration of appropriate antimicrobials. Gram stains should fail to reveal bacteria after 2–3 days of drainage and medication.
   a. **Tube thoracostomy** (see Chapter 7 IV D 1 d) should be performed as soon as possible.
      (1) Usually, a single tube is sufficient although bilateral thoracostomy tubes may be required if the fluid is loculated.
      (2) Use of continuous suction with a water seal is recommended.
   b. **Exploratory thoracotomy.** Failure to respond to treatment or persistence of a consolidated lung lobe on radiographs may be an indication for exploratory thoracotomy, performed through a median sternotomy. Consolidated lung lobes may require partial or complete **lobectomy.**

5. **Prognosis** is fair to good, depending on the chronicity of the problem and the overall health and immune status of the animal. Early, aggressive treatment in an immunocompetent animal carries a good prognosis.

C. **Mediastinal masses**

1. **Etiology.** Mediastinal masses may be the result of neoplasia, cysts, abscesses and granulomas, tracheobronchial lymphadenopathy, or encapsulated fluid.
   a. In **cats,** the most common mediastinal mass is **lymphosarcoma.** The cranial region of the mediastinum is most often affected in cats.
   b. In **dogs,** the most common causes of mediastinal masses are **lymphosarcoma, thymoma,** and **lymphadenopathy.**
      (1) Hilar and perihilar masses are more common in dogs, usually the result of enlargement of the tracheobronchial lymph nodes.
      (2) The cranioventral region is also commonly affected.

2. **Clinical signs**
   a. **Respiratory distress and coughing** associated with tracheal and bronchial compression
   b. **Regurgitation and dysphagia** associated with esophageal compression
   c. **Head, neck, and forelimb edema** associated with intrathoracic vein and lymphatic compression
   d. **Horner's syndrome** associated with compression of the sympathetic ganglion

3. **Diagnosis**
   a. **Radiography and ultrasonography**
      (1) Mediastinal widening, soft tissue density, tracheal displacement to the right, and aortic displacement to the left may be observed.
      (2) Increased perihilar density, tracheal compression, and ventral mainstem bronchi displacement are seen in dogs.
   b. **Biopsy.** A fine-needle aspirate biopsy may be taken transthoracically, or a tissue biopsy may be taken during exploratory thoracotomy.

4. **Treatment.** Animals with large mediastinal masses are a poor anesthetic and surgical risk.
   a. The treatment of choice for **lymphoma** is **chemotherapy.**
   b. If **resection** is possible, the prognosis is favorable for animals with **granulomas, cysts,** or **thymomas.**

D. **Pneumomediastinum** is the accumulation of air around the mediastinal structures. In severe cases, the mediastinum may rupture, causing pneumothorax.

1. **Etiology.** Pneumomediastinum may be caused by rupture of the thoracic trachea or esophagus, or from penetrating neck wounds where air dissects along the fascial planes of the neck into the mediastinum.

2. **Clinical signs** may initially include **emphysematous head and neck swelling.** Respiratory distress is uncommon. Cyanosis is usually observed only in severe cases that involve rapid air leakage into the mediastinum.

3. **Diagnosis** is by radiography. Normally indistinct on radiographs, the mediastinal structures are discernible. Air may be present within the soft tissue of the neck with extension caudally into the retroperitoneal space.

4. **Treatment** is usually unnecessary, although correction of the inciting cause is required. Air is resorbed within 2–10 days.

E. **Mesothelioma** is an uncommon, highly effusive tumor that arises from the mesodermal cells of the pleura, pericardium, or peritoneum.

1. **Clinical signs.** Signs of respiratory distress are usually seen because of the presence of large volumes of pleural fluid.

2. **Diagnosis** is by biopsy. Cytologic evaluation of the pleural fluid is often nondiagnostic because reactive mesothelial cells are difficult to differentiate from neoplastic cells.

3. **Treatment** is palliative and focuses on removing the pleural fluid.

4. **Prognosis.** The prognosis for long-term survival is poor because metastatic spread to intrathoracic organs is common.

F. **Diaphragmatic hernias**

1. **Traumatic diaphragmatic hernias,** which are **pleuroperitoneal,** are most common. They are commonly **circumferential**, ventral to the esophagus at the right costomuscular region. Radial tears are less common and the central tendon is rarely affected because of its strength.
   a. **Clinical signs** may not be apparent for days or even years after the injury and are usually referable to the respiratory or gastrointestinal tracts.
      (1) Respiratory compromise exacerbated by stress is the most common sign.
      (2) Pleural effusion may be detected, especially if liver herniation is present. Blood, modified transudate, and chylothorax have all been reported.
   b. **Diagnosis**
      (1) **Survey radiographs**. Characteristic findings include interruption of the diaphragmatic outline, variable degrees of pleural effusion and thoracic trauma, increased soft tissue density in the thorax, and gas-filled intestinal loops cranial to the diaphragm. If the viscera moves freely across the tear, the hernia may not be apparent.
         (a) Removing pleural fluid and repeating the radiographs may be useful. Alternatively, a horizontal beam radiograph with the animal in dorsal recumbency may be diagnostic.
         (b) Positive-contrast radiographic techniques can be used.
            (i) Oral barium studies are associated with a high rate of false-negative results.
            (ii) Alternatively, positive-contrast peritoneography, which involves the injection of water-soluble contrast material into the abdomen, can be used. Diagnostic criteria include positive contrast in the thoracic cavity, absence of a normal liver outline, and most often, incomplete visualization of the normal outline of the abdominal surface of the diaphragm.
         (c) Negative contrast peritoneography can be performed. After air is injected into the abdomen aseptically, the animal is held standing on its hind legs and a ventrodorsal radiographic projection is taken using a horizontal beam. Air normally accumulates between the liver and the diaphragm, outlining the diaphragm. If a diaphragmatic tear is present, air accumulates in the thoracic inlet. If the liver is incarcerated or adhered, the outline of the diaphragm is abruptly interrupted in this location.

(2) Ultrasound is a noninvasive, quick method of confirming a traumatic diaphragmatic hernia.

c. Treatment involves **surgical repair of the diaphragm.**
   (1) Timing
   (a) Emergency situations. If the stomach is herniated and distended with gas, emergency decompression of the stomach by percutaneous trocharization or stomach intubation is required. Definitive evidence of **bowel incarceration, obstruction,** or **rupture,** or **ongoing hemorrhage** also require immediate attention.
   (b) Nonemergency situations. All other diaphragmatic hernias should be repaired only after the animal's condition is stabilized. The mortality rate in animals undergoing surgery within 24 hours of sustaining a traumatic diaphragmatic hernia is significantly higher than that of animals undergoing surgery after 24 hours.
   (2) Anesthesia. Induction of anesthesia in an animal with a diaphragmatic hernia requires minimizing stress and obtaining rapid control of the airway.
   (a) Preanesthetic tranquilization with an agent that does not severely depress cardiovascular and respiratory function is preferred.
   (b) Rapid induction with a barbiturate or propofol allows the animal to be intubated.
   (c) Maintenance of anesthesia with isoflurane is preferred because of its minimal cardiac depressant and dysrhythmogenic effects. Nitrous oxide should not be used because it accumulates and distends closed, gas-filled spaces such as the abdominal viscera.
   (d) Controlled ventilation is required immediately after induction of anesthesia. Peak airway pressures should not exceed 20–30 cm H_2O. Overinflation may cause pulmonary edema to develop.
   (3) Herniorrhaphy is performed through a midline celiotomy, with extension of the incision through the xiphoid and sternum if necessary (Figure 9–3).
   (a) Identification of tear. Once the diaphragm tear is identified, herniated viscera can be returned to the abdominal cavity using gentle traction. The tear can be extended to facilitate reduction of the viscera.
   (b) Examination of viscera. The abdominal and thoracic viscera are examined to determine integrity. The diaphragm is examined for other tears.
   (c) Closure of the diaphragmatic tear
      (i) The free edge of a chronic tear should be débrided.
      (ii) The diaphragm margins are approximated using atraumatic (Babcock) forceps.
      (iii) Many suture patterns and materials are suitable. Working initially from the least accessible dorsal aspect is advised.
      (iv) Most defects, even large ones, can be closed primarily because the diaphragm is exceptionally mobile and elastic. Reconstructive techniques include use of an omental pedicle based on the left or right gastroepiploic artery, a fascia lata graft, prosthetic materials, or sliding and transpositional abdominal muscle flaps from the transverse abdominal muscle.
   (d) Placement of thoracostomy tube. Air must be removed from the thoracic cavity prior to closure of the abdominal incision. Transdiaphragmatic aspiration of air is possible; however, the use of a lateral thoracostomy tube is preferred and provides access for postoperative assessment of pneumothorax or hemothorax. The thoracostomy tube is usually removed within a few hours.
   (4) Thoracic radiographs should be taken several days after herniorrhaphy to examine for pneumothorax and hydrothorax, and to assess lung inflation.

d. Prognosis. Mortality rates for animals with traumatic diaphragmatic hernia after surgical repair range from 10%–35%. The prognosis for long-term survival is good if the animal survives the first 24 hours after surgery.

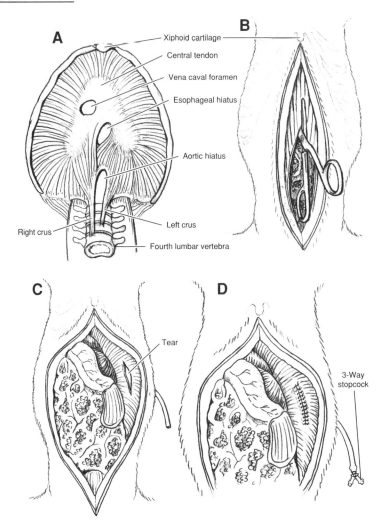

FIGURE 9–3. Diaphragmatic herniorrhaphy. *(A)* Normal anatomic features of the diaphragm. *(B)* A ventral midline celiotomy is made to expose the cranial abdominal cavity and diaphragm. *(C)* The viscera have been retracted through the diaphragmatic tear and placed in the abdomen. The tear can be enlarged to facilitate viscera retraction. A standard thoracostomy tube exits the lateral thoracic wall. *(D)* Closure of the diaphragmatic tear. (Redrawn with permission from Gourley IM, Gregory CR: *Atlas of Small Animal Surgery.* New York, Gower, 1992, p 27:8.)

2. **Congenital diaphragmatic hernias** may be pleuroperitoneal, but are more **frequently peritoneopericardial.** They may be associated with other congenital defects (e.g., cardiac abnormalities, absence of a xiphoid, malformed sternebrae, umbilical hernias).
   a. **Predisposition.** Weimaraner dogs and Persian cats are affected more often than other breeds.
   b. **Etiology.** Peritoneopericardial hernias result from faulty development of the septum transversum, in combination with incomplete fusion of the caudal pleuropericardial membranes.
   c. **Clinical signs** may be of gastrointestinal, respiratory, or cardiac origin.
   d. **Diagnosis** is by **radiography** (Figure 9–4) and **ultrasound.**
      (1) Survey radiographs show enlargement of the cardiac silhouette, dorsal displacement of the trachea, or interruption of the diaphragmatic outline.
      (2) Small intestinal gas patterns over the cardiac silhouette are common and considered pathognomonic.

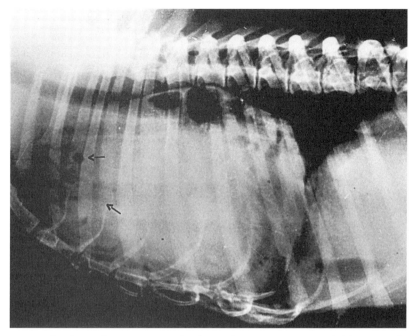

FIGURE 9–4. Lateral radiographic projection of a dog with a peritoneopericardial hernia. Enlargement of the cardiac silhouette with gas-filled loops of bowel (*arrows*) in the pericardial sac are visible.

      e. Treatment. Herniorrhaphy is performed through a midline celiotomy with extension through the xiphoid and sternum if necessary.
          (1) The viscera are reduced and the edges of the diaphragm are débrided and sutured.
          (2) Separating the pericardium from the diaphragm and closing it separately is unnecessary.
      f. Prognosis. The prognosis is good to excellent for long-term survival.

    3. Hiatal diaphragmatic hernias (see Chapter 10 III C 2) may be **sliding** or **paraesophageal** and are considered congenital.

SELECTED READINGS

Anderson M, Payne JT, Mann FA: Flail chest: pathophysiology, treatment, and prognosis. *Comp Cont Educ Pract* 15:65–75, 1993.

Bauer T, Woodfield JA: Mediastinal, pleural, and extrapleural diseases. In *Textbook of Veterinary Internal Medicine*, 4th ed. Edited by Ettinger SJ, Feldman EC. Philadelphia, WB Saunders, 1995, pp 812–843.

Bellenger C: Body cavities and hernias. In *Textbook of Small Animal Surgery*, 2nd ed. Edited by Slatter D. Philadelphia, WB Saunders, 1993, pp 370–399.

Birchard SJ, Sherding RG: *Saunder's Manual of Small Animal Practice.* Philadelphia, WB Saunders, 1994, pp 580–606.

Boudrieau RJ, Fossum TW, Hartsfield SM, et al: Pectus excavatum in dogs and cats. *Compend Contin Educ Pract Vet* 12:341–355, 1990.

Caywood DD (ed): Non-cardiac surgical disorders of the thorax. *Vet Clin North Am* 17(2): 255–503, March 1987.

Gourley IM, Gregory CR: *Atlas of Small Animal Surgery.* New York, Gower, 1992.

Meadows RL, MacWilliams PS: Chylous effusions revisited. *Vet Clin Pathol* 23:54–62, 1994.

Pirkcy-Ehrhart N, Withrow SJ, Straw RC, et al: Primary rib tumors in 54 dogs. *J Am Anim Hosp Assoc* 31:65–69, 1995.

Suess RP, Flanders JA, Beck KA, et al: Constrictive pleuritis in cats with chylothorax: 10 cases (1983–1991). *J Am Anim Hosp Assoc* 30:70–77, 1994.

Chapter 10

Alimentary System

Karen Swalec Tobias

I. OROPHARYNX

A. **Anatomy. Vascularization** and **innervation** of the oropharynx are summarized in Table 10–1.

B. **Surgical considerations**

1. **Wound closure.** Synthetic, monofilament, absorbable sutures are frequently used for closure. Nonabsorbable and absorbable monofilament sutures will slough in several weeks if the knots are left in the oral cavity.

2. **Wound healing. Oral mucosa heals quickly** because of excellent blood supply and rapid epithelialization.

3. **Postoperative considerations. Pharyngostomy** or **esophagostomy tubes** are used for nutritional support when oral feeding is impossible or contraindicated (see Chapter 5 IV B 3, 4).
   a. In order to maintain **lower esophageal sphincter function** (i.e., to prevent gastric reflux), the tube should not extend beyond the midthoracic portion of the esophagus.
   b. After the tube is removed, the neck wound is allowed to **heal by second intention.**

TABLE 10–1. Vascularization and Innervation of the Oropharynx

Region	Arterial Supply	Venous Drainage	Lymphatic Drainage	Innervation
Lips and cheeks	Infraorbital and facial arteries	Facial vein	Mandibular lymph nodes	Facial nerve (motor)
				Branches of the mandibular and maxillary branches of the trigeminal nerve (sensory)
Hard and soft palate	Major palatine artery (hard) Minor palatine artery (soft)	Maxillary vein	Mandibular lymph nodes	Glosso-pharyngeal and vagus nerves
Teeth			Mandibular and medial retro-pharyngeal lymph nodes	
Upper	Caudal, middle, and rostrodorsal alveolar branches of the infraorbital artery	Infraorbital vein into the facial vein		Superior alveolar branch of the infraorbital nerve

(continued)

TABLE 10–1. *(continued)*

Region	Arterial Supply	Venous Drainage	Lymphatic Drainage	Innervation
Lower	Branches of the mandibular alveolar artery	Mandibular alveolar vein into the maxillary vein		Inferior alveolar branch of the mandibular nerve
Tongue	Paired lingual arteries, sublingual artery	Multiple arteriovenous anastomoses	Mandibular lymph nodes	Hypoglossal nerve (motor) Lingual branch of the trigeminal nerve (sensory)
Pharynx	Cranial thryoid artery, external carotid artery	Branches of the linguofacial vein	Mandibular and medial retro-pharyngeal lymph nodes	Glosso-pharyngeal and vagus nerves
Tonsils	Tonsillar arteries	Palatine plexus	Medial retro-pharyngeal and submandibular lymph nodes	Glosso-pharyngeal nerve
Salivary glands			Retropharyngeal lymph nodes	Facial, glossopharyngeal, and vagus nerves
Parotid	Parotid artery	Superficial temporal and greater auricular veins		
Mandibular	Facial artery, caudal auricular artery	Lingual vein		
Sublingual				
Mono-stomatic portion	Facial artery	Facial vein		
Poly-stomatic portion	Lingual artery	Lingual vein		
Zygomatic	Infraorbital artery	Deep facial vein		

C. **Conditions of the tongue treated by surgery**

1. **Traumatic wounds** are treated with débridement; damaged areas may be permitted to slough. Wounds are closed with absorbable suture in an appositional pattern. The animal may need nutritional supplementation through a pharyngostomy, nasogastric, or gastrostomy tube for a short period following surgery.

2. **Eosinophilic granulomas** are seen primarily in cats and occasionally in certain breeds of dogs (e.g., Siberian huskies).

a. **Clinical features.** The lesions appear as raised, firm nodules on the dorsum of the tongue in cats and the sides of the tongue in dogs. They may appear ulcerated.

b. **Treatment.** The most common treatment is local or systemic **corticosteroids. Surgical excision, radiation therapy,** and **cryotherapy** have been used.

3. **Neoplasia.** Lingual tumors are rare. The most frequently reported tumors include **squamous cell carcinoma,** which is most common, granular cell myoblastoma, malignant melanoma, mast cell tumors, and fibrosarcoma.

   a. **Clinical features.** The lesions may appear **infiltrating** or **ulcerating. Squamous cell carcinoma** most frequently occurs **ventrally in the middle third** of the tongue.

   b. **Diagnosis** is by incisional biopsy.

   c. **Treatment**
      (1) **Surgical resection** is the treatment of choice; 40%–60% of the tongue may be removed rostrally or longitudinally.
         (a) **Intraoperative complications** include hemorrhage, incomplete resection, and metastasis.
         (b) **Postoperative complications** include avascular necrosis (if the tongue is transected caudal to the origin of the dorsal branch of the lingual artery), dysphagia, and poor haircoat (in cats).
      (2) **Radiation therapy** and **mitoxantrone** should be used postoperatively for aggressive squamous cell carcinomas.

   d. **Prognosis**
      (1) **Squamous cell carcinoma.** As a result of the high rate of local recurrence or metastasis, only 25% of animals survive 1 year after removal or irradiation of lingual squamous cell carcinoma. Rostral tumors carry a better prognosis.
      (2) **Other lingual neoplasms.** The prognosis is best for granular cell myoblastoma, which is curable in 80% of the animals treated.

D. **Conditions of the teeth treated by surgery**

1. **Indications for tooth extraction** include malocclusion, retained deciduous teeth, caries, complicated fractures, severe periodontal disease, supernumerary teeth, periapical abscesses, odontogenic tumors, and teeth in a fracture line or associated with oral neoplasia.

2. **Extraction of multirooted teeth** is facilitated by crown division with dental burs, disc handpieces, power drills, or handsaws.

3. **Complications** include mandibular or maxillary fractures (especially if chronic disease is present), tooth fracture and root retention, osteitis or osteomyelitis, oronasal fistulae (particularly with upper canine teeth or third incisors), gingival lacerations, temporomandibular joint dislocation, bacteremia, and hemorrhage.

E. **Conditions of the lips treated by surgery**

1. **Lip fold dermatitis**
   a. **Etiology.** Lip fold dermatitis is reported in animals that **drool excessively** (e.g., Saint Bernards, spaniels, setters, Newfoundlands, retrievers). It may also be **secondary to abnormal lip conformation** or **facial nerve paralysis.**
   b. **Treatment** is by lip fold excision **(cheiloplasty)** or modified cheiloplasty. Redundant skin is grasped and resected, taking care to avoid the underlying muscles and oral mucosa. The subcutaneous and cutaneous tissue layers are closed in a routine manner.

2. **Trauma** repair requires careful surgical apposition of the lip margins. Mucosa and skin layers are sutured separately. Drainage or use of skin flaps may be necessary if extensive necrosis occurs after lip avulsion.

3. **Eosinophilic granulomas.** These slowly progressive masses most commonly occur on the maxillary labia midline of middle-aged female cats.
   a. **Treatment** options include systemic or local corticosteroids, radiation therapy, immunotherapy, cryosurgery, and surgical excision.

     b. Prognosis for permanent cure is fair.

   4. Neoplasia. The most frequently reported lip tumors include melanoma, squamous cell carcinoma, fibrosarcoma, basal cell carcinoma, and mast cell tumors.

     a. Treatment of malignant tumors is wide excision.

     b. Complications include damage to salivary ducts and loss of oral mobility.

F. Conditions of the palate treated by surgery

   1. Cleft palate, oronasal fistulae, and **elongated soft palate** are discussed in Chapter 7 III A 4 b and E.

   2. Palatine fractures are discussed in Chapter 19 III A 5.

G. Conditions of the maxilla and mandible treated by surgery

   1. Trauma is discussed in Chapter 19 III A 3–4.

   2. Neoplasia. Oral tumors (Table 10–2) often invade the bone.

     a. Incidence

       (1) Dogs. The most common oral tumors in dogs are **malignant melanoma**, epulides, squamous cell carcinoma, and fibrosarcoma.

       (2) Cats. The most common oral tumors in cats are **squamous cell carcinoma**, fibrosarcoma, and fibromatous epulis. In cats, 89% of oral tumors are malignant.

     b. Predisposing factors. Oral neoplasia is more common in **male** dogs than female dogs. **Cocker spaniels, poodles, German short-haired pointers, weimaraners, golden retrievers,** and **boxers** are commonly affected.

     c. Clinical features. Eighty percent of benign maxillary tumors are rostral; seventy percent of malignant maxillary tumors are caudal.

     d. Clinical signs include an enlarging or ulcerative oral mass, facial deformity, halitosis, ptyalism, dysphagia, anorexia, tooth loss, and oral hemorrhage.

TABLE 10–2. Tumors of the Oropharynx

Type of Tumor	Bone Involvement	Location	Metastasis	Surgical Treatment	Prognosis
Epulides (benign)					
Fibromatous, ossifying	No	Oral cavity	No	Excision, radiation	Excellent
Acanthomatous	Locally invasive	Primary mandible or mandible	No	Radical excision, radiation	Excellent
Malignant melanoma*	Locally invasive	Oral cavity	Spreads early to lungs, lymph nodes	Mandibulectomy, radical surgical excision, intralesional chemotherapy, hyperthermia, radiation	Poor
Squamous cell carcinoma					
Nontonsillar	Locally invasive	Oral cavity	Late	Radical excision, radiation, ± hyperthermia, cryotherapy, phototherapy	Guarded (dogs) Poor (cats)
Tonsillar			Early	See Nontonsillar	Grave
Fibrosarcoma	Locally invasive, osteolytic	Maxilla	Slow	Excision, radiation, hyperthermia	Guarded Poor

* Seen most frequently in dogs older than 12 years of age, small dogs, male dogs, and dogs with pigmented mucosa.

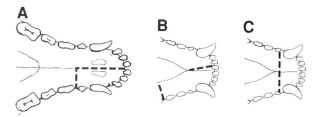

FIGURE 10–1. Maxillectomy and mandibulectomy are useful for treating oral tumors. Additional indications for these techniques include chronic osteomyelitis, oronasal fistulae, and severe oral fractures associated with bone and soft tissue injuries. *(A)* Unilateral rostral maxillectomy is indicated for lesions rostral to the second premolar that do not cross the midline. *(B)* Unilateral rostral mandibulectomy is indicated for tumors or injuries involving the incisors, canines, or first two premolars on one side. *(C)* Bilateral rostral mandibulectomy is indicated for tumors or injuries that cross the midline rostral to the second premolar.

    e. Diagnosis is usually by wedge biopsy. Fine-needle aspiration may also be useful. Lymph node biopsy accompanied by thoracic films, skull films, or computed tomography scans should be used to determine the extent of the disease.
    f. Treatment options include **partial** or **complete maxillectomy** or **mandibulectomy,** radiation therapy, hyperthermia, cryosurgery, and photodynamic therapy. Excisional margins of 1–2 centimeters should be based on physical examination and results of skull radiographs or computed tomography scans.
        (1) Maxillectomy (Figure 10–1) may involve unilateral or bilateral resection along the rostral aspect of the maxilla (premaxillectomy) or unilateral resection along the caudal or rostral aspects of the maxilla.
            (a) Positioning the animal. The animal is placed in dorsal recumbency, and the mouth is held open with an oral speculum.
            (b) Gingival incision. The oral mucosa is incised to the bone, leaving 1-cm margins around the lesion, and soft-tissue attachments are reflected from the bone. Pressure, ligation, or electrocoagulation is used to control hemorrhage.
            (c) Maxillary resection. An oscillating saw, high-speed bur, or osteotome is used to resect the affected portion of the maxilla. The isolated bone segment is removed *en bloc* and bleeding is controlled with bone wax, absorbable hemostatic sponges (Gelfoam), or direct ligation of the major vessels (e.g., the infraorbital artery).
            (d) Closure. The surgical defect is closed with a one- or two-layer closure by undermining the labial and palatal gingival mucosa and suturing the flaps using synthetic absorbable suture (e.g., polydioxanone) in a simple interrupted pattern.
            (e) Postoperative care. The animal should be fed a soft diet for 10–14 days to reduce tension on and contamination of the incision site and promote healing.
            (f) Postoperative complications include local recurrence, dehiscence, oronasal fistula formation, hemorrhage, swelling, dyspnea secondary to nasal cavity obstruction, subcutaneous emphysema, cosmetic facial deformity, drooling, labial ulceration, tooth damage, and anorexia.
                (i) Maxillary dehiscence is highly correlated with the concurrent use of radiation and chemotherapy, tumor location, and tumor recurrence. Eighty percent of dehiscences are associated with caudal maxillectomies.
                (ii) Hemorrhage may be severe, especially with resection of nasal turbinates and the caudal maxilla.
        (2) Mandibulectomy (see Figure 10–1). Resection of the mandible may involve rostral unilateral or bilateral procedures, central or caudal unilateral procedures, or complete removal of the hemimandible.
            (a) Rostral or partial unilateral mandibulectomy. Incision, excision, and clo-

sure of the affected tissues are similar to the procedures outlined for maxillectomy.

(b) Hemimandibulectomy

(i) Incision and elevation. The commissura of the lip is incised, and the caudal mandibular muscles are elevated from the bone medially and laterally. Care should be taken to preserve the major vessels, nerves, and salivary ducts.

(ii) Disarticulation. The mandibular symphysis is separated and the bone pulled laterally to permit disarticulation at the temporomandibular joint.

(iii) Closure. To reduce dead space, the remaining soft tissues, including muscle, are closed in layers with nonabsorbable suture material.

(c) Postoperative care is similar to that for maxillectomy.

(d) Postoperative complications include dehiscence and prehension difficulties, which are more common when a hemimandibulectomy is performed. Other complications include excessive drooling, pain, ranula formation, malocclusion, and lip ulceration.

H. **Conditions of the tonsils treated by surgery. Tonsillar enlargement** may be secondary to tonsillitis caused by *Streptococcus*, *Staphylococcus*, or coliform bacteria, neoplasia (e.g., squamous cell carcinoma, lymphosarcoma), foreign bodies, and cysts.

1. Diagnosis is by biopsy.

2. Treatment

a. Tonsillectomy is indicated for chronic tonsillitis unresponsive to antibiotics, acute tonsillar enlargement with respiratory obstruction, and tonsillar enlargement secondary to neoplasia.

(1) The animal is positioned in ventral recumbency, and the mouth is held open with an oral speculum.

(2) The enlarged tonsils are grasped with Allis tissue forceps and scissors are used to remove the tonsil at the base, following ligation of the tonsillar artery.

(3) Complications include hemorrhage and airway obstruction as a result of tissue swelling. Corticosteroid therapy is useful for reducing postoperative edema.

b. Chemotherapy may be used to treat lymphosarcoma.

I. **Conditions of the salivary glands treated by surgery**

1. Salivary mucoceles. Damage to the salivary duct or gland leads to leakage and the formation of "pockets" of saliva in adjacent tissues.

a. Predisposed breeds include toy and miniature poodles, dachshunds, and Australian silky terriers.

b. Diagnosis is by examination, aspiration, and, occasionally, sialography (particularly for postoperative recurrence). Gold or blood-tinged viscous mucus can be aspirated from the mucocele and will stain positively with a mucus-specific stain (e.g., periodic acid-Schiff).

c. Treatment

(1) Sialoadenectomy (i.e., mandibular and sublingual salivary gland resection) is indicated for cervical mucoceles and recurrent sublingual or pharyngeal mucoceles (ranula).

(a) The animal is placed in lateral recumbency, and a skin incision is made at the junction of the maxillary and linguofacial veins. The incision courses rostrally over the angle of the mandible.

(b) The mandibular and sublingual salivary glands are dissected from the surrounding fibrous tissue capsule, and the ducts are isolated and ligated as far rostral as possible.

(c) The glands and ducts are removed and the remaining layers of subcutaneous tissue and muscle are apposed to reduce dead space. Penrose drains are often used to prevent seroma formation.

(2) Marsupialization can be used to treat oral ranula. The salivary cyst is opened and the edges are sutured to the oral mucosa, allowing permanent drainage into the mouth.

    d. Prognosis. Recurrence is less than 5% with surgical resection of affected glands; recurrence is common with drainage alone.

2. Neoplasia is **rare** in dogs and cats. It is most frequently found in the **mandibular salivary gland** in animals over 10 years of age. Most tumors are **adenocarcinomas**.
  a. Diagnosis is by wedge biopsy.
  b. Treatment is surgical excision. Facial nerve paralysis occurs routinely after *en bloc* resection of the parotid gland.
  c. Recurrence usually occurs within 1–6 months of surgical excision and is common (because of the locally aggressive nature of the tumor). Radiation may be effective in treating recurrence after surgery.
  d. Metastasis to regional lymph nodes and beyond is common.

3. Salivary fistulae
  a. Etiology. Salivary gland or duct injury may result in fistula formation and leakage of clear, thin fluid.
  b. Treatment options include duct diversion, duct reconstruction or ligation if the parotid gland is the source, or gland removal if the zygomatic gland is affected.

4. Sialoliths may occur in canine parotid salivary ducts and result in painful swelling.
  a. Diagnosis is by palpation or radiography.
  b. Treatment is removal of the stone following incision of the duct over the obstruction. The intraoral incision does not require suturing.

J. **Conditions of the pharynx treated by surgery. Cricopharyngeal achalasia** is caused by failure of the cricopharyngeal muscle to relax, or by incoordination of the cricopharyngeal sphincter and pharyngeal contraction.

1. Clinical signs include dysphagia that begins at weaning, coughing, gagging, and food expulsion from the mouth.

2. Diagnosis. Fluoroscopy demonstrates failure of the sphincter to open or failure of pharyngeal contraction and sphincter relaxation to synchronize. Cricopharyngeal achalasia must be differentiated from pharyngeal-phase swallowing disorders.

3. Treatment is **cricopharyngeal myotomy.**
  a. The animal is placed in dorsal recumbency and the extrinsic muscles of the larynx are exposed.
  b. The larynx is rotated 180°, and the cricopharyngeal muscles on the dorsal aspect of the larynx are incised along the median raphe. Perforation of the esophageal and pharyngeal mucosa should be avoided.

II. **ESOPHAGUS**

A. Anatomy

1. Vascularization
  a. Arteries
    (1) The **cervical esophagus** is supplied by the **thyroid** and **subclavian arteries** and by **esophageal branches of the carotid artery.**
    (2) The **thoracic esophagus** is supplied by the **bronchoesophageal artery** and **esophageal branches of the distal thoracic aorta.** Near the cardia, the esophagus is supplied by **esophageal branches of the left gastric and phrenic arteries.**
  b. Veins. The **external jugular vein** drains the proximal portion of the esophagus. **Branches of the azygous vein** drain the distal esophagus.

    c. Lymphatic drainage proceeds to the retropharyngeal, cervical, mediastinal, bronchial, portal, gastric, and splenic lymph nodes.

2. Innervation
    a. Striated muscle is supplied by visceral efferent fibers from the **pharyngoesophageal nerve, recurrent laryngeal nerve,** and **dorsal and ventral vagal trunks.**
    b. Smooth muscle is innervated by **general visceral efferent fibers.**
    c. The esophagus also receives **parasympathetic** and **sympathetic fibers** of the autonomic nervous system.

B. Surgical procedures

1. General considerations. Several factors complicate wound healing in the esophagus.
    a. The esophagus lacks a serosal covering to prevent leakage and dehiscence.
    b. The blood supply of the esophagus is segmental.
    c. The esophagus is mobile and poorly tolerates longitudinal stretching and tension.

2. Esophageal resection and anastomosis
    a. Circular partial thickness (circumferential) myotomy. An incision around the esophagus is made through the outer longitudinal muscle layer and left unsutured. Circular partial thickness myotomy reduces tension at the suture line, improves survival rate, and allows resection of a greater length of esophagus than full-thickness incisions alone.
    b. Anastomosis
        (1) Suturing. Synthetic monofilament suture is usually used for esophageal closure. **Double-layer simple interrupted closure** provides the best healing, tissue approximation, and strength.
            (a) The mucosa and submucosa are apposed and closed in a simple interrupted pattern with 3-mm bites. The sutures are placed 2–3 mm apart. The submucosa is considered the holding layer of the esophagus; careful apposition of the mucosa and submucosa is required to avoid leakage and protect the blood supply.
            (b) The muscularis is closed using a simple interrupted pattern. Knots are placed in the lumen and in the thorax.
            (c) Suture lines can be reinforced with diaphragmatic or intercostal muscle, pericardium, or omentum. These tissues can also be used as patch grafts to fill defects.
        (2) Stapling. Closure with an end-to-end anastomotic stapler results in less leaks than manual anastomosis.

3. Esophageal reconstruction may be necessary when a large portion of the esophagus must be resected (e.g., because of injury, neoplasia, strictures, or diverticula).
    a. Techniques include replacement with skin tubes, gastric wall, intestine, or muscle.
    b. Complications are frequent and include stricture, dehiscence, ischemic necrosis, and infection.

4. Esophagotomy is usually performed to remove foreign objects not easily retrieved by endoscopy or with forceps through a gastrostomy.
    a. Incision. A full-thickness longitudinal incision is made in healthy esophageal tissue cranial or caudal to the obstruction.
    b. Closure. Following removal of the foreign body, the mucosal and submucosal layers are approximated with nonabsorbable or synthetic absorbable suture in a continuous pattern. The muscularis is closed with similar sutures in a simple interrupted pattern.

C. Conditions treated by surgery

1. Megaesophagus may be classified as primary (most commonly idiopathic) and secondary.
    a. Etiology. Disorders leading to **surgically treatable secondary megaesophagus** include:

(1) **Obstructive diseases** such as neoplasia, lymphadenopathy, vascular ring anomalies (see Chapter 8 II B 4), extraesophageal masses, esophageal strictures, granulomas, and foreign bodies

(2) **Thymoma**

(3) **Esophagitis** (from vomiting)

(4) **Mediastinitis**

(5) **Bronchoesophageal fistulae**

(6) **Pyloric stenosis** (in cats)

b. **Clinical signs.** Regurgitation is the major clinical sign. Poor growth rate, ptyalism, respiratory distress, coughing, and signs of aspiration pneumonia may also be seen.

c. **Diagnosis.** Survey thoracic radiographs can be used to diagnose megaesophagus, and contrast studies and fluoroscopy help determine the etiology and may give information on prognosis, especially in regard to motility.

d. **Treatment**

(1) Surgical treatment of **secondary megaesophagus** focuses on treating the primary cause.

(2) Surgical treatment of **primary megaesophagus** is controversial and may be of no therapeutic value.

e. **Prognosis** for recovery from megaesophagus is guarded to poor, depending on the etiology.

2. **Vascular ring anomalies** [e.g., persistent right aortic arch (PRAA), aberrant left or right subclavian artery, persistent right ligament or ductus arteriosus, double aortic arch, aberrant intercostals] occur with abnormal development of the vasculature derived from the embryonic aortic arches, resulting in entrapment and obstruction of the esophagus.

a. **Aberrant subclavian artery** and **double aortic arch** are treated by ligation and division or division and reanastomosis of the obstructing vessel, depending on the extent of collateral blood supply.

b. **PRAA** is discussed in Chapter 8 II B 4.

3. **Esophageal foreign body obstruction and perforations.** Perforations are seen in 17% of dogs with esophageal foreign bodies.

a. **Predisposing factors.** Small breed dogs, particularly terriers and Chihuahuas, are at increased risk for esophageal foreign body obstruction.

b. **Clinical features**

(1) **Objects. Bones** are the most common type of esophageal foreign body.

(2) **Locations.** Foreign bodies usually are trapped in the thoracic esophagus at the diaphragmatic esophageal hiatus or heart base, but they may also be trapped at the thoracic inlet or at the level of the cricopharyngeal sphincter.

c. **Clinical signs** include regurgitation (usually undigested food), ptyalism, anorexia, dysphagia, fever, depression, dehydration, septicemia, coughing, dyspnea, cervical swelling, subcutaneous emphysema, and weight loss. Megaesophagus and aspiration pneumonia may occur secondary to obstructions.

(1) Regurgitation occurs quickly after swallowing if the obstruction is high, and may not occur for hours if a chronic partial obstruction is present.

(2) Persistent and recurrent clinical signs may imply a perforation.

d. **Diagnosis**

(1) **Radiography, fluoroscopy,** or **endoscopy.** Esophagrams help to diagnose perforations, but they miss 56% of all perforations when performed before foreign body removal.

(a) Radiographs demonstrate radiopaque foreign bodies or esophageal distention, and help to diagnose secondary aspiration pneumonia.

(b) Extensive fluid density around the foreign body, loss of detail around the margins of the mass, or obliteration of the caudal vena cava shadow is suggestive of mediastinitis and perforation.

(2) **Blood work.** Neutrophilia is present; increases in immature neutrophils may be suggestive of a perforation.

e. Treatment
  (1) Removal of foreign bodies. A variety of approaches may be taken:
    (a) Forceps retrieval through an endoscope, rigid proctoscope, or gastrostomy
    (b) Advancement of the foreign body into the stomach (with subsequent removal by gastrotomy if the object is indigestible)
    (c) Retrieval via thoracotomy and esophagotomy cranial to the object
  (2) Perforations can be managed conservatively if they are not accompanied by leakage. If leakage is present, the perforation should be débrided and sutured using a two-layer closure technique.
  (3) Postoperative considerations. Food should be withheld for 24–72 hours after surgery; a gastrostomy tube or parenteral feeding may be necessary for animals recovering from perforations.
  (4) Postoperative complications
    (a) Esophageal body removal. Marked ulceration and distal esophagitis are seen in 26% of dogs after foreign body removal.
    (b) Perforation repair is associated with leakage leading to mediastinitis or pleuritis, pneumothorax, and stricture.
f. Prognosis. The overall mortality rate of animals with esophageal perforations that are treated surgically is 57%.

4. Esophageal stricture
  a. Etiology. Acquired strictures can result from corrosive chemicals, trauma, foreign bodies, surgical resection and anastomosis, or gastric reflux esophagitis.
  b. Clinical signs include regurgitation, dysphagia, and coughing.
  c. Diagnosis is by contrast radiography and endoscopy.
  d. Treatment is by **bougienage** or **balloon catheter dilation** under anesthesia.
    (1) Multiple treatments may be necessary.
    (2) Ranitidine or cimetidine are administered for 2–3 weeks to treat reflux esophagitis. Decreasing doses of prednisone or prednisolone are administered for 10–14 days to decrease fibrosis.

5. Esophageal diverticulum
  a. Types
    (1) Pulsion diverticulum is a protrusion (outpouching) of mucosa through a defect in the muscularis in the esophagus.
    (2) Traction diverticulum is an outpouching of all layers of the esophagus.
  b. Clinical signs include regurgitation, dysphagia, and coughing.
  c. Diagnosis is by contrast radiography; motility should be evaluated as well.
  d. Treatment is via **resection of the diverticulum.** The wound is closed using the two-layer closure technique.

6. Esophageal fistulae are abnormal communications between the esophagus and the respiratory tract; esophageal–epidermal fistulae have also been reported.
  a. Etiology. Esophageal–respiratory tract fistulae may be congenital or acquired; usually they occur secondary to trauma.
  b. Clinical signs include coughing, fever, anorexia, lethargy, weight loss, and crepitus in the cervical region.
  c. Diagnosis. Air is seen within the esophagus on plain radiographs. Contrast studies using propyliodone oil or barium sulfate suspensions may delineate the fistula.
  d. Treatment is usually by **lung lobectomy** (see Chapter 7 IV D 1 b). Endobronchial intubation or high-frequency jet ventilation may be necessary to avoid intraoperative gastric distention and maintain anesthesia and oxygenation.

7. Neoplasia is rare in dogs and cats. **Squamous cell carcinoma, leiomyomas, leiomyosarcomas, fibrosarcomas, osteosarcomas,** and **plasmacytomas** have been reported. Fibrosarcomas and osteosarcomas of the esophagus have been related to *Spirocerca lupi* parasitism in the Southwest United States.
  a. Clinical signs include regurgitation, dysphagia, and weight loss.
  b. Diagnosis is by contrast radiography and esophagoscopy.
  c. Treatment is **excision** or **resection and anastomosis.**
  d. Prognosis is poor, especially with esophageal resection. Failure of the anastomosis is more likely if a portion greater than 2 centimeters in length is resected.

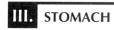

III. STOMACH

A. Anatomy

1. **Vascularization**
   a. **Arteries.** The **splenic, left gastric,** and **hepatic branches of the celiac artery** supply the stomach.
   b. **Veins** are paired with corresponding arteries.
   c. **Lymphatics** drain into the **splenic, gastric,** and **hepatic nodes.**

2. **Innervation** is by parasympathetic fibers of the vagi and sympathetic fibers of the celiac plexus.

B. Surgical procedures

1. **General considerations**
   a. **Contamination.** The bacterial content of the stomach is low except when food or obstructions are present.
      (1) Prophylactic antibiotics may be used at induction if contamination is expected.
      (2) The stomach should be isolated from the rest of the abdominal contents with moist laparotomy pads before incising; suction should be available to remove gastric contents. Instruments and gloves are changed if contaminated.
      (3) If contamination of the abdominal cavity occurs, vigorous lavage should be performed and therapeutic antibiotics (e.g., first-generation cephalosporins) may be used postoperatively.
   b. **Wound closure**
      (1) **Sutures.** A two-layer inverting continuous suture pattern is frequently employed, using 2-0 or 3-0 synthetic absorbable monofilament suture.
      (2) **Staples.** Gastrointestinal or thoracic surgical autostaplers may also be used for closure. Advantages include less time in surgery and reduced risk of gastric spillage.
   c. **Wound healing.** The stomach heals rapidly because of its extensive blood supply, rapid mucosal regeneration, extensive submucosa, well-developed serosa, and proximity to the omentum. The omentum is useful for visceral sealing and, because of its rich vascularization, is helpful for wound healing in wounds with a compromised blood supply.
   d. **Postoperative care.** Animals should be given small amounts of water the day after surgery; if no vomiting occurs, small amounts of a bland, highly digestible diet may be introduced.

2. **Gastrotomy** is performed most frequently for removal of foreign objects not retrievable by endoscopy.
   a. **Approach.** A **cranial ventral midline celiotomy** is performed, and the stomach is isolated to reduce intra-abdominal contamination.
   b. Stay sutures or Babcock forceps are used to maintain traction while a **stab incision** is made to gain access to the lumen.
   c. **Closure.** Following removal of the foreign object, the stomach is closed with a two-layer technique using synthetic absorbable suture material.
      (1) The **mucosal** and **submucosal layers** are closed in a continuous appositional or inverting pattern.
      (2) The **muscularis** and **serosa** are closed in a continuous inverting pattern.
   d. **Omental coverage/serosal patch grafting.** Omentum or an adjacent bowel loop can be sutured over the gastrotomy incision to promote healing and prevent dehiscence.

3. **Billroth I (pylorectomy and gastroduodenostomy).** In this procedure, the diseased portion of the pylorus is removed and the duodenum is connected directly to the body of the stomach.
   a. **Approach.** The approach is similar to that used for a gastrotomy.
   b. **Resection.** Stay sutures are placed proximal and distal to the diseased tissue, and

the area to be resected is isolated and removed. Noncrushing intestinal forceps may be used to reduce reflux of gastrointestinal contents following resection of affected tissue.

   c. **Anastomosis.** A single-layer interrupted appositional suture pattern using nonabsorbable or synthetic absorbable (polydioxanone) suture material is used for anastomosis. Alternatively, a gastrointestinal or thoracic autostapler can be used.

4. Billroth II (gastrojejunostomy) may be necessary when extensive resection of the duodenum and distal aspect of the stomach is required.
   a. The stomach and jejunum are connected using a side-to-side or an end-to-end technique.
   b. If the duodenal segment of the common bile duct opening is not preserved, the gallbladder can be connected to the jejunum via a cholecystenterostomy.

5. Partial gastrectomy is often indicated for the removal of tumors or necrotic areas of the stomach.
   a. **Approach.** The stomach is approached and isolated as for a gastrotomy. Stay sutures or Babcock forceps are used to retract healthy segments. Blood vessels supplying the affected area are ligated.
   b. **Aspiration.** Prior to resection, the gastric contents should be aspirated to reduce the risk of abdominal contamination.
   c. **Closure.** A simple interrupted or continuous pattern using synthetic absorbable or nonabsorbable suture material is used to close all four stomach wall layers, and then a second inverting pattern is used on the outer two layers. Alternatively, the gastrectomy incision may be stapled using a gastrointestinal or thoracic autostapler.

6. Gastropexy is the surgical fixation of the stomach to prevent displacement.
   a. **Tube gastropexy**
      (1) Procedure. A gastrostomy tube is placed in the stomach at the junction of the body and antrum and exits the right ventrolateral body wall. The gastric wall and body wall are then sutured together around the tube.
      (2) Advantages. Tube gastropexy provides continuous postoperative decompression.
      (3) Disadvantages. Entry into the gastric lumen and significant postoperative care are required. Tube gastropexy inhibits aboral motility for 48–168 hours.
      (4) Complications (e.g., infection, tube dislodgment) are seen in 17% of animals treated.
   b. **Incisional (muscular) gastropexy**
      (1) Procedure. Incisions are made through the peritoneum of the right ventrolateral body wall and the seromuscular layers of the stomach at the junction of the stomach body and antrum. The incision sites of the body wall and gastric wall are then sutured to each other.
      (2) Advantages. Incisional gastropexy requires minimal postoperative care and is easy to perform.
      (3) Complications (e.g., vomiting, weight loss) are seen in 7.6% of the animals treated.
   c. **Circumcostal gastropexy**
      (1) Procedure. A seromuscular flap of the gastric wall at the junction of the body and antrum is elevated and sutured around the ventral portion of the twelfth or eleventh rib.
      (2) Advantages. Circumcostal gastropexy results in strong adhesions with less inflammation and complications than tube gastropexy.
      (3) Disadvantages include a long procedure duration, possible rib fracture, and the potential for pneumothorax formation if the diaphragm is incised.
   d. **Belt loop gastropexy**
      (1) Procedure. A "belt loop" is formed in the transverse abdominal muscle by making two transverse stab incisions approximately 3 centimeters apart. A seromuscular flap is elevated from the gastrointestinal wall, passed through the "belt loop," and sutured back to the stomach.

(2) **Advantages.** Although belt loop gastropexy is also a fairly lengthy procedure, strong adhesions are produced.

(3) **Complications** are minimal.

e. **Incorporation of the pyloric antrum.** The gastric wall is included in the cranial abdominal wall closure. This technique has not been evaluated for adhesion strength.

C. **Conditions treated by surgery**

1. **Gastroesophageal intussusception** is an uncommon, often fatal condition in which the stomach herniates into the esophagus. Young animals are most frequently affected.

   a. **Clinical signs** include dyspnea, shock, vomiting, regurgitation, hematemesis, dehydration, abdominal pain, and weight loss.

   b. **Diagnosis** is by plain and contrast radiographs and fluoroscopy. Radiographs reveal esophageal dilation and an epiphrenic mass in the distal esophagus.

   c. **Treatment** includes supportive therapy and **emergency laparotomy** and **gastropexy** of the gastric body to the left body wall.

2. **Hiatal hernia** is a protrusion or herniation of any structure, usually the stomach, through the esophageal hiatus of the diaphragm. It may be **sliding** (i.e., the diaphragm moves up and down on the esophagus) or **paraesophageal** (i.e., the esophagus is in normal position but the stomach herniates adjacent to it).

   a. **Clinical signs** include vomiting, regurgitation, dyspnea, hypersalivation, weight loss, and signs of pneumonia.

   b. **Diagnosis.** Megaesophagus may be seen on plain films, along with a gas-filled soft tissue density in the caudal thorax, absence of the right diaphragmatic crus, and lobar alveolar consolidation. Fluoroscopy may reveal gastroesophageal reflux or hypomotility.

   c. **Treatment**

   (1) **Medical treatment.** Dietary modification and administration of antacids and metoclopramide should be attempted for 1 month in animals with signs of gastroesophageal reflux or asymptomatic animals. If there is no improvement, surgery should be considered.

   (2) **Surgical treatment.** The goal of surgery is to return the lower esophageal sphincter and distal esophagus to the abdominal cavity and maintain them there. **Esophagopexy, gastropexy,** and **diaphragmatic crural apposition** may be used to close the esophageal hiatus and fix the lower esophageal sphincter in the abdomen.

   d. **Prognosis** with medical or surgical therapy is good in cats and asymptomatic dogs. In symptomatic dogs, improvement has been seen with medical and surgical therapy; however, between 11% and 22% of the dogs treated die in the immediate postoperative period of complications related to the disease.

3. **Pyloric stenosis** is a congenital thickening of the pyloric sphincter that results in delayed gastric emptying of solid foods.

   a. **Predisposing factors.** Young male dogs and brachycephalic dogs are predisposed.

   b. **Clinical signs.** Vomiting usually starts after weaning; growth may be retarded.

   c. **Diagnosis** is by contrast studies, ultrasonography, or exploratory laparotomy. Contrast studies may show gastric distention and delayed emptying.

   d. **Treatment.** Surgical options are designed to correct outflow obstruction and include **Fredet-Ramstedt pyloromyotomy** (Figure 10–2A) or **Heineke-Mikulicz pyloroplasty** (Figure 10–2B).

   e. **Prognosis.** Good results are seen after surgery in over 50% of animals.

4. **Pyloric hyperplasia.** Acquired antral pyloric hypertrophy (chronic hypertrophic pyloric gastropathy) is a benign disease that results in mucosal and muscular pyloric hyperplasia and prolonged gastric emptying.

   a. **Predisposing factors.** Middle-aged to older small breed dogs such as Lhasa apso, shih tzu, miniature poodle, and Pekingese are often affected. Males are affected twice as often as females.

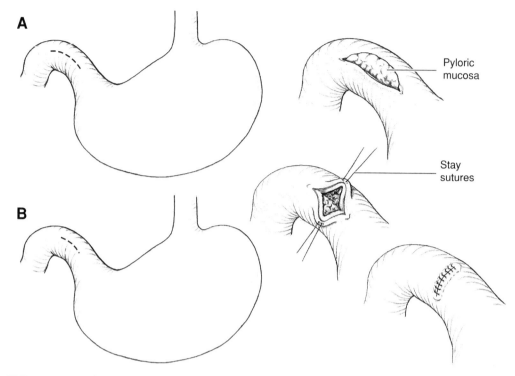

FIGURE 10–2. Pyloroplasty procedures. *(A)* Fredet-Ramstedt pyloromyotomy. A longitudinal incision is made through the serosa, muscularis, and submucosa layers to permit bulging of the gastric mucosa, relieving the restriction and allowing the passage of food. Because the incision does not penetrate all four layers of the pyloric wall, the risk of abdominal contamination is lessened. The incision is not sutured closed. *(B)* Heineke-Mikulicz pyloroplasty. A longitudinal incision is made through the entire wall of the pylorus and sutured transversely to widen the luminal outflow tract.

      b. Clinical signs include chronic intermittent vomiting, anorexia, weight loss, and occasionally, abdominal distention.

      c. Diagnosis is by endoscopic evaluation and mucosal biopsy, contrast upper gastrointestinal studies, and exploratory laparotomy.

         (1) Contrast gastrograms may show severe gastric distention, delayed emptying, intraluminal pyloric filling defects, or a thickened pyloric canal with a narrow beak-like outlet.

         (2) Diagnosis is confirmed by full-thickness biopsy during surgery.

      d. Treatment. Pyloroplasty is used to widen the area. Pyloric removal using a **Billroth I procedure** is also effective.

      e. Prognosis. The overall response to surgery is good or excellent in 85% of animals treated. Results are good to excellent in 100% of animals treated with gastroduodenostomy and in 74% treated with pyloroplasty.

    5. Gastric foreign bodies. Ingestion of foreign bodies becomes a significant problem when gastrointestinal obstruction or perforation occurs, or when toxicity results from partial digestion of the foreign body (e.g., lead toxicity from curtain or fishing weights; zinc toxicity from pennies).

      a. Clinical signs. Frequent or intermittent vomiting is seen with pyloric obstruction.

      b. Diagnosis is by abdominal palpation. Survey films reveal radiopaque and large objects. Contrast studies or endoscopy may also be useful.

      c. Treatment is based on the size and shape of the object.

         (1) Smooth, small objects may be expelled during induced vomiting. **Apomorphine** and **xylazine** have been used to induce vomiting in dogs and cats, respectively.

(2) **Small foreign bodies** may be removed with **grasping forceps during endoscopy.**

(3) **Large, long,** or **rough foreign bodies** can be removed by **gastrotomy.**

6. **Gastric dilation/volvulus** is a life-threatening syndrome in which the stomach becomes dilated and displaced along its long axis, permitting gaseous distention from aerophagia but preventing release of gases through the pylorus or esophagus.

   a. **Pathogenesis.** Excessive or prolonged distention compromises the intramural gastric blood supply and compresses the portal vein and caudal vena cava.

      (1) Reduction of venous return to the heart from caudal vena cava compression eventually results in hypovolemic shock with clinical signs of tachycardia; weak, thready, pulses; pale mucous membranes; prolonged capillary refill time; hypothermia; and collapse.

      (2) Venous stasis may lead to fundic ischemia, mucosal necrosis, splanchnic hypoxia, endotoxic shock, disseminated intravascular coagulation (DIC), myocardial injury, and death.

   b. **Predisposing factors**

      (1) **Signalment.** Gastric dilation/volvulus is usually seen in large or giant, deep-chested, middle-aged dogs, especially Great Danes, weimaraners, Saint Bernards, Gordon setters, Irish setters, and standard poodles.

      (2) **History.** Ingestion of large quantities of food or water, dietary change, postprandial exercise, and hospitalization have all been anecdotally associated with the onset of gastric dilation/volvulus. However, in research studies, feeding habits, type of food, gastroesophageal sphincter pressures, and gastrin levels have not been correlated with development of the syndrome.

   c. **Clinical signs.** Restlessness, panting, abdominal distention, retching, ptyalism, weakness, depression, signs of shock, and acute collapse or death are seen.

   d. **Diagnosis** is based on clinical signs and physical examination, but may be confirmed by radiography. Survey films of the abdomen taken in right lateral recumbency reveal a displaced, air-filled pylorus and gastric distention.

   e. **Treatment** should be initiated before the diagnosis is confirmed if gastric dilation/volvulus is suspected.

      (1) **Stomach decompression.** The stomach is decompressed with an orogastric tube, percutaneous gastrocentesis, or surgical decompression through a gastrotomy.

      (2) **Surgical derotation** and **permanent gastropexy** (to prevent recurrence) are necessary in most cases. Anesthetics for surgery should be reversible or have minimal cardiovascular effects.

         (a) In most cases, the pylorus moves ventrally and to the left and the body of the stomach moves dorsally and to the right. Following a cranial ventral midline celiotomy, the stomach is gently untwisted in a counterclockwise motion while manually supporting the stomach and spleen.

         (b) It may be necessary to pass a stomach tube or perform gastrocentesis during surgery.

      (3) **Partial gastrectomies** are necessary in 10.5% of cases. Nonviable portions of the gastric wall, usually associated with thrombosis of branches of the short gastric or left gastroepiploic vessels, should be resected or invaginated and oversewn.

      (4) **Splenectomy** is necessary if splenic torsion and vascular thromboses are present; the organ should be removed without derotating it (see Chapter 15 IV C).

   f. **Prognosis.** The mortality rate following surgery is 23%–43%; if partial gastrectomy is necessary, the rate increases to 33%–63%.

7. **Gastric ulceration.** Upper gastrointestinal bleeding is rare in small animals and is usually secondary to drugs or other disease conditions.

   a. **Clinical signs** include hematemesis, weight loss, abdominal pain, and shock if perforation occurs. Anemia may be present.

   b. **Diagnosis** is by contrast radiography, endoscopy, and scintigraphy.

c. **Treatment. Surgical excision** of the ulcer via **partial gastrectomy** is required for perforated ulcers or in cases where hemorrhage is severe or the animal does not respond to medical management.

8. **Neoplasia** is uncommon; older animals are affected most often. **Leiomyomas** are the most common benign tumor in dogs. **Adenocarcinoma** and **lymphosarcoma** are the most common malignant gastric tumors in dogs and cats, respectively.
   a. **Clinical signs** include chronic vomiting, hematemesis, anorexia, weight loss, and abdominal pain. Ascites, jaundice, or dyspnea may be seen with metastasis.
   b. **Diagnosis.** Contrast films may show filling defects, delayed gastric emptying, mucosal thickening, loss of normal rugal folds, and ulceration. Endoscopy is occasionally diagnostic; however, exploratory laparotomy and biopsy are often necessary to confirm the diagnosis and determine the extent of disease.
   c. **Treatment** options include **gastrectomy,** a **Billroth I procedure,** or chemotherapy (for lymphoid neoplasia). Extensive pyloric neoplasia is treated with a **Billroth II** procedure.
      (1) If outflow from the common bile duct is affected, the gallbladder is anastomosed to the duodenum or proximal jejunum (**cholecystoenterostomy**).
      (2) If the pancreatic ducts are obstructed or resected, the animal must be treated for pancreatic exocrine insufficiency postoperatively.
   d. **Prognosis.** Animals are often euthanized during exploratory surgery because of the size and aggressiveness of malignant gastric neoplasia. Prognosis following surgery is also poor because of the high rate of recurrent and metastatic lesions.

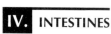

IV. INTESTINES

A. Anatomy

1. **Vascularization**
   a. **Arteries**
      (1) The **small intestine** is vascularized by **branches of the cranial mesenteric artery.** Most of the small intestinal blood supply is **arcuate** with short vasa recta.
      (2) The **large intestine** is vascularized primarily by **branches of the cranial and caudal mesenteric arteries.**
      (3) The blood supply to the **colon** is **segmental.**
   b. **Veins.** Blood from the intestines empties into **branches of the portal vein.**
   c. **Lymphatics.** Lymph is collected primarily by the **mesenteric lymph nodes,** with some drainage into the **hepatic and colic lymph nodes.**

2. **Innervation.** Autonomic innervation is received from the **cranial and caudal mesenteric plexuses.**

B. Surgical procedures

1. **General considerations**
   a. **Preoperative considerations**
      (1) Intravenous fluid therapy and correction of acid–base and electrolyte imbalances may be necessary before surgery.
      (2) Mechanical emptying of the colon before surgery is controversial and in some situations (e.g., perforations, trauma, emergencies) it may be contraindicated.
   b. **Contamination**
      (1) **Prophylactic antibiotics** are used if contamination or complications are expected and are continued as necessary in compromised patients. Animals can be treated preoperatively with oral medications (e.g., metronidazole, neomycin) or intravenously at induction with cephalosporins, ampicillin, metronidazole, gentamicin, or various combinations of these drugs to provide broad-spectrum coverage.

    (2) Gloves and **instruments should be changed** after closure of the intestines is complete to decrease contamination.

  c. Wound closure. The submucosa is the main holding layer of the gastrointestinal tract.

    (1) Small intestine

      (a) Appositional closure of incisions with synthetic monofilament absorbable or nonabsorbable sutures in a simple interrupted pattern **is preferred over crushing, inverting,** or **everting techniques.**

        (i) Crushing suture patterns result in more microhemorrhage, tissue necrosis, tissue eversion or overlap, and inflammatory response than approximating techniques.

        (ii) Mucosal eversion delays healing because of increased necrosis and ischemia and prolonged inflammation; eversion also promotes adhesion formation and reduces early bursting and tensile strength. Prolonged inflammation from mucosal eversion narrows the intestinal lumen.

        (iii) Inversion decreases the intestinal lumen diameter by approximately 65% and compromises blood supply, resulting in edema, necrosis, and delayed mucosal healing.

      (b) Staplers have been used for end-to-end intestinal anastomosis. No long-term complications are reported, but early postoperative complications include leakage and abscess formation.

    (2) Large intestine. End-to-end anastomotic staplers have been used successfully and result in less tissue reaction and greater strength than suture closures.

    (3) Omental coverage (i.e., suturing the omentum over the incision) or **serosal patch grafting** (i.e., suturing of affected intestine to normal intestine) can provide added protection to intestinal incisions.

  d. Wound healing

    (1) Small intestine

      (a) Sutures provide the main wound support for the first 3–4 days following small intestinal surgery; by 10–17 days after surgery, the incision site in the small intestines is rapidly approaching its normal bursting strength. With accurate apposition, mucosal reepithelialization occurs within 3 days.

      (b) The risk of **dehiscence** following small intestinal surgery is greatest after surgery for foreign bodies and traumatic injuries, especially penetrating trauma. Dehiscence is more common if peritonitis is present or if the band neutrophil count is elevated 4–6 days after surgery.

    (2) Large intestine. Colonic **healing is delayed** compared to the rest of the gastrointestinal tract, and **dehiscence is more likely.**

      (a) Collagen lysis exceeds synthesis for 3–4 days after surgery and increases the risk of dehiscence.

      (b) The segmental blood supply, mechanical stress from solid feces, and high bacterial content (primarily anaerobic gram-negative rods) result in higher morbidity and mortality rates.

      (c) Careful aseptic technique, proper suture tension, and judicious use of prophylactic antibiotics reduce the likelihood of dehiscence.

  e. Complications of intestinal surgery include dehiscence, peritonitis, adhesions secondary to ischemia or inflammation, ileus, stricture, and maldigestion/malabsorption secondary to extensive bowel resection (short-bowel syndrome).

2. Intestinal resection and anastomosis is performed to remove diseased segments of bowel associated with trauma, neoplasia, intussusception, volvulus, or infiltrative disorders.

  a. A **midline abdominal approach** is used for most small and large bowel resections. It permits examination of all the abdominal viscera and is therefore especially important in cases involving neoplasia, sepsis, or trauma.

    (1) Approach. A midline ventral abdominal incision is made, and the affected bowel segment is isolated. Mesenteric arteries supplying the area to be re-

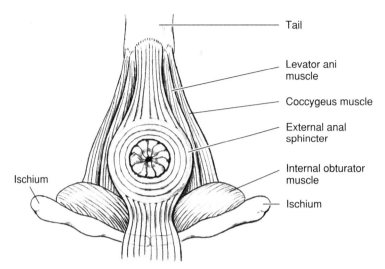

FIGURE 10–3. Perineal muscles that form the pelvic diaphragm.

sected are ligated, and the intestinal contents are "milked" proximally and distally away from the site.

(2) Resection. Crushing clamps are placed on the tissue to be resected, and noncrushing clamps are placed on viable intestinal segments. To correct for luminal disparity after intestinal resection, the narrower segment is cut at an angle or incised longitudinally along the antimesenteric border before intestinal anastomosis.

(3) Anastomosis. Following resection, a full-thickness simple interrupted appositional suture pattern is used to anastomose the two ends. An end-to-end anastomosis can also be rapidly performed using a gastrointestinal autostapler.

b. A **dorsal rectal approach** (i.e., through the perineum) is infrequently used to gain access to the rectum. The rectococcygeal muscle is incised, and the levator ani and external oral sphincter muscles (Figure 10–3) are separated.

c. A **rectal pull-through approach** is used for anastomosis of colonic segments within the pelvic canal. The procedure requires an abdominal approach to isolate and resect the affected colonic segment, and a per rectal approach to evert and anastomose the remaining colonic segments. An **ischiopubic osteotomy** may be required to gain access to the affected intrapelvic segments.

3. Typhlectomy is performed to remove the cecum in cases of neoplasia, impaction, or inversion.

a. Following isolation of the cecum and ligation of the cecal vessels, the base of the cecum is double-clamped with noncrushing intestinal forceps.

b. The cecum is resected between the two clamps, and the remaining stump is oversewn with synthetic absorbable or nonabsorbable suture in an inverting pattern. Typhlectomy can also be performed using a gastrointestinal or thoracic autostapler.

4. Enterotomy/colotomy is often indicated for the removal of obstructive foreign bodies.

a. The affected segment of the bowel is isolated and the intestinal contents are milked away proximally and distally.

b. A linear incision is made in viable tissue on the antimesenteric border of the bowel.

c. The small intestine can be closed using a single-layer simple interrupted appositional suture pattern. For colonic incisions, a second reinforcing row of inverting sutures can be placed in the seromuscular tissues.

5. Colectomy is performed primarily for relief of constipation associated with idiopathic megacolon in cats. Following a ventral midline celiotomy, the ileum and colon are isolated and mesenteric vessels are identified and ligated.

  a. Subtotal colectomy

   (1) Technique. The colon is resected distal to the ileocolic valve and an end-to-end colocolic anastomosis is performed using an intestinal stapler or full-thickness simple interrupted appositional sutures.

   (2) Complications include recurrence, constipation, stricture, dehiscence, and infection. With the exception of recurrence of clinical signs, complications are seen in less than 3% of cats.

   (a) Constipation is the most frequent postoperative complication and in most cases can be managed successfully with medical or dietary therapy.

   (b) Postoperatively, cats may have tenesmus and tarry feces for 3 months.

  b. Total colectomy

   (1) Technique. The colon, cecum, and ileocolic valve are resected and an end-to-end ileocolic anastomosis is performed.

   (2) Complications. As a result of small bowel bacterial overgrowth, **diarrhea** and **weight loss** may occur. Cats may have occasional **hematochezia** or **perineal soiling.** Bowel adaptation (i.e., by increasing villus and enterocyte height and density) occurs within 24 weeks to improve ileal water absorption.

C. **Conditions treated by surgery**

 1. Intestinal obstruction can be caused by foreign bodies, masses (e.g., neoplasia, granulomas, abscesses), intussusception, strangulation, and herniation.

  a. Clinical signs depend on the site and severity of the obstruction and the effect of the obstruction on intestinal blood supply (Table 10–3). Animals with untreated complete distal intestinal obstruction survive longer than those with complete proximal intestinal obstruction (i.e., 5–7 days versus 3–4 days).

  b. Diagnosis is by abdominal palpation, radiography, or exploratory laparotomy.

   (1) Survey radiographs may show radiopaque foreign bodies or gas distention proximal to the obstruction.

   (2) Contrast studies may indicate the site of obstruction (Figure 10–4). Contrast studies should not be performed if a perforation is suspected or if the diagnosis can be made with survey films or on the basis of patient history or physical examination.

  c. Treatment

   (1) Exploratory laparotomy provides a definitive diagnosis of the obstruction and permits treatment.

   (a) Foreign bodies are removed by **enterotomy.**

TABLE 10–3. Clinical Signs of Intestinal Obstruction

Type of Obstruction	Clinical Signs
Complete obstruction	
Proximal to bile and pancreatic duct openings	Acute vomiting, dehydration, hypokalemia, metabolic alkalosis
Distal to bile and pancreatic duct openings	Metabolic acidosis, gas and fluid distention of the intestines, endotoxemia
Partial obstruction	Chronic weight loss and diarrhea (from bacterial overgrowth and maldigestion or malabsorption)
Strangulating obstruction	Hemorrhagic and endotoxemic shock (from venous obstruction), peritonitis and intestinal perforation (from arterial obstruction)
Colonic obstruction	Anorexia

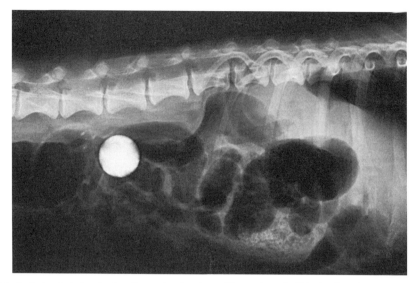

FIGURE 10–4. Lateral abdominal radiograph of a dog with a rubber ball lodged in the jejunum. Dilated bowel loops are located proximal to the obstruction. Colonic distention occurred secondary to an enema.

          (b) Neoplasia and vascular compromise are treated by **resection and anastomosis.**
      (2) Early oral or enteral alimentation after surgery is important to prevent villous atrophy and encourage resolution of ileus. In anorectic dogs, intraoperative placement of a jejunostomy tube allows nutritional support.
    d. Prognosis. Strangulation obstruction carries a grave prognosis, but acute or partial obstructions that do not cause severe systemic changes have a more favorable prognosis.
  2. Intussusception is the inversion of one segment of the intestines (intussusceptum) into another (intussuscipiens). It is most often seen in the ileocolic region of young dogs.
    a. Etiology. Intussusceptions may be associated with intestinal parasitism, foreign bodies, enteritis, or abdominal surgery.
    b. Clinical signs. The clinical course is rapid in high (proximal) intestinal intussusception and may be prolonged in low intussusception.
      (1) Vomiting is frequent in high intestinal intussusception and infrequent in low intussusception. Abdominal pain, bloody mucoid diarrhea, and a palpable abdominal mass are also noted.
      (2) Hematochezia, anorexia, intestinal prolapse through the rectum, and tenesmus may occur with low intussusceptions.
    c. Diagnosis is based on clinical signs, abdominal palpation, radiography, and ultrasonography.
      (1) A soft tissue mass and gas- and fluid-distended bowel loops proximal to the obstruction may be seen on survey radiographs.
      (2) Contrast upper gastrointestinal studies may delineate the intussusception; however, ileus may prevent contrast material from reaching the site.
      (3) Barium enemas are used to diagnose enterocolic and cecocolic intussusceptions.
    d. Treatment
      (1) Reduction of the intussusception may be attempted if the vascular supply and intestines are not compromised. Otherwise, **resection and anastomosis** is performed.
      (2) Alternatively, **enteroplication** may also be performed. The small intestine, from the duodenocolic ligament to the ileum, is folded back and forth in gentle loops, and adjacent walls are sutured to each other.

(3) For **cecal inversion,** the typhlectomy site may be oversewn or closed with a stapler.
  e. Complications
    (1) **Recurrence** occurs in approximately 20% of animals treated and is usually seen within 3 days of surgery. Enteroplication may reduce recurrence rates.
    (2) **Adhesions.** Cats develop adhesions at the intussusception site more frequently than dogs.
    (3) **Dehiscence** after intestinal anastomosis for intussusceptions occasionally occurs.

3. Linear foreign body is a common condition in cats in which continued peristalsis over a fixed linear foreign body results in plication, obstruction, erosion, and vascular compromise of the intestines.
  a. Clinical signs include vomiting, depression, anorexia, abdominal pain, and a palpable abdominal mass. In many cases, the linear foreign body is fixed around the base of the tongue, but it may be difficult to see because it embeds into the tissue.
  b. Diagnosis. Abnormal gas and fluid patterns, intestinal plication, and filling defects are seen on radiographic contrast studies.
  c. Treatment
    (1) **Conservative therapy** involves cutting the string from around the tongue and letting it pass through the intestines.
    (2) **Surgical therapy** involves cutting the string from around the tongue and removing it from the intestines through an **enterotomy.**
      (a) **Indications for surgery** include peritonitis, severe clinical signs, septicemia, persistence or progression of clinical signs following conservative treatment, and lack of movement of radiopaque foreign bodies on serial radiographs.
      (b) **Techniques**
        (i) **Single enterotomy.** The string may be removed via a single enterotomy by sewing the foreign body to a red rubber catheter and milking the catheter through the intestines so that it can be retrieved by an assistant at the anus.
        (ii) **Multiple enterotomies** are frequently needed to remove the string lodged in the mesenteric side of the intestinal wall in order to avoid further laceration of the intestines.
  d. Prognosis. Conservative therapy does not adversely affect outcome if animals are watched closely; 25% of cats with linear foreign bodies can be treated conservatively without complications.

4. Mesenteric volvulus results from excessive rotation of the small intestine along its mesenteric axis, causing vascular compromise, tissue ischemia, luminal obstruction, hypovolemic and endotoxic shock, and death.
  a. Predisposing factors
    (1) German shepherds are predisposed to this condition.
    (2) Other associated factors include vigorous exercise, recent surgery, trauma, pancreatic exocrine insufficiency, enteritis, dietary indiscretion, concurrent gastric dilation/volvulus, intestinal masses, or obstruction. Most animals have a previous history of gastrointestinal disorders, with up to 50% having a prior bout of gastric dilation.
  b. Clinical signs include peracute to acute onset of vomiting or retching, hematochezia, abdominal distention, abdominal pain, shock, or death.
  c. Diagnosis
    (1) **Physical examination** reveals gaseous abdominal distention that is not relieved by passage of a stomach tube.
    (2) **Radiographs** confirm gaseous distention of the small intestines; the stomach and distal colon are usually not affected.
    (3) **Blood work** may reveal hypoproteinemia, hypoalbuminemia, hypokalemia, and abnormal white blood cell count.

    d. Treatment. Mesenteric volvulus is a serious surgical emergency that requires **detorsion** of the intestines; treatment should not be delayed by diagnostics.

    e. Prognosis. The mortality rate is 95%–100%. Dogs that survive this condition are usually surgically treated within 30 minutes of the occurrence of the torsion.

5. Cecal–colic volvulus is a rare condition that occurs when the cecum, ascending colon, and transverse colon rotate around the cranial mesenteric root.

    a. Clinical signs include depression, abdominal distention, tenesmus, diarrhea, and vomiting. Animals may be dehydrated or in shock.

    b. Diagnosis. Radiographs reveal gas-distended bowel loops, suggesting intestinal obstruction.

    c. Treatment. Emergency celiotomy is performed to permit derotation and decompression of affected bowel.

    d. Prognosis depends on the severity of vascular compromise, which may be related to the degree of volvulus. Animals may die from large bowel ischemia, peritonitis, or DIC.

6. Neoplasia (e.g., **adenocarcinoma, lymphoma, lymphosarcoma, leiomyosarcoma, adenomatous polyps, colorectal leiomyoma**) most commonly involves the rectum and colon in dogs and the small intestines in cats. Of nonlymphoid intestinal neoplasia, 88% of tumors in dogs and 100% in cats are malignant.

    a. Clinical signs include weight loss, vomiting, anorexia, and depression. Acute collapse secondary to hemorrhage and hypovolemic shock has been reported. Patients with colorectal tumors may present with hematochezia, tenesmus, dyschezia, and intermittent anal eversion or rectal prolapse.

    b. Diagnosis is by digital rectal or abdominal palpation, survey films, gaseous distention contrast studies, ultrasonography, endoscopy or colonoscopy, and exploratory laparotomy and biopsy.

    c. Treatment

        (1) Adenocarcinoma, lymphoma, and **leiomyosarcoma** are treated by **surgical resection** via a midline abdominal, dorsal rectal, or rectal pull-through approach.

        (2) Lymphosarcoma should be treated with chemotherapy unless obstruction or perforation is present.

        (3) Adenomatous polyps that are palpable on a digital rectal exam may be viewed by prolapsing the rectum out of the anus and are removed by **surgical excision, electrocautery,** or **cryosurgery.** Duodenal polyps are removed by complete excision of the base of the mass and surrounding mucosa.

        (4) Colorectal leiomyomas, benign tumors of the smooth muscle, are removed by **blunt dissection** from the colorectal wall. Intestinal resection and anastomosis are unnecessary.

    d. Complications. Dehiscence occurs after intestinal anastomoses for neoplastic resection in 11.8% of animals treated.

7. Idiopathic megacolon is reported primarily in adult cats (average age, 5 years) that have colonic distention but no evidence of functional or mechanical obstruction.

    a. Clinical signs include chronic or recurrent constipation. Vomiting, anorexia, and weight loss are also reported.

    b. Diagnosis is based on the persistence of constipation despite appropriate medical treatment.

        (1) Digital rectal exam, abdominal palpation, and plain abdominal films demonstrate colonic enlargement.

        (2) Other causes of constipation such as anorectal disease, pelvic trauma, neoplasia, stricture, foreign body, neurologic dysfunction, endocrine dysfunction (e.g., hypothyroidism), metabolic disorders (e.g., dehydration), and drugs should be ruled out.

    c. Treatment

        (1) A **conservative approach** (e.g., laxatives, diet change, enemas) may be taken initially.

        (2) Nonresponsive patients should undergo **colectomy** or **subtotal colectomy.** Cats that have undergone a subtotal colectomy defecate more frequently, but they do not suffer as much diarrhea and weight loss as cats that have undergone total colectomies do.

    d. Prognosis. Surgery results in complete resolution of signs in 64% of animals treated and decreased frequency of signs in 18% of animals treated.

8. Peritonitis is a diffuse inflammation of the peritoneal cavity caused by hematogenous infection, chemical irritation, or septic contamination.

    a. Etiology. The most common cause of peritonitis is surgical dehiscence; other causes include trauma, abscesses, foreign body perforation of the gastrointestinal tract, and gastrointestinal neoplasia.

    b. Clinical signs include depression, anorexia, vomiting, abdominal pain, unusual posturing, abdominal distention, and signs of sepsis or shock (e.g., pale or hyperemic mucous membranes, prolonged capillary refill time, tachycardia, weakness, collapse, dehydration, pyrexia, hypothermia).

    c. Diagnosis

        (1) Survey films reveal loss of detail, a "ground glass" appearance, gas-distended intestines, and free gas.

        (2) Abdominocentesis. Toxic degeneration of neutrophils with extracellular and intracellular bacteria indicates septic peritonitis.

        (3) A **complete blood count** may reveal neutrophilia, increases in the number of immature neutrophils, and anemia.

    d. Treatment includes intravenous fluids and antibiotics followed by exploratory laparotomy, abdominal culture, and drainage. Open peritoneal drainage results in faster and more complete drainage than use of a sump-Penrose drain, which is rapidly encapsulated by the omentum.

        (1) After correction of the primary problem and extensive abdominal lavage, the rectus sheath is sutured loosely with monofilament nonabsorbable suture, leaving a 3–4-centimeter gap between the edges of the rectus sheath.

        (2) The skin and subcutaneous tissue are left open, and sterile bandages are placed over the incision.

        (3) Bandages are changed at least every 24 hours to prevent strike-through of abdominal fluid.

        (4) Most incisions can be closed after 3–5 days of open peritoneal drainage; closure is performed when the quantity of fluid decreases, the quality of fluid changes to sanguineous or serosanguineous, and cells become more normal in appearance. Most abdomens have positive bacterial cultures at the time of closure.

    e. Complications of open peritoneal drainage include partial omental occlusion of the incision, omental herniation, hypoproteinemia, anemia, electrolyte changes, dehydration, and nosocomial infection.

        (1) Postoperatively, patients frequently are hypotensive and tachycardic. Pancreatitis, peripheral edema, and DIC may develop.

        (2) Hypoalbuminemia will develop after surgical treatment of peritonitis, regardless of the technique used.

    f. Prognosis

        (1) Peritonitis has a poor prognosis if the following occur: refractory hypotension, cardiovascular collapse, DIC, or the development of respiratory diseases (e.g., pneumonia, pleural effusion).

        (2) The mortality rate is 33%–48% with open abdominal drainage and 68% without abdominal drainage. The incidence of mortality is highest when the large intestine is the source of contamination.

9. Short-bowel syndrome may occur after resection of 70% or more of the small intestine. The syndrome is diagnosed when nutritional, medical, or surgical therapy is required to control diarrhea and maintain body weight after intestinal resection.

    a. Clinical signs include diarrhea and weight loss.

    b. Diagnosis. Contrast radiographs are used to estimate the length of the bowel; radiographic magnification falsely increases bowel length by 10%–25%. Normal bowel length is approximately five times the length of the trunk.

     c. Treatment. Surgery has been used to slow intestinal transit time or increase the absorptive surface area. Because of limited success, surgery should be attempted only if medical and dietary therapy fail. Techniques include the following:

       (1) Formation of antiperistaltic segments by transposing a reverse segment of bowel

       (2) Formation of valves by intussuscepting a portion of bowel

       (3) Formation of recirculating loops by creating a side-to-side jejunal anastomosis

       (4) Colonic transposition (i.e., interposing a segment of colon in the small intestinal tract)

       (5) Intestinal transplantation

V. RECTUM AND ANUS

A. Anatomy

1. Vasculature

    a. Arteries

      (1) The **intra-abdominal portion of the rectum** is supplied by the **cranial rectal branch of the caudal mesenteric artery.**

      (2) The **retroperitoneal portion and anus** are supplied by the **middle** and **caudal rectal branches** of the **internal pudendal artery.**

    b. Veins. The **cranial rectal vein** drains into the portal vein, while the **caudal rectal vein** drains into the caudal vena cava.

    c. Lymphatic drainage is primarily into the **medial iliac lymph nodes.**

2. Innervation

    a. The **rectum** is innervated by parasympathetic fibers from the **pelvic nerves** and sympathetic fibers from the **hypogastric nerves.**

    b. Anus. The **caudal rectal nerve** and **perineal branches of the pudendal nerve** provide motor and sensory innervation, respectively, to the external anal sphincter.

B. Surgical procedures

1. General considerations

    a. Diagnostic tools. Digital rectal examination, proctoscopy, and barium enemas are useful for diagnostic purposes.

    b. Patient preparation for anorectal or perineal surgery is controversial.

      (1) Generally, enemas are not given within 12 hours of surgery.

      (2) Food may be withheld for 24–72 hours before surgery and prophylactic antibiotics are frequently administered.

      (3) Rectal packing with gauze and purse-string suture closure of the anus are used to decrease contamination in perineal surgeries.

    c. Surgical approaches

      (1) The **distal third of the rectum** may be approached caudally by a rectal pull-through approach or anoplasty.

      (2) The **middle third of the rectum** may be approached by a dorsal perineal incision.

      (3) The **cranial third of the rectum** is approached through a caudal abdominal incision; pubic osteotomy may be necessary to improve exposure.

    d. Wound closure. Rectal incisions are closed with a single layer of simple interrupted appositional sutures using synthetic, monofilament material. Closure with the end-to-end anastomotic stapler results in fewer leaks than manual anastomosis.

    e. Complications of anal and rectal surgery include incontinence secondary to damage of the caudal rectal nerve or anal sphincter, hemorrhage, infection, tenesmus, stricture, and dehiscence.

      (1) Incontinence is seen in 40% of dogs after rectal resection. Resection of 6 centimeters or more of rectum will result in incontinence because of loss of reservoir function.

    (2) Leakage and abscess formation are common with the rectal pull-through approach.

  2. Rectal amputation is performed to resect necrotic, prolapsed segments of the rectum.

    a. The animal is placed in sternal recumbency in the perineal position and a lubricated syringe case is placed in the rectum.

    b. Four full-thickness stay sutures are placed circumferentially around the prolapsed tissue and 180 of the rectum is resected.

    c. Simple interrupted appositional sutures are used to close the cut tissue layers, and the other half of the rectum is amputated and closed in a similar fashion. The rectum is then gently pushed into the pelvic canal.

  3. Anal sacculectomy

    a. Anatomy. The anal sacs are located at approximately the 4 and 8 o'clock positions around the anus. The ducts open at the mucocutaneous junction in dogs and a few millimeters lateral to the junction in cats.

    b. Technique

      (1) Open technique. A groove director or scissor blade is inserted into the duct, and an incision is made through the caudal wall of the anal sac and duct and the overlying tissues. The sac and duct are removed with blunt dissection, and the wound is closed or left to heal by second intention.

      (2) Closed technique. To facilitate removal using a closed technique, the sac may be packed with string, melted wax, plaster, latex, or acrylic.

    c. Complications of anal sacculectomy include:

      (1) Draining sinuses, fistulae, and persistent infection from incomplete surgical resection

      (2) Incontinence from caudal rectal nerve damage

      (3) Intraoperative hemorrhage

      (4) Postoperative tenesmus and dyschezia from inflammation, stricture, or scar formation

C. **Conditions treated by surgery**

  1. Congenital abnormalities (e.g., **atresia ani**)

    a. Types

      (1) In type 1 atresia, the anus is strictured.

      (2) In type 2 atresia, the anus is imperforate.

      (3) In type 3 atresia, the rectum is discontinuous with an imperforate anus.

      (4) In type 4 atresia, the cranial rectum is discontinuous with a normal terminal rectum or anus.

    b. Clinical signs include progressive unthriftiness, abdominal enlargement, tenesmus, and lack of feces. Feces may pass through the vaginal cleft if a rectovaginal fistula is also present.

    c. Diagnosis is by physical examination and radiography.

    d. Treatment is based on the type of defect.

      (1) Type 1 atresia may be treated by bougienage, resection of the skin overlying the anus, or removal of stenotic tissue.

      (2) Types 2 and 3 atresia. The anus is incised over the anal dimple and a rectal pull-through is performed.

      (3) Type 4 atresia may necessitate an abdominal approach and rectal anastomosis.

      (4) Rectovaginal fistulae must be ligated and transected.

    e. Prognosis. Because of prolonged megacolon or associated developmental defects, animals may be incontinent even with surgical reconstruction.

  2. Rectal prolapse occurs most frequently in young, heavily parasite-infested animals with diarrhea and tenesmus; however, it can be associated with rectal polyps, neoplasia, foreign bodies, urolithiasis, dystocia, constipation, congenital defects, prostatic disease, and perineal hernia repair. In cats, rectal prolapse can be extensive, including all of the rectum and part of the colon.

    a. Diagnosis. The inability to pass a blunt probe between the rectal wall and prolapsed tissue differentiates rectal prolapse from prolapsed intussusception.

    b. Treatment. Along with surgical management of the prolapse, the primary cause of tenesmus should be identified and treated.

       (1) Reducible prolapse can be treated with an anocutaneous purse-string suture tied loosely enough to allow passage of soft stools. Purse-string sutures can normally be removed in 4–5 days.

       (2) Necrotic, friable, severely edematous prolapses should be treated by **amputation** and **rectal anastomosis.** Recurrence can be treated with purse-string suture and tranquilization, amputation, or colopexy.

       (3) Extensive prolapse requires **abdominal colopexy.**

3. Rectal perforations

    a. Etiology. Rectal perforations may occur secondary to penetrating foreign bodies or pelvic fractures.

       (1) Rectal perforations from pelvic fractures are caused by lacerations from bone fragments, rectal avulsion, or forcible compression.

       (2) Perforations associated with pelvic fractures are usually located within 4 centimeters of the anus, where the rectum is fixed and less distensible.

    b. Clinical signs related to the perforation may be obscured by the effects of the originating trauma. Eventually, animals develop signs of septicemia, shock, and DIC.

    c. Diagnosis

       (1) Perforations from pelvic fractures are digitally palpable per rectum in 75% of dogs.

       (2) Fresh blood in the rectum is noted in 50% of cases.

       (3) Free gas in the abdomen or gas within perirectal soft tissues may be noted on abdominal radiographs.

    d. Treatment is immediate exploratory surgery and closure of the perforation via an abdominal, perineal, or anal approach.

    e. Prognosis. Prognosis is grave when diagnosis and treatment are delayed or when septicemia or DIC is present.

4. Anal sacculitis is inflammation of the anal sacs, resulting in impaction, infection, or abscessation and rupture of the sac.

    a. Predisposing factors. Anal sacculitis is frequently reported in toy and miniature poodles, Chihuahuas, and German shepherds. Predisposing factors may include improper diet, soft stools, lack of exercise, and perianal fistulae.

    b. Clinical signs include tail-biting, excessive grooming, "scooting," tenesmus, diarrhea, behavioral changes, and pain.

    c. Diagnosis is by digital rectal examination.

       (1) Anal sac material is examined after gentle manual expression. Impacted material is thick, dark, and pasty; infected or abscessed anal sacs produce malodorous, purulent secretions.

       (2) Ventrolateral draining tracts may be present if the sacs have ruptured.

    d. Treatment depends on the severity of the disease.

       (1) Conservative treatment includes frequent anal sac expression, gentle irrigation, and infusion of antibiotic ointment.

       (2) Surgical treatment

         (a) Recurrent disease should be treated with **anal sacculectomy** and **open drainage** or **primary wound closure.**

         (b) Anal sac rupture associated with cellulitis is treated with systemic antibiotics, open drainage, and lavage; surgery is performed once acute inflammation has subsided.

5. Perianal fistulae are multiple, ulcerated sinus tracts in the perineal region associated with inflammation, fibrosis, and drainage.

    a. Predisposing factors. German shepherds and Irish setters may be predisposed to this condition. Affected animals are usually middle-aged, intact, and male.

    b. Clinical signs are related to pain and inflammation; tenesmus, dyschezia, hemorrhage, malodorous discharge, and excessive grooming may be seen.

    c. Diagnosis is by physical examination and digital rectal palpation.

d. Treatment
   (1) Conservative therapy (i.e., antibiotics, antiseptic irrigation, tail braces) provides only temporary relief.
   (2) Nonconservative options include:
      (a) Surgical excision and open drainage
      (b) Cryosurgery
      (c) Chemical cauterization using 75% silver nitrate, 80% liquefied phenol, or 10% Lugol's solution
      (d) Deroofing and fulguration (i.e., incising the tract and destroying the lining with a high-frequency current)
      (e) Excision of fistulae using laser therapy [neodymium:yttrium aluminum garnet (ND:YAG)]
      (f) Anal sacculectomy
      (g) Tail amputation
      (h) Partial or complete excision of the anus and sphincter (in severe cases)
e. Complications of nonconservative therapy include recurrence, anal stenosis, flatulence, tenesmus, diarrhea, stricture, and fecal incontinence.
   (1) Cryosurgery relies on tissue necrosis and sloughing, and results in swelling, malodorous discharge, and increased risk of anal stenosis.
   (2) Radical resection allows rapid healing (as compared to cryosurgery and deroofing and fulguration) but carries a greater risk of incontinence.
   (3) Deroofing and fulguration carries a high risk of recurrence; therefore, this technique should not be used in cases where more than half of the anus circumference is affected.
   (4) Laser therapy is effective for relieving pain, but may cause fecal incontinence.
f. Prognosis. Successful outcomes are reported in 48%–97% of cases. Prognosis depends on the severity of the disease and the type of treatment used.

6. **Neoplasia** (e.g., **perianal adenomas, rectal or anal adenocarcinoma, anal sac adenocarcinoma**). Perianal neoplasia is more common in male dogs than females, except for anal sac adenocarcinoma. In male dogs, 80% of perianal tumors are benign adenomas.
   a. Perianal adenomas usually occur in intact males in the perineal region; they may also occur on the prepuce or tailhead.
      (1) Clinical signs include an enlarging mass that may be ulcerated.
      (2) Treatment
         (a) In some cases, **castration** alone may result in remission and cure.
         (b) Adenomas are also responsive to **cryosurgery** or **surgical excision.**
         (c) Radiation is effective but is more expensive, takes longer, and entails a greater risk of morbidity.
      (3) Prognosis is excellent, and recurrence is less than 10% with complete excision and castration.
   b. Rectal or anal adenocarcinoma is the most common malignant tumor type of the perianal region. Tumors may be **infiltrative, ulcerative,** or **pedunculated.**
      (1) Clinical signs include dyschezia, hematochezia, diarrhea, obstipation, tenesmus, and pain. Circumferential infiltrative adenocarcinoma may result in a "napkin ring" stricture of the affected area.
      (2) Treatment is discussed in IV C 6 c (1).
   c. Anal sac adenocarcinoma is seen most frequently in female dogs.
      (1) Clinical signs. Up to 90% of females have paraneoplastic syndrome (i.e., hypercalcemia and renal failure); hypercalcemia is very rare in males.
      (2) Treatment is **aggressive surgical resection.** Because of rapid metastasis, females should also undergo abdominal exploration to evaluate the medial iliac lymph nodes; **lymphadenectomy** should be performed if necessary.
      (3) Prognosis is very poor in females, particularly if they are hypercalcemic; death usually results from hypercalcemia or local disease.

7. **Perineal hernia**
   a. Predisposing factors
      (1) Male dogs and cats are predisposed to rectal sacculation or deviation result-

ing from failure of the pelvic diaphragm (i.e., the levator ani and coccygeus muscles; see Figure 10–3).

(2) Prior perineal urethrostomy is associated with an increased risk of perineal hernia in cats.

b. **Clinical signs** include perineal swelling, constipation, tenesmus, dyschezia, and diarrhea. Swelling and herniation are present bilaterally in 95% of cats. Bladder retroflexion occurs in up to 20% of dogs and results in stranguria or anuria.

c. **Diagnosis** is by digital rectal examination. Perineal centesis with creatinine analysis of fluid may confirm bladder entrapment.

d. **Treatment**

(1) **Medical treatment** (i.e, dietary therapy, enemas) is successful in 15% of treated cats.

(2) **Surgical treatment** involves **reconstruction of the pelvic diaphragm** with suture, muscle, or prosthetic implants. Fixation of the deferent ducts and colopexy have been used to treat retroflexion of the bladder and rectal sacculation, respectively.

e. **Complications** include recurrence, infection, tenesmus, fecal incontinence, sciatic nerve damage, rectal prolapse, hemorrhage, iatrogenic urethral injury, rectal or anal sac fistulae, urinary bladder necrosis, and transient or persistent cystic atony or urinary incontinence.

8. **Fecal incontinence** is the inability to retain feces.

a. **Types**

(1) **Reservoir incontinence** involves the colon or rectum; defecations are conscious and frequent.

(2) **Sphincter incontinence** involves the anus or nervous system; defecations are involuntary.

b. **Diagnosis and therapy** should focus on localizing and treating the primary lesion.

(1) **Diagnostic tools** include neurologic examination, colonoscopy, radiography, and electromyography.

(2) **Treatment.** Symptomatic surgical treatments include fascial slings and silicone elastomer sling implants.

SELECTED READINGS

Bojrab MJ: *Disease Mechanisms in Small Animal Surgery,* 2nd ed. Philadelphia, Lea & Febiger, 1993, pp 187–291.

Bone DL: Surgical correction of canine perineal disorders. *Vet Med* 87:127–138, 1992.

Ellison GW, Bellah JR, Stubbs WP: Treatment of perianal fistulas with ND:YAG laser—results in 20 cases. *Vet Surg* 24:140–147, 1995.

Evans HE, Christensen GC: *Miller's Anatomy of the Dog,* 3rd ed. Philadelphia, WB Saunders, 1993, pp 385–462.

Evans KL, Smeak DD, Biller DS: Gastrointestinal linear foreign bodies in 32 dogs: a retrospective evaluation and feline comparison. *J Am Anim Hosp Assoc* 30:445–450, 1994.

Hosgood G: Gastric dilatation-volvulus in dogs. *J Am Vet Med Assoc* 204:1742–1747, 1994.

Klausner JS, Hardy RM: Alimentary tract, liver, and pancreas. In Lorenz MD, Cornelius LM: *Small Animal Medical Diagnosis,* 2nd ed. Philadelphia, JB Lippincott, 1993 pp 247–322.

Leib MS: Gastroenterology: the 1990s. *Vet Clin North Am* 23, 1993, pp 513–530, 547–554, 587–594, 609–624.

Matthiesen DT: Gastrointestinal system. In Slatter D (ed): *Textbook of Small Animal Surgery,* 2nd ed. Philadelphia, WB Saunders, 1993, pp 483–677.

Raffan PJ: A new surgical technique for repair of perineal hernias in the dog. *J Small Anim Pract* 34:13–19, 1993.

Sweet DV, Hardie EM, Stone EA: Preservation versus excision of the ileocolic junction during colectomy for megacolon: a study of 22 cats. *J Small Anim Pract* 35:358–363, 1994.

Wylie KB, Hosgood GH: Mortality and morbidity of small and large intestinal surgery in dogs and cats. *J Am Anim Hosp Assoc* 30:469–474, 1994.

Chapter 11

Hepatobiliary System

Karen Swalec Tobias

I. INTRODUCTION

A. Liver

1. Anatomy

  a. **Location.** The liver, which accounts for nearly 3.5% of the total body weight in dogs, is located below the diaphragm and cranial to the stomach.

  b. **Lobes and lobules**

   (1) The liver consists of **seven lobes:** the right lateral, right medial, left medial, left lateral, and quadrate lobes; and the caudate and papillary processes of the caudate lobe (Figure 11–1).

   (2) The liver is organized into hepatic **lobules,** each containing a **central vein** and **sinusoids. Bile canaliculi** are found between hepatocytes, which radiate in rows away from the central vein.

  c. **Vasculature.** Interlobular connective tissue contains **portal triads**—the interlobular bile duct and branches of the hepatic artery and portal vein—and lymphatics.

   (1) **Blood supply** is from the portal vein (80%) and hepatic artery (20%).

    (a) The portal vein, located at the dorsal boundary of the epiploic foramen, divides into seven branches to supply liver lobes.

    (b) Branches of hepatic arterioles and portal venules drain into hepatic sinusoids, where arterial and venous blood mixes.

   (2) **Drainage**

    (a) **Sinusoid blood** drains toward the central vein and is collected by interlobular veins, which eventually form hepatic veins that empty into the caudal vena cava.

    (b) **Lymph** is collected from interlobular vessels and drains into hepatic and splenic lymph nodes.

   (3) **Innervation** is by sympathetic fibers from splanchnic nerves, celiac ganglia, and the celiac plexus, and by vagal fibers.

2. Functions of the liver

  a. **Synthesis.** Products synthesized by the liver include **albumin; glycogen; glucose** from amino acids, glycogen, galactose, and fructose; **plasma proteins** and **amino acids; clotting factors; triglycerides** from excess carbohydrates and protein; **urea** from ammonia; and **ketone bodies.**

  b. **Secretion of bile.** Components of bile include bilirubin, electrolytes, cholesterol, bile salts synthesized from cholesterol (e.g., cholic acid, chenodeoxycholic acid), phospholipids, water, and various products of hepatic metabolism. Bile salts, the most abundant substances secreted in bile besides water, emulsify fat particles and aid in absorption of lipids.

  c. **Excretion of bilirubin.** The liver excretes bilirubin, an end product of hemoglobin decomposition.

  d. **Storage.** The liver stores vitamins A, D, K, and B_{12}; iron; lipids; and carbohydrates (in the form of glycogen).

  e. **Biotransformation.** Toxic substances, drugs, hormones, and metabolites are biotransformed by synthesis or conjugation reactions in the liver to alter toxicity, reduce activity, and facilitate elimination.

  f. **Metabolism.** Lipids, proteins, carbohydrates, vitamin D, and hemoglobin are metabolized in the liver. Bilirubin is conjugated to glucuronic acid before it is actively transported into bile.

  g. **Phagocytosis.** Reticuloendothelial cells lining sinusoids are phagocytic and bactericidal.

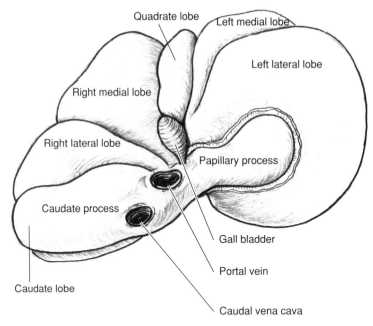

FIGURE 11–1. Visceral surface of a canine liver *in situ.*

B. **Gallbladder and biliary tree**

1. **Anatomy.** The **gallbladder,** a sac-like organ located between the quadrate and right medial liver lobes, collects and drains bile through the **cystic duct.**
   a. The **cystic duct** from the gallbladder is joined by **hepatic bile ducts** from the liver lobes to form the **common bile duct.**
   b. The terminal portion of the common bile duct runs intramurally in the proximal duodenal muscularis and **drains at the major duodenal papilla.** In cats, the duodenal entrance of the common bile duct is located close to that of the major pancreatic duct.
   c. **Vasculature.** The gallbladder is supplied by the **cystic artery,** a branch of the hepatic artery.
   d. **Innervation.** Parasympathetic innervation to the gallbladder is from vagal nerve fibers, and sympathetic innervation is from splanchnic nerves. Parasympathetic stimulation relaxes the sphincter and contracts the gallbladder; sympathetic stimulation produces the opposite effect.

2. **Functions of the gallbladder and biliary tree** include storage, concentration, and delivery of bile, which aids in fat digestion and absorption and acid neutralization in the small intestines.

II. **SURGICAL PROCEDURES**

A. **General considerations**

1. **Regenerative capacity of the liver.** Because the liver has tremendous regenerative capabilities, 70%–80% of its mass may be resected in healthy animals.
   a. **Regenerative hyperplasia** and **hepatic hypertrophy** result in restoration of 70% of the liver mass within 6 weeks of a 70% hepatectomy.

b. **Metabolic derangements.** Resection of 70% of the liver mass results in transient hypoglycemia for 3–6 hours, bilirubinemia for up to 1 week, and increases in alanine aminotransferase and alkaline phosphatase for up to 6 weeks. Other changes include increased glucagon level, hyperammonemia, hypoproteinemia, and hypoalbuminemia. Animals undergoing massive hepatectomies should receive intraoperative intravenous dextrose and should be monitored for early postoperative hypoglycemia.

2. **Maintenance of blood flow and bile excretion**
    a. **Hepatic artery ligation. Collateral circulation** and the portal vein provide adequate blood flow in many animals following ligation of the hepatic artery.
    b. **Hepatic duct ligation** results in atrophy of the affected lobe and hypertrophy of the remaining liver, or **rerouting of bile drainage** through an **auxiliary retroportal biliary network** to maintain bile excretion.
    c. **Portal vein ligation** results in death.

3. **Antibiotic therapy.** Antibiotics are frequently used prophylactically or therapeutically with hepatic and biliary surgeries.
    a. **Commonly encountered organisms**
        (1) *Clostridium* has been cultured from the livers of healthy dogs. Death from *Clostridium* proliferation leading to gangrenous hepatic necrosis frequently can be prevented by antibiotic administration.
        (2) *Escherichia coli, Streptococcus faecalis, Proteus,* and *Klebsiella* have been associated with biliary tract disease.
    b. **Antibiotic selection.** Hepatobiliary function and routes of antibiotic metabolism and excretion should be taken into consideration when selecting an antibiotic. Antibiotics commonly used for patients with hepatobiliary disease include **cephalosporins** and **chloramphenicol,** which reach high concentrations in the bile and liver, respectively.

4. **Blood pressure should be monitored** carefully during surgery because retraction of the liver frequently results in decreased caudal vena cava and portal flow.

5. **Hemorrhage** may be a serious complication of hepatic surgery.
    a. Fifty percent of animals with hepatobiliary disease have abnormal one-stage prothrombin time, and seventy percent have abnormal activated partial thromboplastin time. These indicators should be evaluated preoperatively.
    b. Vitamin K therapy with or without cryoprecipitate transfusion may be warranted.

B. **General surgical approach.** Surgery of the liver and biliary tract is performed through a cranial **ventral midline celiotomy.**

1. **Sternal splitting** and **diaphragmatic or right paracostal incision** may also be necessary.

2. **Resection of the triangular ligaments** facilitates exposure of the hepatic veins and the cranial portion of the hepatic parenchyma.

C. **Specific procedures**

1. **Liver**
    a. **Biopsy**
        (1) **Percutaneous biopsy.** Liver biopsies may be taken percutaneously via a **transthoracic or transabdominal approach** when diffuse disease (e.g., hepatic lipidosis) is suspected.
        (2) **Surgical biopsy.** To ensure accurate sampling and adequate hemostasis, surgical biopsies are performed via a **celiotomy.**
            (a) **Marginal lesions** can be biopsied with a **guillotine technique,** in which a suture loop is used to ligate the tip of a lobe, which is then excised (Figure 11–2). Alternatively, the liver can be sutured at the periphery to provide a triangular piece of tissue (see Figure 11–2).
            (b) **Central lesions** may be biopsied with a **wedge technique** or a **Keyes biopsy punch.** Hemostasis is achieved by pressure or by packing with absorbable gelatin foam.

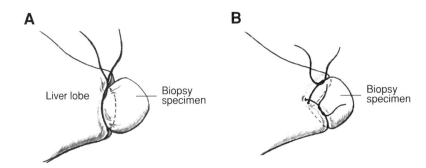

FIGURE 11–2. Liver biopsy techniques. *(A)* Guillotine technique. Suture material is placed around the liver proximal to the affected site. The suture is manually tightened to cut through (guillotine) the parenchyma and surround the vessels, thus ligating them. The sample is harvested following resection of the tissue distal to the ligature. *(B)* Suture technique. Hepatic parenchyma is ligated using nonabsorbable or synthetic absorbable suture material placed in a through-and-through simple interrupted pattern. In this technique, the parenchyma is crushed, not lacerated. The affected tissue is resected distal to the ligatures.

    b. Lobectomy
        (1) Techniques. Lobectomy can be performed by **mass ligation,** particularly in small animals, or by **stapling** with a thoracoabdominal stapler.
            (a) Mass ligation of the vascular and biliary pedicles with a crushing synthetic absorbable or nonabsorbable ligature results in less complete resection and more parenchymal hemorrhage, necrosis, inflammation, and postoperative adhesions than stapling, but it is less expensive.
                (i) Hepatic vein ligation results in hepatic congestion, ischemia, and necrosis, but usually is not fatal.
                (ii) Ligation of a branch of the portal vein to the affected lobe is not fatal.
            (b) Stapling takes less time and results in less inflammation, hemorrhage, and necrosis than ligation.
                (i) Resection of the triangular ligament is necessary to allow easier positioning of the stapler and to ensure adequate resection.
                (ii) Minor arterial hemorrhage may occur from the stump.
        (2) Considerations
            (a) Skeletalization of branches of the portal vein, hepatic vein, and **hepatic artery** (i.e., removal of hepatic parenchyma, leaving the vessels intact) may be necessary in large dogs or when removing the entire right or central portion of the liver.
            (b) Dissection of hepatic parenchyma from the caudal vena cava is necessary with right or central lobectomies.
  2. Biliary tract. Synthetic absorbable suture is used to close incisions in the gallbladder or bile duct.
    a. Cholecystotomy is performed to remove biliary calculi or to flush the gallbladder and common bile duct of inspissated or infected bile.
        (1) Approach. A cranial ventral midline celiotomy is performed and the gallbladder isolated. Stay sutures or Babcock forceps are used to stabilize the gallbladder while an incision is made into the lumen.
        (2) The **contents** of the gallbladder and duct are **removed,** submitted for histologic or microbiologic analysis, and the **tissues flushed** with saline. The **duct** can be **cannulated** to ensure patency.
        (3) Closure. The gallbladder incision is closed with absorbable suture in a continuous two-layer inverting pattern.
    b. Cholecystectomy is performed following gallbladder trauma, infection, or neoplasia.
        (1) Approach. A cranial ventral midline celiotomy is performed and the gallbladder isolated with moistened laparotomy sponges.
        (2) The **gallbladder is** gently **dissected away from the liver** using sterile cotton-

tipped applicators. Dissection should proceed distally to free the cystic duct as well.

(3) The cystic duct and artery are ligated and clamped and the **gallbladder is removed** following transection of the tissues between the clamps.

(4) Omental adhesions cover the exposed surfaces soon after the abdominal incision is closed.

c. **Tube cholecystostomy** is used to achieve biliary decompression.

(1) The gallbladder is mobilized and a Foley catheter is placed through the right ventrolateral body wall and the gallbladder fundus, and secured in the gallbladder with a purse-string suture. A cholecystopexy is performed to encourage adhesion and decrease the chance of bile leakage.

(2) Alternatively, the gallbladder is left in its hepatic fossa, and the catheter is inserted through several layers of omentum before entering the gallbladder. A cholecystopexy is unnecessary with this technique.

d. **Choledochotomy** is performed to remove an obstruction of the bile duct.

(1) Two stay sutures are used for traction, and a longitudinal incision is made in the duct to permit removal of the obstruction and flushing of the duct.

(2) The incision is closed with small-gauge absorbable sutures placed in a simple continuous or interrupted pattern.

e. **Cholecystoduodenostomy** (bile flow diversion) is performed to bypass bile duct injury or obstruction when the gallbladder is normal.

(1) The gallbladder is mobilized, and a 2.5–4 cm incision is made in the fundus and in the antimesenteric surface of the duodenum.

(2) A single-layer, full-thickness continuous closure is used to anastomose the gallbladder to the duodenum. Leakage is most likely to occur at the ends of the incisions.

III. CONDITIONS TREATED BY SURGERY

A. **Hepatic trauma.** Hepatic parenchymal fractures resulting from abdominal trauma are usually not a significant problem. However, substantial fractures may result in severe hemorrhage requiring emergency surgery.

1. **Diagnosis** is by clinical signs of hemorrhagic and hypovolemic shock, lack of response to fluid therapy, abdominocentesis, and exploratory laparotomy.

2. **Treatment. Digital inflow occlusion** of the portal vein and the hepatic artery ventral to the epiploic foramen may be necessary to slow hemorrhage until **vascular ligation** is accomplished. The duration of inflow occlusion should not exceed 10–15 minutes.

B. **Hepatic abscesses** are rare but may occur secondary to biliary tract disease, bacteremia, foreign bodies, or trauma. Predominant bacteria isolated include *Escherichia coli, Klebsiella, Proteus,* and *Enterobacter* species.

1. **Clinical signs** include pyrexia, abdominal pain, depression, anorexia, and weight loss.

2. **Diagnosis** is by ultrasonography or exploratory laparotomy.

3. **Treatment** includes appropriate **systemic antibiotics** based on bacterial culture and antimicrobial sensitivity testing, and **surgical drainage.**

a. **Individual abscesses** may be **incised** or perforated and digitally emptied.

b. A **large single abscess** may be treated with **hepatic lobectomy.**

c. If **continued purulent drainage** is expected or **peritonitis** is present, **open abdominal drainage** should be established (see Chapter 10 IV C 8 d).

C. **Extrahepatic biliary obstruction**

1. **Etiology.** Causes include inspissated bile, neoplasia, cholangitis, pancreatitis, duodenal inflammation, liver fluke infestation, cysts, diaphragmatic hernia, and congenital atresia.

    a. Periductal fibrosis from pancreatitis is a major cause of extrahepatic biliary obstruction in dogs.

    b. Cholelithiasis and cholecystitis are discussed in III E.

2. Pathophysiology. Extrahepatic cholestasis may result in impaired function of the reticuloendothelial system, endotoxemia, coagulopathies, platelet dysfunction, and increased risk of postoperative renal failure.

3. Clinical signs are chronic and progressive and may wax and wane. They include depression, lethargy, weight loss, vomiting, diarrhea, icterus, abdominal pain, abdominal enlargement, fever, and acholic feces.

4. Diagnosis is usually based on results of blood work, radiographs, ultrasonography, scintigraphy, abdominocentesis, and exploratory surgery.

    a. Blood work. Prolonged clotting times may occur from decreases in vitamin K–dependent factors. Increased levels of alkaline phosphatase, γ-glutamyl transpeptidase, bile acids, and total bilirubin may be seen.

        (1) Bilirubinemia is primarily caused by increased conjugated bilirubin, although unconjugated bilirubin may also be increased.

        (2) Bilirubinuria. Excess conjugated bilirubin is excreted in the urine. In cats, bilirubinuria is usually considered abnormal. In dogs, however, low levels of bilirubinuria are normal.

    b. Radiographs or ultrasound may demonstrate choleliths, gallbladder enlargement, and increased abdominal fluid. Ultrasonography is particularly useful for demonstrating gallbladder and hepatic duct enlargement and for determining the cause of biliary obstruction.

    c. Abdominocentesis or diagnostic peritoneal lavage and cytology aid in diagnosing biliary leakage and septic or chemical peritonitis.

    d. Hepatobiliary scintigraphy with radiolabeled technetium has been used to confirm the presence of extrahepatic biliary obstruction.

5. Treatment

    a. Supportive therapy with intravenous fluids, antibiotics, vitamin K_1, whole fresh blood transfusion, and treatment of electrolyte or acid–base abnormalities are often necessary before surgical exploration.

    b. Surgical treatment

        (1) Cholecystotomy. Cystic or common bile duct obstructions resulting from inspissated bile or stones may be relieved with cholecystotomy and flushing of the duct.

        (2) Cholecystectomy may be used to treat gallbladder neoplasia, irreparable damage to the gallbladder or cystic duct, chronic cases of cystic duct obstruction or calculi, and nonresponsive cases of inflammation.

        (3) Cholecystoenterostomy or **choledochoenterostomy.** Anastomosis of the gallbladder or cystic duct to the intestine (**cholecystojejunostomy/duodenostomy** and **choledochojejunostomy/duodenostomy,** respectively) may be performed to relieve extrahepatic biliary obstruction.

            (a) Cholecystojejunostomy should be avoided whenever possible because of postoperative weight loss—possibly resulting from lipid maldigestion—and duodenal ulceration resulting from increased gastric acid secretion and decreased duodenal pH.

            (b) Because the original stoma contracts by 50%, stricture of the gallbladder anastomotic site and subsequent cholangitis may be avoided by creating a long incision (i.e., greater than or equal to 2.5 cm).

        (4) Tube cholecystostomy can be used for temporary decompression of the biliary tract. The tube may be pulled 5–10 days after placement.

        (5) Pancreatectomy, Billroth II, and cholecystoduodenostomy/jejunostomy. In cases of extensive neoplasia (e.g., pancreatic or proximal gastrointestinal adenocarcinoma), pancreatectomy, Billroth II gastroduodenal resection with gastrojejunal anastomosis, and cholecystoduodenostomy may be attempted. Alternatively, cholecystojejunostomy may be used as a palliative procedure.

(6) Prognosis. Survival of animals with cholelithiasis is greater after cholecystectomy than cholecystotomy, and lowest with choledochotomy.

D. **Biliary tract rupture**

1. **Etiology**
   a. **Trauma** causes 98% of bile duct ruptures and 6% of gallbladder ruptures.
   b. **Necrotizing cholecystitis** (see III E 2) causes 30% of gallbladder ruptures.
   c. **Cholelithiasis** (see III E 1) causes 2% of bile duct ruptures and 64% of gallbladder ruptures.

2. **Pathogenesis.** The usual cause of death in animals with biliary tract disruption is bile peritonitis due to bile salt toxicity and subsequent tissue necrosis and bacterial replication.

3. **Clinical features.** The **common bile duct** is the most frequent site for ductal rupture. Less frequent sites are the termination of the common bile duct on the duodenum and, occasionally, the junction of the common bile duct with the hepatic ducts.

4. **Clinical signs** include anorexia, lethargy, vomiting, depression, abdominal pain, fever, icterus, abdominal distention, ascites, and, possibly, acholic feces. Clinical signs are more chronic and subtle for ductal rupture than for gallbladder rupture.

5. **Diagnosis.** Bile-colored fluid may be obtained on abdominocentesis. Elevated levels of total bilirubin, alkaline phosphatase, and alanine aminotransferase may be present, as well as bilirubinuria. Anemia, hypoproteinemia, dehydration, electrolyte imbalances, and erythrocyte lysis may result from retention of hyperosmolar, alkaline bile salts in the abdominal cavity.

6. **Treatment.**
   a. **Supportive therapy** is similar to treatment for biliary tract obstruction [see III C 5a].
   b. **Surgical treatment. Surgical exploration** is the treatment of choice.
      (1) Abdominal lavage should be used in all cases.
      (2) Open abdominal drainage is used if peritonitis is present (see Chapter 10 IV C 8 d).
      (3) Tears in biliary tract
         (a) Primary closure. Small tears in the biliary tract can sometimes be closed directly. A latex rubber T tube can be used as a stent to prevent stricture after suturing the common bile duct; however, the small size of the duct usually inhibits primary repair or the use of stents.
         (b) Biliary diversion is less technically demanding than primary bile duct repair.
            (i) Cholecystoduodenostomy is called for to treat avulsion or irreparable tears of the common bile duct.
            (ii) Choledochoduodenostomy is not recommended except in cases of severe duct dilation where a 2.5-cm stoma can be created.
      (4) Torn hepatic ducts are ligated.
      (5) Necrotizing cholecystitis is treated with **cholecystectomy.**

E. **Cholelithiasis and cholecystitis** are uncommon conditions in small animals.

1. **Cholelithiasis**
   a. **Etiology.** Biliary stasis, cholecystitis, trauma, infection, and altered bile composition as a result of dietary changes can lead to cholelithiasis. Female, older, small-breed dogs are predisposed.
   b. **Clinical signs.** Affected animals are often asymptomatic but will develop clinical signs if biliary obstruction, biliary tract rupture, or cholelithiasis is present (see III C 3, D 4, E 1 c).
   c. **Diagnosis**
      (1) Blood work abnormalities include leukocytosis, neutrophilia with a shift to the left, elevated hepatic enzymes, hypoalbuminemia, and hyperbilirubinemia.

     (2) Radiography. Choleliths, which may be large, organized concretions or sand-like sediment and are frequently composed of calcium bilirubinate, are radio-dense in up to 48% of animals.

     (3) Ultrasonography will confirm the disease in most animals.

  d. Treatment entails **cholecystotomy, duodenotomy,** or, if the bile duct is severely dilated, **choledochotomy.** Because bacterbilia is found in 75% of affected animals, bile should be submitted for culture and sensitivity testing, and appropriate antibiotic therapy should be initiated.

  e. Prognosis. The survival rate is greatest following cholecystectomy (86%). Cholecystotomy and choledochotomy carry survival rates of 50% and 33%, respectively.

2. Cholecystitis may be **necrotizing, acute,** or **chronic.**

  a. Etiology. Sources of bacteria, commonly *E. coli* and *Klebsiella,* include duodenal reflux and hematogenous spread.

  b. Predisposing factors. Biliary stasis may be a predisposing factor. Hepatic necrosis, fibrosis, or degeneration may also be present.

  c. Clinical signs include vomiting, anorexia, abdominal pain, and fever.

  d. Diagnosis. Radiographic evidence of cholecystic emphysema is suggestive of cholecystitis.

  e. Treatment. Cholecystectomy is the treatment of choice.

  f. Prognosis. Survival rates are inversely proportional to age, the severity of preoperative clinical signs, and the duration of presurgical hospitalization.

F. | **Hepatic and biliary tract neoplasia** is usually seen in animals 10 years of age or older. Metastatic hepatic tumors are more common than primary hepatic tumors.

1. Clinical signs may be absent, nonspecific, related to the primary tumor, or suggestive of hepatic failure. Ascites, vomiting, and hepatomegaly are seen frequently in dogs, while anorexia, lethargy, and hepatomegaly are common in cats. Weight loss, weakness, abdominal enlargement, a palpable mass, and jaundice may also be seen.

2. Diagnosis. Definitive diagnosis is by **exploratory laparotomy** and biopsy.

  a. Blood work. Elevated liver enzymes (particulary alanine aminotransferase), bilirubinemia, anemia, hypoglycemia (in dogs), azotemia (in cats), and decreased clotting factors may be seen.

  b. Imaging. Hepatic masses may be visible with radiography, ultrasonography, and computed tomography.

  c. Techniques of intraoperative hepatic biopsy include instrument or finger fragmentation, wedge, punch, needle, and guillotine techniques. Percutaneous needle biopsy may be diagnostic.

3. Treatment. Surgical excision (hepatic lobectomy) is the treatment of choice for resectable masses.

4. Specific tumor types

  a. Hepatocellular adenoma is a benign tumor that occurs more frequently than malignant primary liver tumors.

    (1) Appearance. It usually occurs as a single mass, but may be hard to differentiate from nodular hyperplasia.

    (2) Prognosis is good with complete removal.

  b. Hepatocellular carcinoma is the most common type of malignant primary hepatic tumor in cats or dogs. It is seen primarily in older animals—the mean age of affected dogs is 12 years.

    (1) Clinical signs include an abdominal mass, polyuria and polydipsia, vomiting, anorexia, and weight loss. Clinical signs are absent in 28% of patients.

    (2) Blood work. Elevations in liver enzymes and white blood cell count are often seen on blood work. Hypoglycemia may be present.

    (3) Prognosis is usually poor because of the extent of disease seen at the time of surgery.

      (a) The **metastatic rate** in dogs is high with diffuse and nodular adenocarcinoma but less with the massive form, which is the most common type of hepatocellular carcinoma. The metastatic rate in cats is 28%.

(b) The **average length of survival** with complete resection by lobectomy is 308 days, with many dogs dying from unrelated diseases.

c. **Bile duct carcinoma** is the second most common type of primary malignant hepatic tumor in dogs. Intrahepatic bile duct carcinoma occurs more commonly than extrahepatic or cholecystic bile duct carcinoma.

(1) **Predisposing factors.** It is seen more frequently in females, mixed-breed dogs, and Labrador retrievers.

(2) **Appearance.** Grossly, bile duct carcinoma may look like nodular hyperplasia, chronic active hepatitis, or cirrhosis.

(3) The **metastatic rate** is high in dogs and cats. Tumors spread primarily to the lymph nodes and lungs.

(4) **Prognosis** is poor.

G. **Portosystemic shunts** are vascular anomalies that divert blood from the portal circulation into the systemic circulation, bypassing the liver (Figure 11–3).

1. **Pathophysiology.** Liver growth is poor. Liver functions such as protein and urea production and ammonia clearance decrease because of diminished hepatic mass and blood supply. Hepatic encephalopathy may develop from systemic toxins that alter cerebral metabolism.

2. **Classifications.** Shunts can be congenital or acquired, single or multiple, and intrahepatic or extrahepatic.

a. **Single congenital shunts**

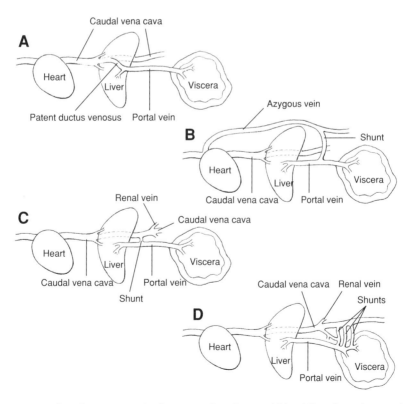

FIGURE 11–3. Examples of portosystemic shunts causing abnormal blood flow from the portal to the systemic venous circulation. *(A)* Intrahepatic shunt. *(B)* Portoazygous shunt. *(C)* Single extrahepatic portacaval shunt. *(D)* Multiple extrahepatic portacaval shunts.

(1) **Dogs.** Single congenital shunts are usually seen in young purebred dogs.
   (a) **Intrahepatic** congenital shunts are usually found in large-breed dogs, such as Labrador retrievers.
   (b) **Extrahepatic** congenital shunts are usually found in small- and toy-breed dogs, such as Yorkshire terriers and miniature schnauzers.
(2) **Cats** can have intrahepatic or extrahepatic congenital shunts.
   b. **Multiple acquired extrahepatic shunts** develop secondary to portal hypertension from hepatic disease or extrahepatic portal vein compression.

3. **Clinical signs.** In general, animals may be underweight or have stunted growth. Signs may be precipitated by the ingestion of meals containing protein or by administration of drugs that are metabolized by the liver, such as anesthetics.
   a. **Neurologic signs** are secondary to toxic effects on the central nervous system (e.g., hepatic encephalopathy) and include abnormal behavior, dementia, seizures, blindness, and circling. Signs of **hepatic encephalopathy** are seen in most animals with portosystemic shunts.
   b. **Urologic signs** result from ammonium biurate crystal and calculus formation and decreased urea production. Hematuria, polyuria, pollakiuria, and stranguria may be seen.
   c. **Gastrointestinal signs** may result from abnormal bile acid metabolism and include vomiting, diarrhea, anorexia, and ptyalism. **Hypersalivation** is the single **most common clinical sign in cats.**
   d. **Ascites and coagulopathies** may be present in animals with multiple acquired portosystemic shunts.

4. **Diagnosis** is based on clinical signs and results of blood work, radiography, ultrasonography, scintigraphy, or exploratory laparotomy.
   a. **Blood work** reveals hypoproteinemia, hypoalbuminemia, low blood urea nitrogen (BUN) and elevations in bile acids and ammonia. Hypoglycemia, leukocytosis, and microcytic anemia may be present.
   b. **Urinalysis.** Specific gravity of urine may be low because of decreased urea production. Ammonium biurate crystalluria and pyuria may be present.
   c. **Radiography.** Microhepatica, renomegaly, and cystic or renal calculi may be seen on survey abdominal films. Calculi are often radiolucent but may be discernible using portography, ultrasonography, or excretory urography.
   d. **Liver biopsy** may show lobule atrophy, decreased distance between portal triads, narrowed portal venules, proliferation of hepatic arterioles, hepatocellular degeneration, and foci of macrophages containing iron-like pigments.
   e. **Definitive diagnosis.** Presence of a shunt may be confirmed with ultrasound, operative mesenteric or transplenic portography, colonic portal scintigraphy, or exploratory laparotomy.
      (1) Mesenteric portography and surgical biopsy may be necessary to differentiate portosystemic shunts from hepatic vascular dysplasia.
      (2) Shunts that are not located on exploratory laparotomy may be identified easily with operative mesenteric portography.
         (a) A jejunal vessel is catheterized and injected with sterile, water-soluble contrast media.
         (b) Operative mesenteric portography is not necessarily predictive of postligation hepatic portal vascularization.

5. **Treatment**
   a. **Medical treatment.** Animals should be stabilized with medical management before surgery.
      (1) Multiple acquired shunts secondary to hepatic fibrosis are usually managed medically.
      (2) Medical therapy may include a low-protein diet, lactulose, and antibiotics.
         (a) Lactulose is a disaccharide that decreases bacterial numbers and reduces the conversion of ammonium to ammonia by decreasing colonic pH. It also acts as a cathartic to decrease bacterial and substrate load.
         (b) Oral antibiotics such as neomycin or metronidazole may also be used to decrease numbers of urease-producing bacteria.

(c) Severely affected animals should be treated with intravenous fluids with dextrose supplementation for hypoglycemia, and with saline or saline/lactulose enemas. Activated charcoal can be administered by stomach tube in nonresponsive animals.

b. **Surgery** to ligate the shunt is the treatment of choice for single congenital shunts to encourage return of hepatic blood supply and regeneration of hepatic tissue, and to discourage progressive liver atrophy and fibrosis. Measures should be taken to prevent hypoglycemia, hypothermia, and overhydration during and after surgery. If necessary, shunts should be partially ligated to prevent portal hypertension.

(1) **Intraoperative monitoring of central venous and portal pressures**

  (a) **Central venous pressure.** The **normal** central venous pressure is **2–7 cm H_2O.** It should not drop more than 1 cm H_2O during ligation of the shunt.

  (b) **Portal pressure.** The **normal** portal pressure **is 8–13 cm H_2O;** in dogs with single congenital shunts it may be lower (4–8 cm H_2O) because of decreased hepatic vascular resistance.

   (i) **Subjective signs of intraoperative portal hypertension** include increased peristalsis, increased vascular pulsation, and pallor and cyanosis of the intestines and pancreas.

   (ii) In animals with high splanchnic compliance, portal pressure may not change, and the degree of shunt ligation must be based on central venous pressure or on subjective signs.

(2) **Surgical technique** depends on the location and type of shunt.

  (a) **Intrahepatic shunts**

   (i) **Identification.** Intrahepatic shunts can be identified by directly visualizing (particularly left hepatic shunts), by palpating a catheter threaded through the portal vein and shunt, or by monitoring portal pressure changes during vascular compression.

   (ii) **Treatment options** include surgical ligation of the hepatic vein draining the shunt or of the portal branch supplying the shunt, intravascular occlusion of the shunt, or ligation of the shunt itself.

   (iii) Potential **complications** during intrahepatic shunt ligation include severe hemorrhage and hepatic congestion.

  (b) **Single extrahepatic congenital shunts** should be ligated as close to their vascular insertion point as possible.

  (c) **Multiple acquired shunts.** Animals with multiple acquired shunts secondary to cirrhosis may be treated with **caudal vena caval banding.**

   (i) The caudal vena cava is partially occluded until its pressure is 1.5–2.5 cm H_2O greater than that of the portal vein, or until the pressures are at least equalized.

   (ii) Portal pressures should be kept below 22 cm H_2O.

(3) Removal of **cystic calculi.** Cystic calculi may be removed after shunt ligation or during a second procedure.

(4) **Dissolution of renal calculi** has been reported after shunt ligation; animals should be monitored after surgery for urinary tract obstruction.

6. **Postoperative considerations**

  a. **Postoperative care** includes continued supportive therapy, a low-protein diet, and close monitoring for signs of portal hypertension and seizures.

  (1) **Diet.** Adult maintenance pet food can be fed when the animal shows signs of improved hepatic function (e.g., increased albumin production), usually after approximately 3 months. Alternatively, the amount of protein can be gradually increased in the diet over 6 months until either a normal maintenance level is reached or clinical signs recur.

  (2) **Portal hypertension. Postligation portal pressure** should not exceed 16–18 cm H_2O and should not be more than 9–10 cm H_2O over baseline.

   (a) **Signs of portal hypertension** include hypovolemic shock, progressive hypothermia, and severe abdominal pain.

      (b) Correction of portal hypertension. Animals that develop postoperative portal hypertension should be taken back to surgery for **ligature removal.** Religation can be performed after the animal has recovered completely from the surgeries and portal hypertension.

    (3) Seizures have been reported to occur 13–72 hours after extrahepatic shunt ligation in up to 11% of animals.

      (a) Predisposing factors. Dogs over 18 months of age may be predisposed.

      (b) Treatment. Seizures **are not correlated with ammonia concentrations** or **degree of shunt ligation** and do not respond to normalization of blood glucose, calcium, or potassium levels. Treatments include **intravenous barbiturates** and **mannitol.**

      (c) Mortality rates are 50%–80%.

  b. Failure of ligation. If clinical signs of the shunt recur, portography should be repeated to assess the success of the ligation and to determine whether a second ligation is needed.

  c. Serum bile acids often continue to be abnormal after shunt ligation; in one study, 75% of dogs had abnormal values a median time of 18.6 months after ligation.

7. Prognosis after surgery depends on the type of shunt. Poorer results are seen with dogs that are over 2 years of age at the time of diagnosis of congenital PSS.

  a. Prognosis is good with single congenital extrahepatic shunts. The survival rate reaches 95% when surgery is quick and portal hypertension is avoided. Transcolonic portal scintigraphy has demonstrated eventual shunt occlusion in 75% of dogs with partially ligated single extrahepatic shunts.

  b. Intrahepatic shunts are associated with a higher mortality rate (25%) because of the difficulty of the surgery.

  c. Clinical improvement is seen in 60% of animals with multiple acquired extrahepatic shunts. Postoperative morbidity is high; ascites and pelvic limb edema may persist for 6 weeks.

  d. Cats may have recurrence of clinical signs and recanalization of the shunt if the original shunt is only partially occluded. Although 59% of cats have no recurrence of clinical signs after shunt ligation, 23% show no improvement and die or are euthanized after surgery.

H. **Hepatic arteriovenous fistula** is a rare congenital or acquired arteriovenous communication seen in young animals, resulting in portal hypertension and multiple acquired extrahepatic portosystemic shunts.

  1. Clinical signs. Acute onset of neurologic and gastrointestinal signs is seen, including depression, lethargy, ascites, vomiting, diarrhea, weight loss, and behavior changes. Arteriovenous fistulae may also decrease arterial blood volume, resulting in increased cardiac output and tachycardia.

  2. Diagnosis. Definitive diagnosis is by angiography, nuclear scintigraphy, or exploratory laparotomy. Blood work reveals anemia, hypoproteinemia, leukocytosis, and low BUN; as well as increases in alanine aminotransferase, alkaline phosphatase, ammonia, and bile acids. Shunting blood is auscultable as a continuous murmur at the abdomen in 71% of animals.

  3. Treatment. Partial hepatectomy is performed to remove the fistula. If portal hypertension is present after hepatectomy, **caudal vena caval banding may be necessary** to improve hepatic perfusion. The heart rate may decrease during shunt closure because of the Branham reflex.

  4. Postoperative care. Low-protein diets are necessary for the many dogs that continue to have hepatic insufficiency.

SELECTED READINGS

Bjorling DE: Surgical management of hepatic and biliary diseases in cats. *Compen Contin Educ Pract Vet* 13(9):1419–1425, 1991.

Bojrab MJ (ed): *Current Techniques in Small Animal Surgery,* 3rd ed. Philadelphia, Lea & Febiger, 1990, pp 291–303.

Bojrab MJ (ed): *Disease Mechanisms in Small Animal Surgery,* 2nd ed. Philadelphia, Lea & Febiger, 1993, pp 292–310.

Evans HE, Christensen GC: *Miller's Anatomy of the Dog,* 3rd ed. Philadelphia, WB Saunders, 1993, pp 451–458, 699–700.

Guyton AC: *Textbook of Medical Physiology,* 8th ed. Philadelphia, WB Saunders, 1991, pp 771–774.

Lorenz MD, Cornelius LM: *Small Animal Medical Diagnosis,* 2nd ed. Philadelphia, JB Lippincott, 1993, pp 275–320.

Martin RA: Congenital portosystemic shunts in the dog and cat. *Vet Clin North Am: Small Anim Pract* 23(3):609–623, 1993.

Martin RA: Liver and biliary system. In *Textbook of Small Animal Surgery,* 2nd ed. Edited by Slatter D. Philadelphia, WB Saunders, 1993, pp 645–677.

Neer TM: A review of disorders of the gallbladder and extrahepatic biliary tract in the dog and cat. *J Vet Int Med* 6:186–92, 1992.

Parchman MB, Flanders JA: Extrahepatic biliary tract rupture: Evaluation of the relationship between the site of rupture and the cause of rupture in 15 dogs. *Cornell Vet* 80:267–272, 1990.

Postorino NC: Hepatic tumors. In *Clinical Veterinary Oncology.* Edited by Withrow SJ, MacEwen EG. Philadelphia, JB Lippincott, 1989, pp 196–200.

Chapter 12

Urogenital System

Elizabeth J. Laing

I. KIDNEY

A. Anatomy. The kidneys are located in the retroperitoneal space ventral to the thoracolumbar vertebrae. The renal arteries and veins and the ureter enter the medial border of each kidney at the hilus.

1. In **cats,** each kidney is usually supplied by a single renal artery and is drained by one or more renal veins.

2. In **dogs,** the right kidney usually has a single artery and vein whereas the left kidney may have multiple arteries. The left renal vein may also receive the ipsilateral ovarian vein.

B. Congenital disorders. The clinical significance of renal anomalies depends on the functional capability of the contralateral kidney.

1. A unilateral missing kidney **(agenesis),** a small kidney **(hypoplasia),** or a deformed kidney **(dysgenesis)** is a concern if renal surgery is anticipated, because renal function is normally maintained by hypertrophy of the unaffected kidney. Renal agenesis is frequently associated with underdevelopment of the ipsilateral genitalia.

2. **Renal ectopia** occurs when the kidney remains in its embryonic position in the caudal abdomen.
   a. **Diagnosis.** Abdominal palpation and radiography reveal a caudal abdominal mass. Renal function is usually normal.
   b. **Treatment. Nephrectomy** is indicated if pressure from the ectopic kidney causes constipation, dysuria, or other organ dysfunction, and if the opposite kidney is anatomically and functionally normal (see I C 3 d).

3. **Renal cysts** can arise during embryonic development or after the kidney is fully formed.
   a. **Solitary cysts,** if small and asymptomatic, rarely require treatment.
   b. **Large or multiple cysts** are predisposed to infection. If only one kidney is affected, nephrectomy may be required. Renal transplantation may be a treatment option if both kidneys are affected.

C. Acquired disorders

1. **Nephrolithiasis.** Kidney stones account for 4% of urinary tract calculi.
   a. **Pathophysiology.** Mineral composition and pathophysiology are discussed in III C 1.
   b. **Clinical presentation.** Clinical signs include hematuria, pyuria, depression, anorexia, and nonspecific lumbar or abdominal pain (renal colic). Animals with bilateral disease may show signs of chronic renal failure (polyuria, polydipsia, weight loss).
   c. **Diagnosis** is based on imaging studies and laboratory testing.
      (1) **Localization of stones. Abdominal radiographs** often reveal radiopaque calculi (struvite and calcium-containing stones). Diagnosis of cystine and urate stones may require **contrast radiography** or **ultrasonography.**
      (2) **Evaluation of renal function.** Serum chemistries, urinalysis, and **excretory urography** are used to evaluate the functional capacity of both kidneys prior to deciding on a course of therapy.
   d. **Treatment**
      (1) **Dietary management** must be based on quantitative mineral analysis. For example, low magnesium diets may be effective in the dissolution or prevention of struvite calculi. However, because these diets cause increased intestinal ab-

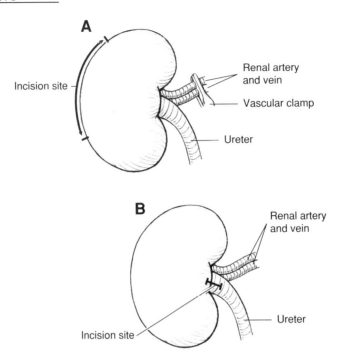

FIGURE 12–1. *(A)* Sagittal nephrotomy. The incision is made in the central body of the kidney and extended by blunt and sharp dissection into the renal pelvis. Hemorrhage is controlled by temporary occlusion of the renal artery and vein. (Some surgeons occlude only the renal artery to permit venous drainage of the kidney.) *(B)* Pyelolithotomy. To avoid damage to the renal blood supply, the kidney is reflected medially and the incision is made through the dorsolateral surface of the renal pelvis.

sorption of calcium, they may enhance the formation of calcium phosphate and oxalate stones.

(2) **Surgical treatment. Nephrolithotomy** is the treatment of choice (Figure 12–1). The kidneys are approached via a cranioventral midline celiotomy. Temporary occlusion of the renal vessels, using vascular forceps or a tourniquet, minimizes hemorrhage and facilitates stone removal.

    (a) **Nephrotomy.** The renal pelvis is usually approached through a **bisectional** or **sagittal nephrotomy,** separating the renal parenchyma in a longitudinal plane along the lateral surface of the kidney. Because surgery temporarily decreases renal function by 20%–50%, unilateral nephrotomies staged several weeks apart may be safer for animals with impaired renal function and bilateral calculi.

    (b) **Pyelolithotomy,** an incision directly into the dorsal surface of the renal pelvis, is reserved for dogs with a dilated proximal ureter and renal pelvis. By minimizing trauma to the renal parenchyma, renal function is less likely to be affected.

  e. **Postoperative care**

    (1) **Urinary tract infections** are treated with antibiotics, based on bacterial culture and antimicrobial sensitivity testing, for a minimum of 4 weeks.

    (2) **Persistent hematuria** may be controlled with hemostatic agents (e.g., aminocaproic acid, tranexamic acid).

    (3) **Calculi** are submitted for quantitative mineral analysis. Appropriate dietary management is instituted to help avoid recurrence.

2. **Renal trauma.** Blunt trauma to the abdomen is the most common cause of renal parenchymal damage.

  a. **Clinical presentation.** Clinical signs reflect the severity of the injury. Mild subcapsular hemorrhage and parenchymal bruising may cause transient hematuria. Severe parenchymal damage or rupture of the kidney may result in hemorrhagic shock and acute renal failure.

b. Diagnosis

   (1) Imaging studies

      (a) Abdominal radiographs and **ultrasound** may show an altered kidney size or shape. Leakage of urine or blood appears radiographically as retroperitoneal swelling, streaking, or mottling.

      (b) Excretory urography best defines the site and degree of injury. However, because renal blood flow is decreased in hypovolemic patients, this procedure should be reserved for animals with normal cardiovascular function and adequate renal perfusion.

   (2) Abdominocentesis may reveal uroperitoneum or hemoperitoneum if the peritoneum is disrupted.

c. Treatment

   (1) Conservative treatment. Mild trauma usually resolves with rest and diuresis.

   (2) Surgical treatment. Indications for surgery include hypovolemic shock unresponsive to medical therapy and uncontrolled intra-abdominal hemorrhage or urine leakage. A **ventral laparotomy** approach allows inspection of the entire peritoneal cavity.

      (a) Small parenchymal **tears are sutured or packed with gelatin sponges.**

      (b) Damage confined to one pole of the kidney may require a **partial nephrectomy** (Figure 12–2). The multiple suture method is preferred over wedge resection to control hemorrhage and minimize the risk of ligature slippage.

      (c) Severe damage to the parenchyma or ureter may require **nephrectomy,** assuming the opposite kidney is functional and undamaged (see I C 3 d).

3. Renal neoplasia. Primary renal tumors are uncommon in small animals, accounting for 2% of all tumors. The kidneys may also be the site of metastatic neoplasms.

a. Classification

   (1) Benign tumors include hemangiomas, adenomas, interstitial cell tumors, papillomas, lipomas, fibromas, and embryonal nephromas.

   (2) Malignant tumors

      (a) In dogs, tubular cell carcinomas are the most common malignancy. In cats, lymphomas are most common. Other malignant tumors include transitional and squamous cell carcinomas, nephroblastomas, hemangiosarcomas, fibrosarcomas, undifferentiated sarcomas, and multiple cystadenocar-

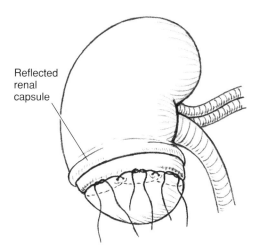

Reflected
renal
capsule

FIGURE 12–2. Multiple suture method of partial nephrectomy. Following reflection of the renal capsule, three separate loops of suture are placed to encircle the kidney parenchyma. Tightening the sutures simultaneously cuts and ligates the tissue.

cinomas. The latter is associated with generalized dermatofibrosis in German shepherds.

    (b) The majority of renal tumors are malignant and spread by local invasion within the abdomen or by metastasis to the lungs.

        (i) Nearly 50% of affected dogs have radiographic evidence of pulmonary metastases at the time of diagnosis.

        (ii) Other common sites for metastasis are abdominal lymph nodes, liver, mesentery, brain, and bone.

  b. Clinical presentation. Clinical signs vary with the location, size, duration, and type of tumor.

    (1) Most **benign tumors** are asymptomatic and are found incidentally at necropsy. The exception is **hemangioma,** which frequently causes gross hematuria.

    (2) Tumors in the renal pelvis usually cause urinary tract changes (e.g., hematuria, hydronephrosis, renomegaly) prior to any systemic signs.

    (3) Tumors of the renal parenchyma usually present with systemic signs, including anorexia, depression, weight loss, fever, and abdominal pain.

    (4) Associated paraneoplastic syndromes include anemia, polycythemia, hypercalcemia, and hypertrophic osteopathy.

  c. Diagnosis should concentrate both on establishing a histologic diagnosis and on clinical staging.

    (1) Abdominal radiographs and **ultrasound** may reveal an enlarged kidney and possibly associated lymphadenopathy.

    (2) Excretory urography confirms the presence of a renal mass and demonstrates the functional status of the other kidney.

    (3) Unless neoplastic cells are found in the urine sediment, **exploratory laparotomy** may be needed to establish a histologic diagnosis. Percutaneous needle biopsy is not recommended because of the risk of potentiating metastasis.

  d. Treatment. Nephrectomy, the surgical removal of the kidney and ureter, is the treatment of choice for animals without apparent metastasis and with a second functional kidney.

    (1) Approach. A ventral midline celiotomy provides the best exposure of the kidneys and renal vessels and allows the entire abdomen to be inspected for signs of metastatic disease.

    (2) Dissection

        (a) The right kidney is exposed by retracting the descending duodenum to the left. Exposure of the left kidney is aided by retraction of the descending colon.

        (b) The peritoneum is incised at the caudal pole and gently reflected until the renal hilus is exposed. Excessive handling or manipulation of the tumor is avoided until the renal vessels are ligated.

        (c) The renal vein is usually ligated first to decrease the risk of tumor embolization and hematologic spread. The branches of the renal artery are then ligated separately.

        (d) The ureter is dissected from the retroperitoneum and ligated close to the urinary bladder.

  e. Prognosis. The average survival time for animals with epithelial malignancy is 8 months following surgery. The survival time for animals with mesenchymal tumors is somewhat shorter.

D. **Renal transplantation** is available on a limited basis for treatment of decompensated renal failure in dogs and cats.

  1. Patient selection. The ideal transplant recipient is in the early stages of decompensated renal failure and has minimal weight loss (less than 20% of normal body weight). In addition, recipients must:

    a. Be free of bacterial and viral infections

    b. Have normal cardiovascular function

    c. Have no history of previous urinary tract infection, inflammatory bowel disease, diabetes, or oxaluria

2. Donor selection. The donor should be a healthy adult of the same body size as the recipient, be free of infectious diseases, and have two functional kidneys.
    a. Cats. Donor selection is based on blood crossmatch compatibility.
    b. Dogs. In addition to blood crossmatch compatibility, the donor must also be compatible on mixed lymphocyte response testing.

3. Immunosuppression is achieved with a combination of cyclosporine and prednisolone. Treatment is started 48 hours prior to surgery and is continued for life. Cyclosporine dosage is based on trough blood levels.

4. Surgical technique
    a. The donor kidney is placed in the iliac fossa of the recipient and the renal artery and vein are attached to the corresponding external iliac vessels.
    b. The ureter is then implanted in the urinary bladder using a ureteroneocystotomy technique (see II B 4 a).
    c. The recipient's kidneys are usually left in place to act as a reserve in case the donor kidney fails to function.

5. Prognosis. The transplanted kidney usually begins working within 3 days of surgery, and lasts an average of 3–5 years. **Transplantation failures** may result from:
    a. Vascular thrombosis
    b. Ureteral obstruction
    c. Urinary tract infection
    d. Graft rejection (acute or chronic)

II. URETER

A. **Anatomy.** The ureters, which transport urine from the kidney to the urinary bladder by myogenic peristalsis, lie in the retroperitoneal space ventral to the sublumbar muscles. They enter the bladder at the trigone through a long submucosal tunnel, the **ureterovesicular junction,** creating a flap valve to prevent vesicoureteral reflux.

B. **Congenital disorders.** The most common congenital ureteral anomaly is **ectopic ureters.**

1. Pathophysiology. Ectopic ureters result from abnormal positioning of the ureteral bud along the mesonephric duct. The ureters may either bypass the urinary bladder completely **(extramural ectopia)** or course within the wall of the bladder to open at the bladder neck, urethra, or vagina **(intramural ectopia).** The condition may be unilateral or bilateral.

2. Clinical presentation. Clinical signs include urinary incontinence, recurrent urinary tract infections, and chronic vulvar dermatitis. Incontinence can be intermittent and positional.

3. Diagnosis
    a. Affected ureters appear dilated and tortuous on **excretory urography,** although the exact site of termination may be difficult to visualize (Figure 12–3).
    b. Concurrent **negative-contrast cystography** or **retrograde vaginocystography** may help identify the point of termination.

4. Treatment. Surgery is required to repair ectopic ureters (Figure 12–4). Because of the high incidence of concurrent urinary tract infections, antibiotic therapy (based on bacterial culture) should be instituted prior to surgery.
    a. Ureteroneocystostomy. Extramural ureters are implanted into the urinary bladder through a short oblique seromuscular tunnel, using a spatulated anastomosis technique.
    b. Neoureterostomy. Intramural ectopia is treated with **intravesicular diversion.** The

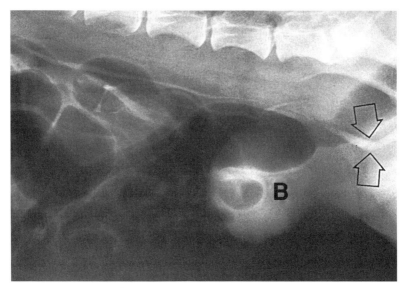

FIGURE 12–3. Ectopic ureter depicted in a lateral view of the caudal abdomen and urinary bladder following excretory urogram. The urinary bladder *(B)* is easily identified by contrast opacification. Segments of the proximal ureters extending from the kidneys to the trigone region are visible. The ectopic ureter courses caudally to bypass the trigone region and enter the pelvic inlet *(open arrowheads).*

intramural ureter is incised and sutured to the surrounding bladder mucosa. The distal portion of the ureter is then ligated or excised.

5. **Complications.** Nearly half of female dogs with intramural ectopia have **persistent urinary incontinence** after surgery.
   a. **Cystic hypoplasia,** in which the bladder is unable to expand sufficiently, usually resolves within 4–6 weeks after surgery.
   b. **Persistent urethral sphincter incompetence** may be treated with exogenous estrogen, α-adrenergic agonists, or both. Delaying ovariohysterectomy in affected dogs for one estrus cycle may also improve urethral sphincter function.

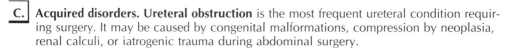

C. **Acquired disorders. Ureteral obstruction** is the most frequent ureteral condition requiring surgery. It may be caused by congenital malformations, compression by neoplasia, renal calculi, or iatrogenic trauma during abdominal surgery.

1. **Clinical presentation**
   a. Unilateral obstruction causes progressive dilation of the renal pelvis and atrophy of the renal parenchyma **(hydronephrosis).** The patient presents with an enlarged kidney and varying degrees of abdominal pain, anorexia, polyuria, and polydipsia.
   b. With bilateral obstructions, **azotemia** usually develops before any significant change in kidney size.

2. **Diagnosis**
   a. **Imaging studies**
      (1) An enlarged kidney shadow is seen on **abdominal radiographs** and **ultrasonography.**
      (2) Depending on the degree of renal function remaining, **excretory urography** reveals a dilated renal pelvis with decreased renal opacification.
   b. **Laboratory testing.** Serum chemistries and urinalysis may show varying degrees of azotemia and isosthenuria.
   c. **Differential diagnosis.** In **cats,** ureteral obstruction must be differentiated from **capsular hydronephrosis,** in which fluid accumulates between the renal capsule

A

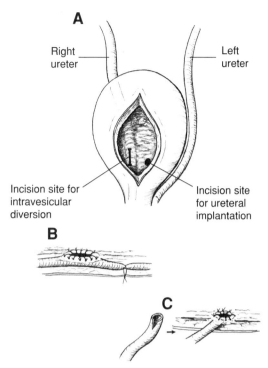

Right ureter

Left ureter

Incision site for intravesicular diversion

Incision site for ureteral implantation

B

C

FIGURE 12–4. Surgical correction of ectopic ureters. *(A)* View of the trigone through a ventral cystotomy in a dog with bilateral ectopic ureters. The right (intramural) ureter can be palpated in the submucosal tissue. The opening of the left (extramural) ureter is distal to the bladder neck and cannot be visualized. *(B)* Neoureterostomy. A ureteral stoma is made by incising and suturing the intramural ureter to the bladder mucosa. The distal ureter is ligated by one or more extramural transfixation sutures. Care must be taken to avoid penetrating the bladder lumen. *(C)* Ureteroneocystostomy. To reimplant the extramural ureter following distal ligation, the free end is spatulated, passed through a short oblique tunnel in the bladder wall, and sutured to the bladder mucosa.

and the parenchyma, forming a pseudocyst. Surgical removal of the cyst wall is usually curative.

3. **Treatment** depends on the duration and degree of the obstruction.
   a. If the obstruction is less than 4 weeks old, or if excretory urography suggests some renal function is present, then treatment is aimed at **restoring urine outflow.**
      (1) **Ureteral stenting.** Using a cystoscope or surgical cystostomy, a ureteral catheter is inserted to bypass the obstruction.
      (2) **Ureteral resection and anastomosis** is used to treat stenotic lesions of the proximal and mid-ureter. It is a technically demanding surgery with a high incidence of postoperative stricture formation.
      (3) Lesions of the distal ureter are most easily treated with **ureteroneocystostomy** (see II B 4 a).
      (4) If surgical repair leaves the ureter too short to reach the urinary bladder, **renal autotransplantation (nephropexy)** can be performed to move the kidney closer to the bladder.
      (5) Other techniques for urinary tract diversion and salvage include bladder pedicle flaps, free autologous tubes, and intestinal conduits.
   b. Complete obstructions lasting longer than 4 weeks usually result in irreversible

renal damage. **Nephrectomy** is recommended to relieve pain and minimize stress on the remaining kidney.

III. URINARY BLADDER

A. **Anatomy.** The urinary bladder varies in size, shape, and position depending on the volume of urine it contains. When empty, it may lie entirely within the pelvic canal. As it fills, it moves cranially to lie along the floor of the abdomen.

1. Urination is initiated by the pelvic parasympathetic nerves that supply the detrusor muscle, causing contraction of the bladder wall.

2. Urination is inhibited by the hypogastric sympathetic nerves supplying the internal urethral sphincter and by the pudendal nerve supplying the external urethral sphincter.

B. **Congenital disorders. Urachal remnants** are the most common congenital anomaly of the urinary bladder.

1. **Pathophysiology.** The urachus is an embryonic conduit connecting the urinary bladder and the allantoic sac. It normally disappears prior to birth. Several types of urachal abnormalities have been described.
   a. A **persistent urachus** is a patent tube connecting the bladder and umbilicus and is often associated with omphalitis and cystitis.
   b. In a **vesicourachal diverticulum,** only the bladder end of the urachus remains patent. This blind pouch at the bladder apex predisposes the animal to recurrent urinary tract infections.
   c. A **urachal cyst** occurs when urachal epithelium persists in isolated segments. If the cyst communicates with the umbilicus, it is called a **urachal sinus.** Urachal cysts are rare and usually asymptomatic.

2. **Diagnosis** is based on clinical **examination** and **double-contrast cystography** (Figure 12–5).

3. **Treatment** is **surgical excision** of the urachal remnant or diverticulum. **Concurrent antibiotic therapy** is based on results of bacterial culture and antimicrobial sensitivity testing.

C. **Acquired disorders**

1. **Cystic calculi** (bladder stones) are a common cause of chronic cystitis in dogs and cats.
   a. **Pathophysiology.** Urinary calculi (uroliths) are organized aggregations of crystals embedded in an organic matrix.
      (1) **Urine characteristics affecting stone formation**
         (a) **Urine pH** influences crystal precipitation and stone formation. Struvite calculi tend to form in alkaline urine, while urate and cystine calculi are associated with acidic urine.
         (b) **Other factors** include the concentration of crystalloids, the presence of crystallization inhibitors, and the proteinaceous matrix.
      (2) **Classification.** Uroliths are classified by the **predominant mineral** present.
         (a) **Magnesium ammonium phosphate (struvite) calculi** are the most common. They are frequently associated with bacterial infections but may also occur in sterile urine.
         (b) **Calcium oxalate calculi.** The pathophysiology of calcium oxalate stone formation is poorly understood but appears to involve hypercalciuria (with or without hypercalcemia).

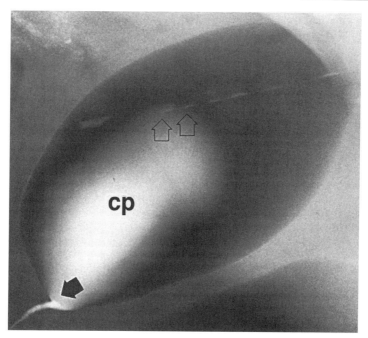

FIGURE 12–5. A lateral view of a double-contrast cystogram demonstrating a urachal diverticulum. The urachal diverticulum can be seen coursing cranioventrally from the apex of the bladder and filled with contrast material *(dark arrowhead)*. The urinary catheter can be seen extending into the dorsal aspect of the urinary bladder and contains air bubbles and residual contrast material *(open arrowheads)*. The contrast pool *(CP)* is within the dependent region of the carbon dioxide–distended urinary bladder.

      (c) Calcium phosphate calculi, less common than oxalate, are associated with hypercalciuria.

      (d) Urate calculi include those composed of **uric acid, ammonium urate,** and **sodium urate.** Dalmatians and animals with portosystemic shunts are at risk.

      (e) Cystine calculi are associated with cystinuria, caused by a genetic inability to absorb cystine in the proximal tubules of the kidney. Dachshunds and English bulldogs are breeds at risk.

      (f) Silica uroliths (jackstones) have been associated with diets high in corn gluten or soybean hulls.

  b. Clinical presentation. Clinical signs usually reflect urinary tract inflammation (e.g., hematuria, stranguria, pollakiuria). Stones are often palpable, especially if the bladder is empty. Dysuria and a distended urinary bladder occur with urethral obstruction.

  c. Diagnosis. Diagnostic work-up is directed at identifying the type of calculi, predisposing cause, and presence of calculi elsewhere in the urinary tract.

    (1) Preliminary identification may be based on crystals in urine sediment. However, quantitative mineral analysis of calculi should be performed once samples are available.

    (2) An underlying infectious etiology is suggested by bacteriuria and a positive quantitative urine culture.

    (3) Radiopaque calculi (struvite and calcium-containing stones) may be seen on abdominal radiographs. Abdominal ultrasonography, excretory urography, or double contrast cystography may be needed to locate radiolucent stone.

  d. Treatment

    (1) Conservative treatment. Struvite, urate, and cystine calculi not causing urine outflow obstruction can be treated with medical dissolution by dietary management.

(2) Surgical treatment. Surgical removal is recommended for other types of calculi, or if medical treatment is unsuccessful after 2 months.

(a) The bladder is exposed via a caudoventral midline celiotomy. A **ventral cystotomy** provides the best exposure of the bladder neck and proximal urethra.

(b) Calculi are removed using a curette, forceps, or small hemostat. Using a urinary catheter, the bladder neck and urethra are flushed to remove small calculi and debris.

(c) The bladder is closed with synthetic absorbable sutures in a two-layer simple continuous or inverting pattern.

2. **Rupture of the urinary bladder** occurs following blunt trauma to the abdomen or pelvis, penetrating abdominal wounds, or traumatic urinary catheterization. The bladder may also rupture spontaneously during prolonged urethral obstruction or secondary to bladder wall necrosis.

   a. **Clinical presentation.** Clinical signs include hematuria, dysuria, anuria, abdominal pain, and ascites. Progressive uremia may cause vomiting and depression.

   b. **Diagnosis**

      (1) Abdominocentesis. Abdominal fluid will have increased concentrations of urea nitrogen and creatinine when compared to serum levels.

      (2) Radiography

         (a) Survey abdominal radiographs reveal ascites, a small or inapparent bladder outline, ileus, and retroperitoneal density changes.

         (b) Positive-contrast cystography confirms the diagnosis. Negative-contrast cystography is not recommended because of the risk of venous air embolization.

   c. **Treatment.** Surgical repair is the treatment of choice.

      (1) Temporary urine diversion may be required until the patient is stable for surgery. Techniques include:

         (a) Bladder drainage using an indwelling urinary catheter

         (b) Bladder drainage using a cystostomy catheter (Foley or balloon) placed through the ventral abdominal wall and into the bladder lumen

         (c) Abdominal drainage using a peritoneal dialysis catheter

      (2) Definitive repair is performed through a ventral celiotomy, débriding necrotic tissue and suturing the bladder wall to prevent further urine leakage. If the bladder wall is friable, the suture line can be reinforced with an omental or serosal patch.

3. **Neoplasms of the urinary bladder**

   a. **Classification.** Carcinomas account for the vast majority of all bladder tumors; transitional cell carcinoma is the most common histologic type. Other bladder tumors include squamous cell carcinoma, adenocarcinoma, fibroma, fibrosarcoma, leiomyoma, leiomyosarcoma, rhabdomyosarcoma, and papilloma.

   b. **Clinical presentation**

      (1) The typical presentation is a middle-aged to older animal with signs of **lower urinary tract disease** (hematuria, stranguria, pollakiuria).

      (2) Urinary incontinence may occur as a result of nerve or muscle damage, or because of decreased bladder capacity.

      (3) Signs of partial or complete **urethral obstruction** are common because two-thirds of all bladder tumors also involve the urethra.

      (4) Occasionally, the primary tumor is **asymptomatic** and the presenting complaint is lameness or respiratory distress resulting from metastatic lesions in the bones or lungs.

      (5) Associated paraneoplastic syndromes include hypercalcemia, cachexia, and hypertrophic osteopathy.

   c. **Diagnosis.** Diagnostic work-up is directed toward establishing a histologic diagnosis and clinical staging.

      (1) Histology

         (a) Examination of **urine sediment** may reveal bizarre malignant cells. However, these must be differentiated from cells altered by severe inflammatory conditions.

   (b) Tissue for histologic diagnosis may be collected by prostatic or urethral washing, urethral biopsy, or fine-needle aspiration of a palpable mass.

(2) Imaging

   (a) Positive- and **double-contrast cystograms** and **ultrasound** may reveal a soft tissue mass arising from the bladder wall.

   (b) Abdominal and **thoracic radiographs** may reveal regional (lumbar) lymphadenopathy, tumor invasion of the lumbar spine or pelvis, or pulmonary metastasis. Approximately one-third of affected animals have detectable metastatic lesions at the time of initial diagnosis.

d. Treatment is based on clinical staging.

   (1) Partial cystectomy. Animals with solitary lesions of the bladder body and no evidence of metastasis may benefit from partial cystectomy.

   (a) Technique. The affected portion of the bladder is excised and the remaining tissues are closed with synthetic absorbable suture in an appositional or inverting manner with a single- or double-layer pattern.

   (b) Prognosis. Nearly two-thirds of the nontrigone bladder can be resected with few complications. However, most dogs with malignant tumors have recurrent disease within 12 months of this surgery.

   (2) Total cystectomy. Excision of solitary tumors of the trigone and bladder neck requires complete excision of the bladder and proximal urethra, and **urinary tract diversion.**

   (a) Depending on the location of the tumor and tissues removed, procedures to restore urine outflow after surgery include **ureterocolonic transposition, trigonal–colonic transposition,** or **bladder substitution** using an isolated ileal or jejunal pouch.

   (b) The clinical applicability of these procedures is limited by the **associated side effects.** Serious complications are frequent and include ascending urinary tract infections, urinary incontinence, electrolyte and acid–base imbalances resulting from absorption of urinary solute, and ureteral stenosis at the site of anastomosis.

   (3) Other treatment modalities include intraoperative radiotherapy, intravesical and systemic chemotherapy, and steroidal and nonsteroidal anti-inflammatory medications.

IV. URETHRA

A. Anatomy. The urethra extends from the neck of the bladder to the urethral meatus.

1. In **males,** the urethra is divided into prostatic, membranous (pelvic), and penile (cavernous) sections. The prostate gland surrounds the proximal urethra in dogs and accounts for the high incidence of urinary outflow problems in prostatic disease.

2. In **females,** the urethra corresponds to the preprostatic portion in males. It enters the genital tract just caudal to the vaginovestibular junction. The shortened urethral length in females may account for the higher incidence of urinary incontinence, especially in dogs.

B. Disorders of the urethra

1. Urethral obstruction

a. Pathophysiology

   (1) Mechanical causes of urethral obstruction include strictures, tumors, and calculi.

      (a) In **male dogs,** stones usually lodge just behind the os penis.

      (b) In **male cats,** the blockage is usually caused by a plug of struvite crystals and mucoid debris, formed as part of the feline urologic syndrome (FUS).

      (c) **Transitional cell carcinoma** is the most frequent tumor associated with urethral obstructions and is the most common cause of urethral obstruction in female dogs.

    (2) **Functional urethral obstruction** is caused by urethral muscle hyperactivity (detrusor–urethral dyssynergia) and may be secondary to either neurogenic or inflammatory stimuli.

  b. **Clinical presentation.** Clinical signs depend on the degree and duration of obstruction.

    (1) Stranguria, dysuria with oliguria or anuria, and abdominal pain are common complaints.

    (2) Depression and vomiting are associated with azotemia.

  c. **Diagnosis.** Urethral obstruction usually is diagnosed clinically on examination and confirmed with urinary catheterization. Further diagnostics are described in III C 1 c.

  d. **Treatment** is aimed at relieving the obstruction, maintaining bladder decompression, and correcting fluid and electrolyte imbalances.

    (1) **Medical treatment.** Inflammatory or neurogenic causes are treated with dietary modification, antibiotics, and anti-inflammatory medications as indicated. Diazepam may provide some relief from dysuria resulting from increased urethral resistance.

    (2) **Urinary catheterization** and **urohydropulsion** are used to mechanically dislodge obstructions caused by calculi and debris. If excessive urine sediment remains after bladder lavage, or if detrusor atony is suspected, a soft indwelling urinary catheter may be needed to maintain bladder decompression.

    (3) **Surgical treatment.** If the obstruction cannot be relieved, surgical decompression is indicated.

      (a) **Prescrotal (prepubic) urethrotomy** provides access to calculi lodged near the os penis and is performed via a ventral midline preputial approach. An incision through the corpus spongiosum penis exposes the urethral lumen. Cystic calculi or calculi lodged in the perineal urethra are removed through a concurrent cystotomy. The urethrotomy may be sutured or left to heal by granulation.

      (b) **Urethrostomy** (i.e., suturing the urethral mucosa to skin to create a permanent stoma) is recommended for animals with recurrent stone formation unresponsive to medical therapy or with secondary urethral strictures.

       (i) **Scrotal urethrostomy** is the recommended procedure for dogs. Although it is associated with fewer complications (e.g., urine scald, urine leakage, stricture formation) than other techniques, it does require that intact males be neutered. **Prepubic urethrostomy** is an alternate technique if castration is not desired.

       (ii) **Perineal urethrostomy** is the recommended procedure in cats. Following removal of the scrotum and prepuce, the pelvic and penile urethral mucosa is sutured to the skin, forming a ventral drain board. To ensure adequate urine flow, the urethral incision should extend proximally through the fascia of the bulbospongiosus muscle.

2. **Urethral trauma** may occur with penetrating abdominal or perineal wounds, blunt abdominal trauma, or as a direct result of pelvic fractures.

  a. **Clinical presentation.** Clinical signs of serious injury include dysuria, anuria, hematuria, and pain, swelling, or discoloration of the perineum. If the urethra has ruptured, perineal swelling and discoloration will progress, although the animal may still void urine normally.

  b. **Diagnosis.** If urethral disruption is suspected, a **positive-contrast urethrogram** is used to confirm the diagnosis and locate the site of leakage.

  c. **Treatment** depends on the degree of disruption.

    (1) If the tear is incomplete and the urethra can be catheterized, an **indwelling urethral catheter** is maintained for 3 weeks while the epithelium regenerates.

(2) If the urethra is transected, **primary surgical anastomosis** is indicated to restore urine outflow and minimize the risk of later stenosis. An indwelling urethral catheter is maintained for 2 weeks following surgery.

3. Urethral sphincter mechanism incontinence
  a. Physiology
    (1) The **internal urethral sphincter** is a functional entity composed of circular rings of smooth muscle. It is located at the junction of the urinary bladder and the urethra and is innervated by the hypogastric nerve.
    (2) The **external urethral sphincter** is an anatomic sphincter composed of striated muscle and innervated by the pudendal nerve.
    (3) In the non-voiding state, the urethra is a high-resistance conduit designed to prevent passage of urine. During urination, reflex inhibition of sympathetic and somatic spinal neurons decreases urethral pressure and thus decreases resistance to urine flow.
  b. Pathophysiology. Any alteration in urethral sphincter innervation or function can result in urinary incontinence. Examples include:
    (1) Neurogenic impairment
    (2) Chronic bladder or urethral disease that decreases urethral distensibility or weakens the pelvic floor muscles
    (3) Anatomic abnormalities
    (4) Hormonal imbalances
  c. Clinical presentation. The most common presentation is **urinary incontinence.** Female dogs are most commonly affected.
  d. Diagnosis
    (1) A thorough **history** is required to eliminate behavioral causes of inappropriate urination.
    (2) **Physical examination, urinalysis,** and **urine culture** may suggest a physical cause for incontinence, such as partial mechanical urethral obstruction, infection, or a neurologic disorder.
    (3) Trial **hormone replacement therapy** may identify estrogen-response incontinence in spayed females.
    (4) **Abdominal** and **contrast radiography** are best-suited for diagnosing anatomic abnormalities.
      (a) The most common abnormality is the **pelvic bladder.** The bladder neck lies caudal to the pecten of the pubis regardless of the degree of bladder distention, resulting in a shortened urethra, decreased urethral sphincter pressure, and, possibly, urinary incontinence.
      (b) Other abnormalities associated with incontinence are **urachal remnants** (see III B) and **bladder wall adhesions.**
    (5) A **urethral pressure profile** can confirm urethral sphincter weakness in the non-voiding state, while a **voiding cystourethrogram** may help diagnose reflex dyssynergia.
  e. Treatment
    (1) Medical treatment
      (a) Infections are treated with appropriate antibiotics and anti-inflammatory agents.
      (b) Exogenous estrogen, α-adrenergic agonists (e.g., ephedrine, phenylpropanolamine), or both may increase the resting urethral pressure.
      (c) Weight loss is recommended in obese animals.
    (2) Surgical treatment is reserved for those animals with adhesions or shortened urethras that are unresponsive to medical management. Several techniques have been described.
      (a) Cranial relocation of the bladder is achieved through creation of a **bladder neck sling,** with the goal of increasing the resting urethral pressure to 50 mm Hg.
        (i) In **colposuspension,** each side of the ovariohysterectomized uterine stump is sutured to the ipsilateral ventral abdominal wall, encircling

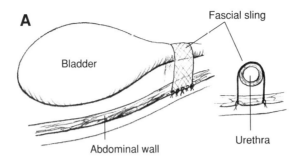

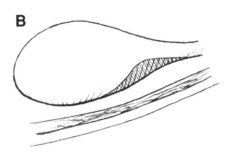

FIGURE 12–6. Surgical methods to repair urethral sphincter mechanism incompetence. *(A)* Bladder neck slings, fashioned from adjacent tissue or synthetic materials, pull the bladder neck cranioventrally and increase resting urethral tone. *(B)* Excision of the ventral bladder neck *(crosshatched area)* increases urethral length, thereby increasing urethral tone.

the bladder neck. If insufficient uterus is available, the proximal vagina may be sutured in a similar fashion **(vaginopexy).**

  (ii) In **cystourethroplasty** (Figure 12–6A), a strip of fascia from the fascia lata or rectus abdominis muscle sheath is placed dorsal to the bladder neck. Each end is then passed through a small incision in the abdominal wall and sutured.

  (b) **Reinforcement of the urethral sphincter.** The urethral sphincter can be reinforced with periurethral injections of polytetrafluoroethylene (Teflon).

  (c) **Lengthening of the functional urethra.** For animals with severe urethral hypoplasia, the functional urethra can be lengthened with a bladder neck flap or partial bladder neck excision (Figure 12–6B).

V. FEMALE REPRODUCTIVE SYSTEM

A. Anatomy

1. Paired **ovaries** are located just caudal to the kidneys. They are attached to the body wall by the **mesovarium,** containing the ovarian artery and vein, and by the **suspensory ligament.**

2. The **oviduct** extends from the ovarian bursa to the uterine horn.

3. The **uterus** is a hollow muscular organ responsible for maintaining and nourishing the fertilized egg.
   a. It is divided into **three parts:** the body, the cervix, and the paired horns.
   b. It lies in the caudal abdomen between the descending colon and urinary bladder.
   c. It is attached by the **mesometrium** to the dorsal body wall and by the **round ligament** to the inguinal canal.
   d. **Blood supply** is via the **ovarian** and **uterine vessels.**

4. The **vagina** is a musculomembranous canal extending from the cervix to the vulva. A vestige of the hymen may be found at the vaginovestibular junction.

5. The **vulva,** or external female genitalia, consists of three parts: the vestibule, clitoris, and labia. The external urethral opening lies on the floor of the vestibule.

B. **Congenital disorders** of the female reproductive tract are uncommon. Although most are incidental findings during ovariohysterectomy, some may cause infertility or dystocia (i.e., abnormal labor).

1. A **supernumerary ovary** is an additional ovary separate from the normal ovary, while an **accessory ovary** develops from a split in the embryonic gonad and is found near or attached to the normal ovary. Failure to remove these structures during ovariohysterectomy may result in signs of recurrent estrus.

2. **Uterus unicornis** is the absence of the uterine horn. The corresponding ovary may be hypoplastic but is usually present and must be removed during ovariohysterectomy.

3. **Segmental defects of the vagina** may be partial (**hypoplasia**) or complete (**aplasia**). A **persistent hymen** may take the form of a vaginal septum or annular ring fibrosis at the vaginovestibular junction. The resultant obstruction may interfere with breeding or cause retention of uterine fluids during estrus. Treatment depends on the degree of obstruction and breeding potential of the animal and may include ovariohysterectomy, vaginectomy, or vaginoplasty to reconstruct the vaginal canal.

C. **Acquired conditions**

1. **Neoplasia**
   a. **Mammary gland tumors** are among the most common tumors in females, although the incidence is significantly reduced in animals spayed before their first estrus.
      (1) Clinical features
         (a) In **dogs,** approximately **50%** of mammary gland tumors are benign. The **caudal mammary glands** are **most often affected** by tumors.
         (b) In **cats,** approximately **90%** of mammary gland tumors **are malignant,** and **all glands** are **equally at risk.**
      (2) Clinical presentation. Clinical signs are usually limited to a soft tissue swelling associated with the mammary tissue. Highly malignant lesions are often ulcerated or inflamed, and may adhere to underlying fascia.
      (3) Diagnosis
         (a) Solitary, small masses (less than 1 cm in diameter) may be diagnosed with **excisional biopsy** prior to further diagnostic procedures.
         (b) Patients with large or multiple tumors should be screened radiographically for chest and lymph node metastases prior to surgery.
         (c) Differential diagnosis. Benign mammary hyperplasia is a general enlargement of mammary tissue seen in cats under the influence of progesterone. Generalized mammary hyperplasia occurs rarely in dogs.
      (4) Treatment. For most animals, surgery is the treatment of choice. The extent of surgery does not appear to influence survival time or cancer-free survival time.
         (a) A **lumpectomy** removes the tumor mass only.
         (b) In a **simple mastectomy,** the tumor and affected gland are removed.
         (c) Regional mastectomy also removes the ipsilateral glands drained by the same lymphatic. *En bloc* **resection** also includes the draining lymph node.
         (d) Unilateral mastectomy removes all glands on one side.
         (e) Bilateral mastectomy removes both mammary chains. However, because of the potential difficulty in skin closure and risk of wound complications, this technique is not often recommended. For animals with bilateral disease, unilateral mastectomies staged several weeks apart may be a safer approach.
      (5) Prognosis depends on the biologic behavior, size, and extent of the tumor.

Adjuvant chemotherapy or radiation therapy may be beneficial for advanced or inoperable tumors.

b. Vaginal and vulvar tumors

(1) Classification

(a) Common **malignant tumors** of the vagina and vulva include leiomyosarcoma and squamous cell carcinoma. Occasionally, transitional cell carcinoma may invade the vulva from the external urethral opening.

(b) Benign tumors include leiomyoma, vaginal polyps (polypoid fibroleiomyoma) and transmissible venereal tumor.

(2) Clinical presentation. The most common presentation is a middle-aged to older animal with a visible mass protruding from the vulva. Vaginal discharge or hemorrhage may be present.

(3) Diagnosis may be tentatively based on the clinical appearance of the lesion, although histologic confirmation is strongly advised.

(a) Transmissible venereal tumors are irregular, friable, and hemorrhagic. They must be differentiated from malignant tumors such as squamous cell carcinoma.

(b) Polyps and benign tumors are smooth and firm and are frequently pedunculated.

(4) Treatment

(a) Transmissible venereal tumors are treated with vincristine chemotherapy or radiation therapy, with or without concurrent surgical excision.

(b) Surgical excision is recommended for other tumor types, using an episiotomy to increase exposure if needed. Vulvovaginectomy and perineal urethrostomy may be required to remove large or malignant tumors. Because estrogen often stimulates growth of vaginal and vulvar tumors, especially fibroleiomyomas, concurrent ovariohysterectomy is recommended.

(5) Prognosis. Most vaginal and vulvar tumors are benign and respond to local excision and ovariohysterectomy. Malignant tumors tend to be locally invasive and carry the risk of early metastasis to regional lymph nodes.

2. Pyometra is a disease of the diestrual uterus.

a. Pathophysiology. Progesterone produced by the corpus luteum stimulates the endometrial glands, resulting in cystic endometrial hyperplasia and increased susceptibility to bacterial infection. The most common bacteria isolated are *Escherichia coli* and *Staphylococcus* species.

b. Clinical presentation

(1) Animals usually have a history of recent estrus or hormonal therapy.

(2) A serosanguineous or purulent vaginal discharge may be visible if the cervix is open. No discharge may be visible if the cervix is closed.

(3) Systemic signs of illness are common and include anorexia, depression, fever, polyuria and polydipsia, vomiting, and diarrhea.

c. Diagnosis

(1) Hematologic studies may reveal a leukogram indicative of inflammation, often with a degenerative left shift. Anemia and azotemia are not uncommon.

(2) Abdominal radiography and ultrasonography reveal an enlarged uterus, visible as a tubular structure of fluid density in the middle-to-caudal abdomen.

d. Treatment depends on the importance of maintaining reproductive function.

(1) Medical treatment. In **breeding females,** medical management has a 40% success rate in terms of permitting future term pregnancies.

(a) Prostaglandins are administered to stimulate luteolysis, decrease serum progesterone levels, and encourage uterine drainage.

(b) Uterine lavage may be necessary to facilitate drainage and to obtain samples for bacterial culture and antibiotic sensitivity testing.

(c) Despite appropriate antibiotic therapy and ancillary supportive care, clinical improvement may not be seen for 48 hours or more. For this reason, medical therapy may not be appropriate in critically ill animals.

(d) The recurrence rate is 70% within 2 years.

(2) Surgical treatment. If reproductive function is not essential or if the animal is severely ill, **ovariohysterectomy** is the surgical treatment of choice. Supportive fluid and antibiotic therapies are provided as needed.

3. **Vaginal edema (hyperplasia) and prolapse** are conditions of the intact cycling female.
   a. **Pathophysiology**
      (1) Vaginal edema results from excessive mucosal folding of the vaginal floor due to estrogen stimulation during the follicular phase of estrus.
      (2) Vaginal prolapse also occurs most commonly during estrus and may be caused by breeding trauma or excessive straining.
      (3) Because both conditions are more common in brachycephalic dogs, a hereditary predisposition has been proposed.
   b. **Clinical presentation.** Edematous mucosal tissue is seen protruding through the vulvar labia.
      (1) In vaginal prolapse, the tissue forms a donut-shaped ring with a patent opening in the center. The cervix and external urethral orifice may be involved.
      (2) In vaginal edema, the tissue originates from the vaginal floor.
   c. **Diagnosis.** Differential diagnoses include tumors of the vagina and vestibule. The presenting signs can be similar, and biopsy is recommended if results of vaginal examination are inconclusive.
   d. **Treatment**
      (1) **Medical treatment**
         (a) Mild cases of edema or prolapse regress spontaneously during diestrus. The exposed tissue should be protected from desiccation or self-trauma until regression occurs.
         (b) Vaginal edema has been treated medically with megestrol acetate or gonadotropin-releasing hormone administered early in the estrus cycle to prevent ovulation.
      (2) **Surgical treatment**
         (a) Vaginal prolapse can be treated by **manual reduction** under general anesthesia using **labial retaining sutures.** An indwelling urinary catheter is placed until the swelling subsides. Recurrent prolapse may require suturing the uterine body or broad ligament to the abdominal wall.
         (b) In cases of prolapse or edema with mucosal necrosis or infection, the **devitalized tissue is surgically resected** and the **vaginal canal reconstructed** with absorbable sutures. An **episiotomy** incision through the dorsal vaginal wall provides additional exposure if needed.
         (c) **Ovariohysterectomy** is recommended for recurrent cases.

4. **Clitoral hypertrophy** may occur in animals with disorders of intersexuality, or secondary to anabolic steroid administration.
   a. **Clinical presentation.** The hyperplastic tissue protrudes out of the labia from the vulvar cleft. A small bone **(os clitoris)** may be present.
   b. **Treatment. Surgical excision** is recommended if the tissue is causing mechanical irritation or for cosmetic reasons. Because the urethral opening is just cranial to the incision site, urinary catheterization is recommended to identify and protect the urethra. An episiotomy may be needed to improve exposure.

5. **Dystocia**
   a. **Etiology.** Both maternal and fetal factors can contribute to dystocia.
      (1) Abnormal fetal size, shape, or presentation increases the risk of birth canal obstruction.
      (2) Maternal causes include narrowing of the pelvic canal, abnormalities of the uterus and caudal reproductive tract, and primary or secondary uterine inertia.
   b. **Diagnosis.** Criteria indicating a need for veterinary evaluation include:
      (1) Prolonged gestation greater than 68 days
      (2) No contractions or delivery following placental separation (signaled by the appearance of lochia, a dark green uterine discharge)
      (3) Strong uterine contractions without delivery in 30 minutes, weak contractions

without delivery in 2 hours, or cessation of contractions without delivery in 4 hours

(4) A puppy or kitten lodged in the pelvic canal

(5) Signs of toxicity (depression, weakness, fever) in a pregnant animal

(6) Abnormal vaginal discharge (foul-smelling, purulent, or hemorrhagic)

(7) Radiographic signs of fetal death (e.g., intrafetal gas accumulation, collapse of the spine or skull), pelvic obstruction, or an oversized fetus

c. **Treatment**

(1) **Nonsurgical therapy** is reserved for cases of nonobstructive dystocia without complete or primary uterine inertia.

(a) Ecbolic agents (e.g., oxytocin) are administered to stimulate uterine contractions, decrease uterine hemorrhage, and promote uterine involution. Additional fluid and electrolyte support is provided as needed.

(b) A rapid response should be apparent if treatment is effective. If not, prompt surgical intervention will improve the chances of delivering viable offspring.

(2) **Cesarean section** is recommended for primary uterine inertia, mechanical or obstructive dystocias, and for secondary uterine inertia unresponsive to oxytocin.

(a) **Anesthesia.** Either general or regional anesthesia may be used—the decision is based on the patient's condition and the personal preference of the surgeon or anesthetist.

(i) Drugs and dosages should be chosen to minimize postanesthetic depression in both mother and offspring.

(ii) Operative speed is important because a long "anesthesia-to-delivery" time is associated with increased fetal morbidity and mortality.

(b) **Technique**

(i) Following a ventral midline celiotomy, each fetus is removed through a single longitudinal incision in the dorsal uterine body and passed to an assistant for resuscitation. The uterus is then inspected to ensure that all placentas have been removed prior to a double-layer inverting closure with absorbable suture material.

(ii) Oxytocin is given at surgery to stimulate uterine contraction. Persistent uterine hemorrhage may necessitate ovariohysterectomy.

d. **Postoperative complications**

(1) Hypovolemia and hypotension are treated with fluid replacement therapy.

(2) Agalactia may be an initial problem, but usually resolves within 24 hours. Oxytocin may help to stimulate milk production.

D. **Ovariohysterectomy** is the surgical removal of the ovaries and uterus.

1. **Indications**. Ovariohysterectomy is a common elective procedure to sterilize young females not intended for breeding. If performed before the first estrus cycle, it decreases the risk of future mammary gland tumors. If surgery is delayed past 2.5 years of age, this protective effect is lost. Other indications for ovariohysterectomy are:

a. Prolonged estrus resulting from ovarian cysts

b. Ovarian or uterine tumors

c. Uterine disease (e.g., metritis, cystic endometrial hyperplasia, pyometra, torsion, or prolapse)

d. Vaginal edema

e. Prevention of hormonal changes that interfere with therapy for diabetes or epilepsy

2. **Surgical technique**

a. **Approach.** Either a ventral midline celiotomy (centered between the umbilicus and pubis) or a paralumbar flank approach may be used. The midline incision allows better visualization and easier removal of the uterine body.

b. **Ligation of the ovarian and uterine pedicles.** The ovaries are exteriorized by stretching or breaking the suspensory ligaments.

(1) A three-clamp technique and absorbable suture material are used to ligate the ovarian and uterine pedicles, severing the latter just proximal to the cervix.

(2) If the broad ligament is vascular, as is often the case in older dogs, one or more ligatures should be placed prior to transection.

3. **Complications** of surgery include:
   a. Hemorrhage from the ovarian or uterine pedicles
   b. Recurrent estrus resulting from residual ovarian tissue
   c. Uterine stump infection
   d. Iatrogenic ureteral trauma
   e. Estrogen-responsive urinary incontinence
   f. Fistulous tracts and granuloma formation resulting from ligatures of nonabsorbable multifilament or nylon cable suture material.

VI. MALE REPRODUCTIVE SYSTEM

A. Anatomy

1. The **testes,** or male gonads, are located external to the abdominal cavity within the **scrotum.** Each testicle is secured to the scrotal wall by the parietal vaginal tunic and caudal ligaments of the epididymis. The other end of the testicle is stabilized by the spermatic cord and vaginal tunics.

2. The **epididymis** stores and transports mature spermatozoa. It is divided into three regions: head, body, and tail. The latter structure continues cranially within the spermatic cord as the **ductus deferens.**

3. The **spermatic cord** extends from the internal inguinal ring to the scrotum. It contains the ductus deferens, the testicular vessels (the veins of which form the **pampiniform plexus**), and the cremasteric vessels and nerves. Once within the abdominal cavity, these structures diverge to their various destinations:
   a. The ductus deferens empties into the prostatic urethra on the dorsal surface of the prostate.
   b. The testicular arteries originate from the aorta at the level of the fourth lumbar vertebra. The testicular veins drain into the caudal vena cava and left renal vein.

4. The **prostate gland** surrounds the proximal urethra and bladder neck in dogs. It is the only accessory sex organ in male dogs, and prostatic secretions provide a vehicle for spermatozoa. Although male cats have a prostate gland, prostatic disease in cats is rare.

5. The **penis,** the male copulatory organ, is divided into three regions:
   a. The **root** is attached to the tuber ischii by the ischiocavernosus muscles and corpus cavernosum.
   b. The **body** consists of the corpus cavernosum, corpus spongiosum, and proximal penile urethra.
   c. The **glans** contains the distal urethra and external urethral opening. In dogs, the glans contains the os penis, a small bone surrounded proximally by the bulbus glandis and caudally by the pars longa glandis.

B. Congenital disorders. Cryptorchidism, the most common congenital anomaly of the male reproductive system, is the failure of one or both testes to descend into the scrotum.

1. **Pathophysiology.** Cryptorchidism is believed to be a hereditary condition. The affected testicle may be found near the scrotum, within the inguinal canal, or within the abdomen. The higher temperature of this atypical environment results in degener-

ation of the germinal epithelium and loss of spermatogenesis. Endocrine function is minimally affected.

2. **Diagnosis** is based on palpation. Because testicular descent may occur at any time up to 6 months of age, a definitive diagnosis cannot be made before that age.

3. **Treatment.** Surgical replacement of the testicle within the scrotum (orchiopexy) is not condoned in veterinary medicine. Instead, **surgical removal** is recommended because the cryptorchid testicle has an increased risk of spermatic cord torsion and testicular neoplasia.
   a. Extra-abdominal testes are removed using standard castration techniques (see VI D).
   b. Abdominal testes may be removed using either a ventral median or parapreputial abdominal incision. Localization is aided by tracing the ductus deferens or testicular vessels.

C. **Acquired conditions**

1. **Prostatic disease** is most common in older intact male dogs, although it also may occur in neutered males. Prostatic disease is rare in cats.
   a. **Pathophysiology**
      (1) **Benign prostatic hyperplasia** is a change due to aging that is seen in male dogs under the influence of either testosterone or estrogen.
         (a) Prolonged exposure to testosterone causes **glandular hyperplasia.**
         (b) Exposure to estrogen causes **squamous metaplasia.**
      (2) **Suppurative prostatitis** occurs when bacteria colonize the prostate gland, usually via an ascending urinary tract infection. If left untreated, microabscesses develop and coalesce, resulting in **prostatic abscess.**
      (3) **Prostatic cysts** result from either ductal occlusion secondary to squamous metaplasia, or from increased secretion by glandular tissue. **Paraprostatic cysts** arise from the uterus masculinus, a remnant of the müllerian duct adjacent to the prostate gland.
      (4) **Prostatic neoplasia** may be primary or secondary to urinary bladder or urethral cancer. Transitional cell carcinoma and adenocarcinoma are most common.
   b. **Clinical presentation.** Clinical signs are usually the result of pressure on adjacent structures and may include:
      (1) Problems with defecation (constipation, tenesmus, dyschezia)
      (2) Urinary tract signs (hematuria, bleeding between urination, urine retention, urinary incontinence)
      (3) Locomotion problems (rear limb stiffness, lameness, or weakness)
      (4) Systemic signs of illness (depression, weight loss, anorexia, fever), especially if the underlying cause is infectious or neoplastic
   c. **Diagnosis**
      (1) **Physical examination.** Digital rectal exam provides information on prostate size, symmetry, texture, and mobility.
         (a) Symmetric prostatomegaly is associated with benign hyperplasia and prostatitis.
         (b) Asymmetric enlargement is more often found with cysts, abscesses, and neoplasia.
      (2) **Imaging studies**
         (a) Abdominal radiographs and ultrasound may reveal cystic areas within the gland as well as lumbar lymphadenopathy.
         (b) If neoplasia is suspected, pelvic and thoracic radiographs are recommended to screen for bone or pulmonary metastases.
      (3) **Laboratory studies**
         (a) Cytologic diagnosis may be obtained from urine sediment, ejaculation and prostatic fluid analysis, prostatic wash, or prostatic needle aspirate. Caution should be used with cysts or abscesses to avoid laceration of the gland and contamination of the abdominal cavity.

(b) Histologic diagnosis may be obtained either by ultrasound-guided percutaneous biopsy or at the time of surgery.

d. Treatment options

(1) Antibiotics based on the results of bacterial culture and sensitivity testing are used to treat bacterial prostatitis. The drug selected must be able to reach therapeutic concentrations within the prostate.

(2) Castration is recommended for hyperplasia and suppurative prostatitis to shrink the gland and decrease glandular secretions. **Estrogen therapy** has a similar effect, but carries the risk of bone marrow suppression and squamous metaplasia of the prostate.

(3) Marsupialization of the prostate gland is a surgical treatment for nonresectable prostatic cysts and large abscesses. In this technique, a fistula is created between the fluid sac and the abdominal wall for drainage.

(a) The stoma heals by granulation over several weeks.

(b) The primary complication is premature healing, which causes recurrence of the cyst or abscess.

(c) Concurrent castration is recommended.

(4) Subtotal (intracapsular) prostatectomy is indicated for multiple cysts and microabscesses. It is also a palliative therapy for prostatic neoplasia. The advantage of intracapsular prostatectomy over complete prostatectomy is that it spares the essential nerves and blood supply to the urinary bladder and urethral sphincter, located along the dorsal surface of the bladder neck and prostate.

(a) Approximately 80% of the diseased parenchyma is removed with electrocautery, leaving a dorsal strip of urethra as a bridge for epithelial regeneration. The prostatic capsule, with a thin rim of the parenchyma, is then sutured to prevent urine leakage (Figure 12–7).

(b) Postoperatively, a urinary catheter is maintained for 5 days to maintain bladder decompression and minimize stress on the suture line.

(5) Complete prostatectomy, while technically feasible, usually results in urinary incontinence. Urine leakage and urethral stenosis are also common complications. These problems, coupled with the poor long-term prognosis for prostatic neoplasia, limit the usefulness of this procedure.

2. Testicular tumors are common in older dogs but rare in cats. Multiple occurrence is common, with 50% of affected dogs having bilateral involvement. Undescended testicles are at increased risk.

a. Classification

(1) Seminoma is the most common neoplastic cause of scrotal enlargement.

(2) Sertoli cell tumors are the most common tumor in retained (cryptorchid) testi-

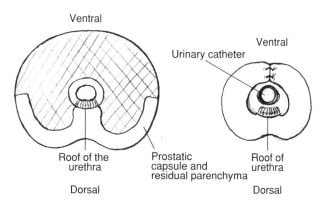

FIGURE 12–7. In an intracapsular prostatectomy, the ventral capsule and parenchyma are removed *(crosshatched area),* leaving a strip of urethral mucosa dorsally and enough capsule to close around an indwelling urinary catheter.

cles. They have the potential to metastasize and to produce estrogen, causing feminization and bone marrow toxicity.

(3) **Interstitial cell tumors** are usually small and asymptomatic, causing neither scrotal enlargement nor feminization.

b. **Clinical presentation**
(1) Scrotal swelling or asymmetry is detected by palpation of the testicles.
(2) Signs of feminization, seen with Sertoli cell tumors, include alopecia, hyperpigmentation, pendulous prepuce, penile atrophy, and gynecomastia.

c. **Diagnosis**
(1) Hematologic work-up may reveal signs of estrogen toxicity (thrombocytopenia, granulocytopenia, anemia).
(2) Metastastic disease may occur in up to 15% of dogs with Sertoli cell tumors, primarily by lymphatic spread.

d. **Treatment**
(1) Castration with removal of the adjacent spermatic cord is the treatment of choice.
(2) Prophylactic antibiotics, platelet rich plasma, and anabolic steroids may be needed in cases of bone marrow suppression.

3. **Penile injury.** Because of its exposed location, the penis is vulnerable to injury from bite wounds, strangulation, blunt and penetrating trauma, and breeding injuries.
a. **Clinical presentation** depends on the extent of injury.
(1) Hemorrhage is the most common clinical sign and may be intermittent or profuse.
(2) Dysuria and hematuria may be seen with rupture of the penile urethra or fracture of the os penis.
(3) Hair or foreign material wrapped around the base of the penis will result in a strangulated appearance, with tissue edema and pain and necrosis.

b. **Diagnosis** is based primarily on clinical examination. Survey and contrast radiography help define the extent of any urethral damage.

c. **Differential diagnoses** include **paraphimosis** (inability to retract the penis into the prepuce), **priapism** (persistent erection), and **penile tumors** (transmissible venereal tumor).

d. **Treatment**
(1) **Mild lacerations and bite wounds** are allowed to heal by granulation. Deep wounds with persistent hemorrhage require suture repair of the tunica albuginea and penile mucosa.
(2) **Fractures of the os penis** are treated conservatively with urinary catheterization and rest. Rarely, open reduction and fixation is required for unstable fractures.
(3) **Incomplete urethral disruption** also responds well to urinary catheterization and rest. Complete urethral transection requires anastomosis and postoperative catheterization for 2–3 weeks.
(4) **Severe trauma** with extensive infection or necrosis may require partial penile amputation or amputation with scrotal or perineal urethrostomy.

D. **Orchiectomy** (castration) is the surgical removal of the testicles.

1. **Indications.** Castration is a common elective procedure to sterilize young males not intended for breeding, or to modify certain male behavioral characteristics. Other indications include:
a. Cryptorchidism
b. Testicular neoplasia
c. Severe testicular or scrotal trauma
d. Chronic orchitis or epididymitis

2. **Surgical principles**
a. **Cats.** The testicles are removed through bilateral scrotal incisions. The spermatic cords are ligated with absorbable sutures or tied in a figure-eight knot.
b. **Dogs.** A single prescrotal incision is used in dogs. The ligation technique depends on the surgeon's preference and the size of the patient.

    (1) In a **closed castration,** the vaginal tunic is removed with the testicle. This technique causes minimal scrotal swelling and is used for dogs weighing less than 20 kg.

    (2) In an **open castration,** the testicle is removed through an incision in the vaginal tunic. The ligatures around the spermatic cord are more secure with this method. For this reason, this technique is recommended for large dogs or if the surgeon is inexperienced. Open castration is associated with an increased incidence of scrotal swelling and hematomas.

    c. If the scrotum is severely traumatized or necrotic, concurrent **scrotal ablation** is performed.

SELECTED READINGS

Allen SW, Mahaffey EA: Canine mammary neoplasia: Prognostic indicators and response to surgical therapy. *J Am Anim Hosp Assoc* 25:540–546, 1989.

Bjorling, DE (ed): Urinary System. In *Textbook of Small Animal Surgery,* 2nd ed. Edited by Slatter DS. Philadelphia, WB Saunders, 1993, pp 1368–1495.

Bjorling DE, Petersen SW: Surgical techniques for urinary tract diversion and salvage in small animals. *Comp Cont Ed Prac Vet* 12:1699–1708, 1990.

Bjorab MJ (ed): *Current Techniques in Small Animal Surgery,* 3rd ed. Philadelphia, Lea & Febiger, 1990, pp 367–430.

Gregory CR: Renal transplantation in cats. *Comp Cont Ed Prac Vet* 15:1325–1338, 1993.

Harari J, Dupuis J: Surgical treatments for prostatic diseases in dogs. *Semin Vet Med Surg* 10: 43–47, 1995.

Holt PE: Surgical management of congenital urethral sphincter mechanism incompetence in eight female cats and a bitch. *Vet Surg* 22:98–104, 1993.

Norris AM, Laing EJ, Valli VEO: Canine bladder and urethral tumors: A retrospective study of 115 cases. *J Vet Int Med* 6:145–153, 1992.

Stone EA (ed): Reproductive System. In *Textbook of Small Animal Surgery,* 2nd ed. Edited by Slatter DS. Philadelphia, WB Saunders, 1993, pp 1293–1367.

Stone EA, Barsanti JA (eds): *Urologic Surgery of the Dog and Cat.* Philadelphia, Lea & Febiger, 1992.

Stone EA, Mason LK: Surgery of ectopic ureters: Types, method of correction, and postoperative results. *J Am Anim Hosp Assoc* 26:81–88, 1990.

Withrow SJ, MacEwen EG (eds): *Clinical Veterinary Oncology.* Philadelphia, JB Lippincott, 1989, pp 283–324.

Chapter 13

Endocrine and Exocrine Glands

Elizabeth J. Laing

I. ADRENAL GLANDS

A. Anatomy

1. The paired, retroperitoneal adrenal glands are located cranial and medial to each kidney. The capsule of the right adrenal gland may be continuous with the external tunic of the caudal vena cava.

2. Each gland consists of an outer **cortex** and inner **medulla.** The cortex can be further divided into three functional zones. Each area is responsible for producing a different class of steroid hormone.
   a. The outermost portion of the cortex, the **zona glomerulosa,** produces **mineralocorticoids** such as aldosterone.
   b. The intermediate portion of the cortex, the **zona fasciculata,** produces cortisol and other **glucocorticoids.**
   c. The inner portion of the cortex, the **zona reticularis,** produces **androgens** and **estrogens.**
   d. The **medulla** produces the **catecholamines** epinephrine and norepinephrine.

B. Disorders treated by surgery

1. **Hyperadrenocorticism** (Cushing's syndrome)
   a. **Pathophysiology.** Hyperadrenocorticism is a systemic disease resulting from **excessive secretion of cortisol** by the adrenal gland.
      (1) The most common cause of spontaneous disease in dogs is **pituitary-dependent adrenocortical hyperplasia (Cushing's disease).** This bilateral condition results from increased production of adrenocorticotropic hormone (ATCH) by the adenohypophysis, because of either a pituitary adenoma or the oversecretion of corticotropin-releasing factor by the hypothalamus.
      (2) **Adrenocortical tumors** can produce large amounts of cortisol independent of ACTH production. Tumors may be benign (adenomas) or malignant and locally invasive (carcinomas). Bilateral tumors are uncommon.
      (3) **Iatrogenic hyperadrenocorticism** results from overtreatment with glucocorticoid medication.
   b. **Clinical presentation.** Because of the systemic effects of cortisol, many organs are affected.
      (1) **Polydipsia** and **polyuria** are the most common signs cited by owners and result from increased renal blood flow and from inhibition of antidiuretic hormone release.
      (2) **Skin changes** include bilaterally symmetric alopecia, hyperpigmentation, thin skin, and calcinosis cutis.
      (3) A **pendulous abdomen** results from hepatomegaly and obesity (caused by polyphagia).
      (4) **Muscle weakness** results from the catabolic effects of cortisol. **Myotonia,** with its characteristic stiff gait, occurs less commonly.
   c. **Diagnosis** is based on laboratory testing and radiography.
      (1) Laboratory findings suggestive of hyperadrenocorticism include neutrophilia, eosinopenia, lymphopenia, and elevated levels of alkaline phosphatase and plasma lipids. Hyperglycemia and glucosuria caused by concurrent diabetes mellitus occur in 10%–20% of patients.
      (2) Specific laboratory and radiographic tests are needed to confirm and localize the disease.
         (a) ACTH stimulation, low-dose dexamethasone suppression, and urine corti-

coid–creatinine ratios can usually confirm a diagnosis of hyperadrenocorticism.
  (b) Measurement of endogenous plasma ACTH concentration and high-dose dexamethasone suppression testing may help distinguish between pituitary-dependent hyperadrenocorticism and adrenal neoplasia.
  (c) Approximately 50% of adrenal tumors are calcified and can be seen with abdominal radiographs, ultrasound, or computerized tomography.
  d. Medical management is the treatment of choice for pituitary-dependent adrenal hyperplasia in dogs. It may also reduce the risks of complications associated with adrenalectomy when used prior to surgery.
  (1) Mitotane (*o,p´*-DDD) causes selective destruction of the zona fasciculata and reticularis. Because the zona glomerulosa is spared, mineralocorticoid production is usually not affected. Mitotane has also been used to treat malignant adrenocortical tumors in patients with metastatic disease to avoid the high morbidity and mortality associated with surgery.
  (2) Ketoconazole suppresses serum cortisol concentration and the adrenal response to ACTH in dogs. It is not effective in cats.
  e. Surgery is recommended for animals with adrenal tumors, for cats with pituitary-dependent hyperplasia, and for dogs with pituitary-dependent hyperplasia unresponsive to medical management.
  (1) Adrenalectomy is the surgical removal of one or both adrenal glands.
    (a) Approaches
      (i) A **ventral midline approach** allows access to both glands, as well as evaluation of the rest of the abdomen. The disadvantage of this approach is that surgical excision may be difficult in obese or deep-chested animals.
      (ii) The **retroperitoneal approach** uses a grid incision just caudal to the last rib. This approach provides better exposure of a single gland, but requires that the lesion be localized prior to surgery.
    (b) Dissection. Careful attention must be paid to **hemostasis** during adrenalectomy, and care must be taken to preserve the **blood supply to the adjacent kidney.**
      (i) Adrenal tumors can be vascular and invasive; hemostatic clips should be used as necessary.
      (ii) Thrombi or tumor invasion of the caudal vena cava requires venotomy.
    (c) Closure. Because hyperadrenocorticism can cause delayed wound healing, nonabsorbable sutures are used for wound closure to minimize the risk of dehiscence.
    (d) Complications
      (i) Mineralocorticoid and glucocorticoid deficiencies may develop rapidly after unilateral or bilateral adrenalectomy, necessitating exogenous supplementation. In the case of unilateral surgery, the remaining adrenal gland usually resumes function within 2 months.
      (ii) Other complications include fluid and electrolyte imbalances, hemorrhage, renal failure, pancreatitis secondary to iatrogenic trauma, poor wound healing, and infections.
  (2) Hypophysectomy (removal of the pituitary gland) is an alternate treatment for dogs with functional pituitary microadenomas or adenohypophyseal hyperplasia unresponsive to medical management.
    (a) Approach. A trans-sphenoidal (transoral) approach provides better access to the pituitary gland and is associated with decreased morbidity and mortality when compared to an intracranial approach.
      (i) Following transection of the soft palate, the sphenoid bone is trephined in the center of the sella turcica (a small depression on the dorsal surface of the sphenoid bone).
      (ii) This approach is complicated by the lack of reliable anatomic landmarks and by the variation in skull sizes and shapes. Placement of ra-

diographic markers and venous sinus angiography can help identify the trephination site.

    (b) Dissection. The hypophysis is extracted through a stellate incision in the dura mater, using suction ablation.

    (c) Closure. The ostectomy site is closed with bone wax or with a soft palate muscle graft.

    (d) Complications

      (i) Surgical complications including hemorrhage, iatrogenic damage to the hypothalamus or other adjacent structures, wound dehiscence, and infection.

      (ii) Complications resulting from decreased pituitary endocrine function include infertility and transient diabetes insipidus. Vasopressin is used to treat the diabetes, and lifelong low-dose supplementation with corticosteroids and thyroid hormones is usually required.

2. Pheochromocytoma is a functional tumor of the adrenal medulla that secretes catecholamines.

  a. Clinical presentation. Signs depend on the tumor size and on the type and frequency of catecholamine secretion.

    (1) Both α- and β-adrenergic stimulation can occur, causing restlessness, panting, tachycardia, cardiac arrhythmias, collapse, and sudden death.

    (2) Tumor invasion of the vena cava may cause obstructive ascites and edema.

  b. Diagnosis is based on clinical signs, radiographic or ultrasonographic evidence of adrenomegaly, and elevated levels of plasma and urinary catecholamines.

  c. Treatment. Adrenalectomy is the treatment of choice.

    (1) α- and β-**Adrenergic blockers** are administered **prior to surgery** to control hypertension and cardiac arrhythmias.

    (2) Because these tumors may be quite large, a **ventral midline approach** is recommended.

    (3) Postoperative complications include hemorrhage, hypotension, and persistent hypertension.

  d. Prognosis depends on tumor size and the degree of local invasion (e.g., to the kidney or vena cava). Recurrence is common and half of all patients eventually develop lymph node, liver, or lung metastases. A median survival time of 15 months has been reported.

II. THYROID AND PARATHYROID GLANDS

A. Anatomy

1. The **thyroid gland** is divided into two lobes, located adjacent to and on either side of the trachea, just behind the larynx. Many individuals also have ectopic thyroid tissue found along the midline from the hyoid bone to the base of the heart.

2. Two parathyroid glands are associated with each thyroid lobe: an **external parathyroid gland** lies in the fascia at the cranial pole of each lobe, and an **internal parathyroid gland** is embedded within the thyroid parenchyma.

3. The principal **blood supply** to each lobe is from the **cranial thyroid artery,** a branch of the common carotid artery (Figure 13–1). In dogs, the thyroid gland is also supplied by the **caudal thyroid artery.** Venous drainage is via the **cranial** and **caudal thyroid veins.**

B. Thyroid tumors

1. Dogs

  a. Clinical features

    (1) Most thyroid tumors in dogs are **malignant** and **nonfunctional.**

    (2) Adenocarcinomas, the most common histologic type, are characterized by

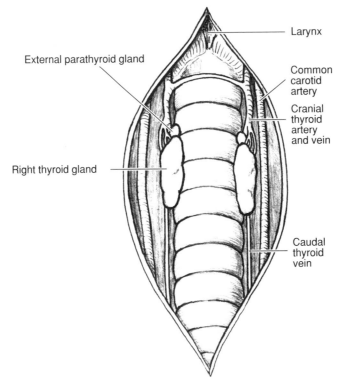

FIGURE 13–1. Ventral view of the cervical anatomy in a cat with bilateral thyroid enlargement. Blood supply to the glands can be quite variable. To ensure adequate supply to the external parathyroid glands, vessels should be ligated close to the thyroid capsule.

rapid and invasive growth (Figure 13–2). Metastasis to cervical lymph nodes and the lungs is common.
b. **Clinical presentation**
   (1) The most common sign is a **ventral neck mass.** Large masses may descend the trachea to the thoracic inlet.

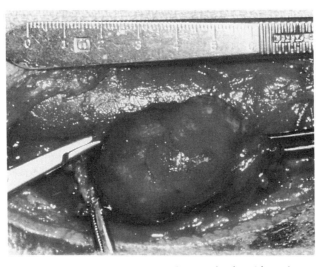

FIGURE 13–2. Intraoperative ventral cervical view of a thyroid carcinoma in a dog.

(2) Compression of lymphatic or venous drainage may cause **facial edema.**

(3) Respiratory signs (e.g., coughing, dyspnea) may result from pressure or invasion of the larynx and trachea, or they may be secondary to pulmonary metastasis.

c. Diagnosis

(1) Fine-needle aspiration of the mass may reveal neoplastic cells, although dilution by hemorrhage is frequent. A needle biopsy may be necessary if cytology is inconclusive.

(2) Thoracic radiographs and radioisotope scanning are useful in identifying metastatic lesions.

(3) Thyroid function should be evaluated in dogs showing signs of hypo- or hyperthyroidism.

d. Treatment. Surgical removal is the treatment of choice.

(1) Thyroidectomy is performed via a ventral cervical approach.

(a) Because the tumors are highly vascularized, **strict hemostasis is essential** to avoid serious blood loss. Careful dissection is required to avoid damaging the vagosympathetic trunk and the recurrent laryngeal nerve.

(b) Approximately 30% of thyroid carcinomas are bilateral, necessitating removal of both thyroid glands. After surgery, these animals are both hypothyroid and hypoparathyroid and require daily supplementation with thyroid hormone, calcium, and vitamin D.

(2) Supplemental therapy. Adjuvant chemotherapy (e.g., with doxorubicin) or radiation therapy may be beneficial when treating large or invasive tumors. In some cases these modalities may be used instead of surgery.

e. Prognosis depends on tumor size, type, and resectability. The median survival time following surgical excision is 7–8 months; however, animals with benign tumors or small carcinomas (< 7 cm in diameter) may have a better outcome.

2. Cats

a. Clinical features. Functional adenomas and **adenomatous hyperplasia** (Figure 13–3 are most common in cats; thyroid carcinomas are rare.

(1) These tumors produce excessive **thyroxine.**

(2) Bilateral involvement occurs in approximately 70% of affected cats.

b. Clinical presentation

(1) Hyperthyroidism results in tachycardia, hyperactivity, weight loss, polyphagia, diarrhea, polyuria, and polydipsia.

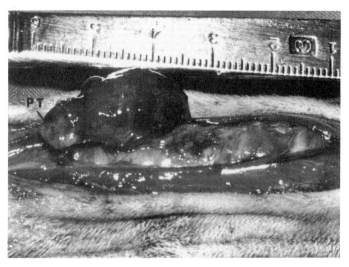

FIGURE 13–3. Adenomatous hyperplasia of the thyroid in a cat. The external parathyroid (*PT*) is cranial to the affected thyroid lobe.

(2) Less commonly, **apathetic hyperthyroidism** occurs. Signs include profound depression, decreased appetite, and muscle weakness.
(3) Secondary hypertrophic cardiomyopathy or, less frequently, dilated cardiomyopathy may produce signs of heart failure.

c. Diagnosis
  (1) Physical examination. Palpation frequently reveals a small, movable nodule adjacent or dorsal to the cervical trachea.
  (2) Laboratory studies
    (a) Elevated serum triiodothyronine (T_3) and thyroxine (T_4) levels are diagnostic.
    (b) The T_3 suppression test is used in cats that show clinical signs of hyperthyroidism but have normal or borderline serum thyroid hormone (T_3 and T_4) levels.
    (c) Other laboratory abnormalities include leukocytosis, elevated liver enzyme values, hyperglycemia, and azotemia.
  (3) Imaging studies
    (a) Radioisotope thyroid scanning, using technetium-99m, shows increased radionucleotide accumulation and enlargement of affected glands.
    (b) Cardiac ultrasonography is used to evaluate heart function in cats with suspected cardiomyopathy.

d. Treatment is aimed at controlling clinical signs by medication, by removing the hyperactive thyroid tissue, or by destruction with radioactive iodine.
  (1) Medical treatment. The goal of medical therapy is to restore the cat to a euthyroid state, either as primary therapy or to stabilize the patient prior to surgery.
    (a) Antithyroid drugs commonly used include methimazole and carbimazole, which block thyroid hormone synthesis, and propranolol, a β-adrenergic blocker that blocks the systemic effect of thyroxine.
    (b) Side effects of medical therapy include gastrointestinal upset, hematologic abnormalities, and hepatopathy.
  (2) Radioactive iodine (^{131}I) concentrates in and destroys the hyperfunctioning thyroid tissue. The parathyroids and atrophic thyroid tissue are spared.
  (3) Thyroidectomy, the surgical removal of one or both thyroid glands, is performed via a ventral cervical approach (see Figure 13–1).
    (a) Modified intracapsular technique. The thyroid parenchyma is separated from its capsule by blunt dissection. Most of the capsule is then removed, leaving a small piece attached to the external parathyroid gland.
    (b) Extracapsular technique. The external parathyroid gland is separated from the thyroid gland by blunt and sharp dissection, preserving the associated blood supply. Dissection is then continued caudally to remove the thyroid gland.

e. Complications
  (1) Hypocalcemia occurs in 6%–10% of cats undergoing bilateral thyroidectomy as a result of damage to the parathyroid glands.
    (a) Clinical signs of weakness, muscle tremors, and seizures usually occur if the serum calcium level drops below 6 mg/dl.
    (b) Calcium and vitamin D supplements maintain normal serum calcium levels until the parathyroid glands recover.
  (2) Cats undergoing bilateral thyroidectomy or ^{131}I therapy occasionally develop signs of **hypothyroidism,** necessitating thyroid hormone replacement therapy.
  (3) Cats with **concurrent renal insufficiency** may experience an exacerbation of clinical signs following treatment, resulting from decreased renal blood flow.

f. Prognosis. Depending on the age of the patient and the severity of hyperthyroidism and associated organ dysfunction (e.g., of kidney, heart, liver), prognosis ranges from fair to good. Regrowth of hyperplastic thyroid tissue has been reported in 8%–10% of cats undergoing either surgery or ^{131}I therapy. The average time until recurrence is 23 months.

C. **Primary hyperparathyroidism** is excessive secretion of parathormone (PTH), resulting in persistent hypercalcemia.

1. **Etiology.** Primary hyperparathyroidism is most often the result of a functional parathyroid adenoma; parathyroid carcinomas are rare. Parathyroid adenomas usually affect a single gland.

2. **Clinical presentation.** Signs result from hypercalcemia and include polydipsia and polyuria, listlessness, decreased appetite, and muscle weakness.

3. **Diagnosis**
   a. The most consistent hematologic abnormality is persistent **hypercalcemia** with or without hypophosphatemia. Chronic or severe hypercalcemia may cause significant renal impairment and azotemia.
   b. **PTH radioimmunoassay** may help to differentiate primary hyperparathyroidism from other causes of hypercalcemia.
      (1) Animals with primary hyperparathyroidism usually have increased PTH levels.
      (2) Animals with hypervitaminosis D or hypercalcemia associated with malignancy usually have low to normal PTH levels.

4. **Treatment. Parathyroidectomy,** the surgical removal of one or more parathyroid glands, is the treatment of choice.
   a. Animals in hypercalcemic crisis are stabilized prior to surgery with saline diuresis and corticosteroids.
   b. If the tumor is not readily visible at surgery, identification may be enhanced with intravenous administration of methylene blue, a vital dye selectively taken up by the parathyroid tissue. Methylene blue, which may cause Heinz-body anemia in cats, is contraindicated in this species.
   c. A ventral cervical approach is used. The external parathyroid gland is excised by gently separating it from the thyroid capsule. If the excision appears incomplete, or if the internal parathyroid gland is affected, concurrent thyroidectomy is recommended.
   d. **Complications. Postoperative hypocalcemia** is the most common complication of surgery. If signs of hypocalcemia develop, supplemental calcium and vitamin D therapy are given until the remaining parathyroid glands resume functioning.

III. PANCREAS

A. Anatomy

1. The pancreas comprises three anatomic regions.
   a. The **right lobe** lies in the mesoduodenum. Its blood supply, the **cranial pancreaticoduodenal artery,** is shared with the proximal descending duodenum.
   b. The **left lobe** lies within the greater omentum and is supplied by the **pancreatic branch of the splenic artery.**
   c. The **body** of the pancreas lies within the angle created by the pyloric region of the stomach and the duodenum.

2. The pancreas can also be divided into two functional areas, the exocrine and endocrine regions.
   a. The **acinar cells** of the **exocrine pancreas** secrete enzymes responsible for protein, lipid, and polysaccharide degradation. Although variations exist, the exocrine pancreas is usually drained by two ducts.
      (1) The **accessory pancreatic duct** opens adjacent to the common bile duct on the major duodenal papilla.
      (2) The more distal **pancreatic duct** opens on the minor duodenal papilla.
   b. The **endocrine pancreas** is composed of the **islets of Langerhans,** anatomically

distinct regions dispersed throughout the exocrine pancreatic tissue that produce and release hormones directly into the blood stream. Cell types with known functions are:

(1) **Alpha cells,** which produce glucagon
(2) **Beta cells,** which produce insulin
(3) **Delta cells,** which produce somatostatin in adults and gastrin during fetal development
(4) **F cells,** which produce pancreatic polypeptide

B. **General surgical principles.** Meticulous surgical technique and knowledge of the regional anatomy and underlying disease processes are essential.

1. **Access to the pancreas** is gained via a **cranioventral midline celiotomy.**

2. **Excessive tissue handling should be avoided** to prevent enzyme leakage.

3. **Suture material.** Nonreactive synthetic absorbable sutures (e.g., polydioxanone) or nonabsorbable sutures (e.g., nylon, polypropylene) should be used to minimize tissue inflammation.

4. In general, food and medication are not given orally in the immediate postoperative period. Rather, intravenous fluid and electrolyte supplements are used.

C. **Disorders of the endocrine pancreas treated by surgery**

1. **Insulinoma (pancreatic beta cell or islet cell tumor)**
   a. **Pathophysiology.** Beta cell tumors produce excessive amounts of insulin, resulting in hypoglycemia. These malignant tumors frequently metastasize to the liver and adjacent lymph nodes.
   b. **Clinical presentation.** Signs result both from hypoglycemia and from increased catecholamine release.
      (1) Intermittent weakness, disorientation, restlessness, muscle tremors, collapse, and focal or grand mal seizures are common.
      (2) Symptoms are often triggered by fasting or occur after events that stimulate insulin secretion, such as eating or exercise. The severity of signs depends on the rate, degree, and duration of hypoglycemia.
   c. **Diagnosis**
      (1) **Whipple's triad.** To confirm a diagnosis of **clinical hypoglycemia,** three criteria must be met:
         (a) spontaneous hypoglycemia
         (b) neurologic signs consistent with hypoglycemia
         (c) resolution of those signs with glucose administration
      (2) **Laboratory studies**
         (a) **Hematologic studies** are recommended to screen for other causes of hypoglycemia, such as hypoadrenocorticism, hepatic disease, glycogen storage disease, extra-pancreatic neoplasia, juvenile or hunting dog hypoglycemia, sepsis, and starvation.
         (b) **Immunoreactive insulin assay.** Diagnosis of insulinoma is confirmed by demonstrating elevated plasma insulin levels in conjunction with hypoglycemia. Blood samples are most likely to be diagnostic if collected during a clinical episode or after a prolonged fast.
   d. **Treatment.** Early surgical intervention is the treatment of choice.
      (1) Prior to surgery, serum glucose levels are stabilized with frequent feedings, supplemental intravenous dextrose, and corticosteroids.
      (2) To control clinical signs, the primary tumor and all metastatic lesions must be removed.
         (a) Lesions involving the left or distal right lobe are removed with a **partial pancreatectomy,** using a dissection and ligation technique or a suture fracture technique (Figure 13–4).
         (b) Lesions of the body or proximal right lobe are removed with **local excision** (enucleation) to avoid damage to the adjacent ductal and vascular tissue.

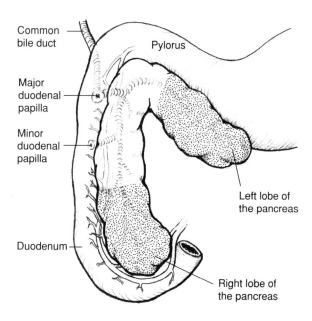

Common
bile duct

Pylorus

Major
duodenal
papilla

Minor
duodenal
papilla

Left lobe of
the pancreas

Duodenum

Right lobe of
the pancreas

FIGURE 13–4. Areas available for partial pancreatectomy are marked by *stippling.* Surgery in the body of
the pancreas is complicated by the bile and pancreatic ducts, and shared blood supply with the proximal
duodenum. Partial pancreatectomy may be performed by either bluntly separating the lobules and ligating
the ducts (dissection and ligation technique) or by encircling the gland with a monofilament suture that
dissects when tightened (suture fracture technique).

      (c) Methylene blue may be administered intravenously to identify both pan-
creatic and metastatic tissue at surgery. Methylene blue may induce
Heinz body anemia and should not be used in cats.
   (3) Complications
      (a) Persistent hypoglycemia indicates incomplete surgical resection and the
need for additional medical management.
        (i) Corticosteroids increase plasma glucose levels by stimulating hepatic
gluconeogenesis and interfering with insulin receptors.
       (ii) Diazoxide, a nondiuretic benzothiazide, increases plasma glucose by
inhibiting insulin secretion, increasing hepatic gluconeogenesis, and
increasing epinephrine secretion.
      (b) Transient postoperative hyperglycemia, resulting from the suppression of
normal beta cells, may require temporary insulin therapy.
      (c) Iatrogenic pancreatitis results from leakage of pancreatic enzymes at the
surgery site. The severity of pancreatitis may be minimized with gentle tissue handling, abdominal lavage during surgery, and withholding food
and water for 36–48 hours following surgery.
  e. Prognosis. Even with complete surgical excision, tumor recurrence is common.
The average survival duration is 18 months following complete excision, and 7–8
months following incomplete excision with persistent hypoglycemia.

2. Zollinger-Ellison syndrome (gastrinoma)
  a. Pathophysiology. These non–beta endocrine tumors produce excessive quantities
of **gastrin,** a hormone that stimulates secretion of gastric acid, resulting in gastric
and duodenal ulceration. Both pancreatic and extrapancreatic gastrinomas have
been reported.
  b. Clinical presentation. Chronic gastrointesinal ulceration results in vomiting, hematemesis, diarrhea, steatorrhea, anorexia, and weight loss.
  c. Diagnosis
    (1) Gastric ulceration is confirmed with endoscopy and biopsy.

(2) Radioimmunoassay reveals increased serum gastrin concentrations in conjunction with hyperchlorhydria.

d. Treatment

(1) Medical treatment. Gastrin secretion may be decreased by H_2 antagonists such as cimetidine and ranitidine. Sucralfate promotes healing of active ulcers.

(2) Surgical treatment. Removal of the tumor is the treatment of choice; however, the presence of extensive metastatic disease often precludes complete tumor excision.

(a) A **partial pancreatectomy** is recommended for animals that respond favorably to preoperative medical management.

(b) Total gastrectomy may be required for animals that have extrapancreatic disease or are unresponsive to medical treatment.

D. **Disorders of the exocrine pancreas treated by surgery**

1. Pancreatitis

a. Pathophysiology. Pancreatitis is characterized by premature activation and release of proteolytic and lipolytic enzymes, causing autodigestion of the gland. Inflammation of the pancreas may be acute, recurrent, or chronic.

(1) Dogs. In dogs, **acute pancreatitis** is usually self-limiting and associated with dietary indiscretion. Other causes include hyperadrenocorticism, glucocorticoid and other drug administration, thoracolumbar spinal cord disease, and trauma.

(2) Cats are more prone to **chronic, low-grade pancreatic inflammation,** with secondary parenchymal atrophy and fibrosis.

b. Clinical presentation. Vomiting, cranial abdominal pain, and diarrhea are the result of paralytic ileus. Varying degrees of weakness and depression occur, depending on the patient's fluid and electrolyte balance.

c. Diagnosis

(1) Hematologic findings may include neutrophilic leukocytosis, hemoconcentration, hyperlipemia, hypercholesterolemia, and elevated serum lipase and amylase levels.

(2) Abdominal radiographs may reveal increased soft tissue opacity in the region of the pancreas, displacement of the duodenum, and generalized ileus.

d. Treatment

(1) Medical treatment. The goals of medical treatment are to reduce pancreatic secretions and restore normal fluid and electrolyte balance.

(a) Oral food and water are withheld for 2–5 days, and fluids are administered parenterally to correct fluid and electrolyte imbalance. Total parenteral nutrition (TPN) may be required if the recovery period is prolonged.

(b) Glucocorticoid and antibiotic therapy are reserved for animals that are febrile or in endotoxic shock.

(2) Surgical treatment may be required for animals that deteriorate despite medical therapy, show signs of persistent bile duct obstruction, or show signs of secondary infection or mass lesions.

(a) Pancreatic necrosis occurs when inflamed areas of tissue become devitalized. While small areas of necrosis may heal spontaneously, large necrotic lesions require surgical **débridement and peritoneal lavage** to remove pancreatic enzymes and inflammatory cells. **Open peritoneal drainage** is indicated if **peritonitis is present.**

(b) Pancreatic pseudocysts are accumulations of enzymatic secretions, necrotic tissue, and blood that develop in areas of induration. Small cysts may resolve spontaneously. Large or persistent cysts require **surgical drainage.**

(c) Pancreatic abscessation develops secondary to necrosis or infection of a pseudocyst. Abscesses may be sterile or contain gram-negative or anaerobic bacteria. Treatment includes **débridement of necrotic tissue, perito-**

neal lavage and open peritoneal drainage, and aggressive supportive care.

(d) **Extrahepatic biliary or gastrointestinal obstruction** is treated as needed with **cholecystoduodenostomy, gastroduodenostomy** (Billroth I), or **gastrojejunostomy** (Billroth II) (see Chapter 10 III B 3, 4).

e. **Prognosis.** Recovery from mild, acute pancreatitis is usually uncomplicated. Severe or chronic inflammation may result in both endocrine and exocrine pancreatic insufficiency.

2. **Neoplasia of the exocrine pancreas**

a. **Clinical features. Adenocarcinoma** is the most common malignant tumor of the pancreas and may originate from either acinar cells or ductal tissue. These tumors frequently cause **mechanical obstruction of the adjacent duodenum and bile duct. Widespread metastasis** is common.

b. **Clinical presentation.** Signs are often vague and include vomiting, anorexia, weakness, and weight loss. Maldigestion and pancreatic insufficiency may result in bulky feces, diarrhea, steatorrhea, and signs of nutritional deficiencies. Icterus may occur secondary to extrahepatic bile duct obstruction.

c. **Diagnosis**

(1) Abdominal radiographs and ultrasonography may reveal a cranial abdominal mass.

(2) Definitive diagnosis is usually made at the time of exploratory surgery. Fine-needle biopsy can be used to differentiate diffuse pancreatic neoplasia from lesions of chronic pancreatitis.

d. **Treatment.** Surgical excision is rarely indicated because of the highly malignant nature of the tumor and the tendency for early metastasis. Surgical resection is only indicated for solitary masses without visible metastasis.

e. **Prognosis** is poor.

SELECTED READINGS

Birchard SJ, Sherding RG (eds): *Saunders Manual of Small Animal Practice.* Philadelphia, WB Saunders, 1994, pp 218–262.

Bojrab MJ (ed): *Current Techniques in Small Animal Surgery,* 3rd ed. Philadelphia, Lea & Febiger, 1990, pp 304–308, 431–437.

Bojrab MJ (ed): *Disease Mechanisms in Small Animal Surgery,* 2nd ed. Philadelphia, Lea & Febiger, 1993, pp 578–615.

Edwards DF, Bauer MS, Walker MA, et al: Pancreatic masses in seven dogs following acute pancreatitis. *J Am Anim Hosp Assoc* 26:189–198, 1990.

Ettinger SJ, Feldman EC (eds): Textbook of Internal Medicine, 4th ed. Philadelphia, WB Saunders, 1995, pp 1422–1603.

Gilson SD, Withrow SJ, Orton EC: Surgical treatment of pheochromocytoma: Technique, complications and results in six dogs. *Vet Surg* 23:195–200, 1994.

Kintzer PP, Peterson ME: Mitotane treatment of 32 dogs with cortisol-secreting adrenocortical neoplasms. *J Am Vet Med Assoc* 205:54–61, 1994.

Nelson RW, Couto CG (eds): *Essentials of Small Animal Internal Medicine,* 1st ed. St. Louis, Mosby Year Book, 1992, pp 525–608.

Slatter DS (ed): *Textbook of Small Animal Surgery,* 2nd ed. Philadelphia, WB Saunders, 1993, pp 678–691, 1496–1544.

Chapter 14

Ear
Joseph Harari

I. **ANATOMY.** The ear consists of three main portions: the external, middle, and inner ear (Figure 14–1).

A. The **external ear** is composed of the pinna and the external canal.

  1. The **pinna** may be upright or pendulous, depending on the size and shape of the **auricular cartilage.**

  2. The **external canal** is composed of the **vertical (lateral) and horizontal (medial) regions** and ends at the **tympanic membrane. Annular cartilage** surrounds the horizontal aspect of the external canal and attaches to the osseous **external auditory meatus.**

B. The **middle ear** is composed of the **tympanic cavity,** which is connected to the nasopharynx via the **auditory (eustachian) tube** and closed to the outside by the **tympanic membrane.**

  1. The tympanic cavity has a large ventral **tympanic bulla** (i.e., a ventral, hemispheric, osseous projection). In the cat, an incomplete bone septum divides the bulla into the small dorsolateral and large ventromedial compartments.

  2. The tympanic cavity contains the **auditory ossicles** and their associated muscles. The auditory ossicles connect the tympanic membrane with the **vestibular window,** which leads to the perilymphatic space of the inner ear.

C. The **inner ear** is composed of ducts filled with endolymph and chambers.

  1. The **cochlear duct** contains the **organ of Corti** and the **cochlear nerve.**

  2. The **semicircular ducts** are connected to the brain by the **vestibular nerve.**

II. **FUNCTIONS.** The ear has evolved as an organ of **hearing** and **balance.**

A. Hearing

  1. The external ear gathers and transmits sound waves to the tympanic membrane.

  2. The auditory ossicles transmit the vibrations striking the tympanic membrane to the vestibular window, which transmits them to the perilymphatic space of the inner ear.
    a. Movement of the ossicles produces cholear fluid flow, which generates nerve impulses in the inner ear that are transmitted by the cochlear nerve to the brain.
    b. Because the cochlea is embedded within the temporal bone, vibrations of the skull can produce fluid motion and perception of sound, explaining residual hearing capabilities in dogs following ablation of the external ear canal.

B. Balance

  1. Movement of fluid within the semicircular ducts stimulates cells, sending impulses to the vestibular nuclei, cerebellum, and brain stem via the vestibular nerve.

  2. Efferent signals are then sent to the spinal cord to stimulate and inhibit muscles in the extremities, thereby controlling equilibrium.

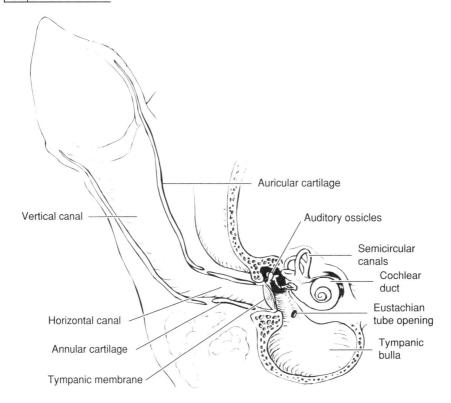

Vertical canal

Horizontal canal

Annular cartilage

Tympanic membrane

Auricular cartilage

Auditory ossicles

Semicircular canals

Cochlear duct

Eustachian tube opening

Tympanic bulla

FIGURE 14–1. Basic anatomy of the ear.

III. **SURGICAL PROCEDURES** are frequently performed on the pinna, external ear canal, and tympanic bulla.

A. **Pinna.** Surgery of the pinna includes **surgical drainage** and **resection.**

1. **Surgical drainage of aural hematoma.** Aural hematoma is an excessive collection of blood within fractured auricular cartilage.
   a. **Cause.** Aural hematoma is caused by auricular vessel trauma related to head shaking or scratching. Discomfort from otitis externa may be a predisposing cause.
   b. **Clinical signs** include a soft, fluctuant swelling on the concave aspect of the pinna. Chronic lesions become firm and fibrotic, and they may contract to produce ear deformation.
   c. **Treatment** is based on identifying the cause of the initial trauma and evacuating the hematoma. Needle aspiration and bandaging of the hematoma frequently lead to recurrence; hence surgical drainage is recommended.
      (1) Surgical drainage can be accomplished by use of **Penrose drains, teat cannulas,** or **silicone rubber drains.**
      (2) Hematomas undergoing fibrinous or fibrous replacement should be treated by excision of affected tissue and suturing to obliterate dead space.
   d. **Prognosis** is good if the underlying cause is identified and corrected, and the hematoma drained before fibrosis and tissue contracture occur.

2. **Resection and epithelial suturing of the pinna** is performed to remove diseased tissue resulting from environmental causes, trauma, or neoplastic diseases.

    a. Environmental causes include **solar dermatitis** in cats and **hypothermia. Treatment** involves partial pinnal resection of affected tissues.

    b. Traumatic injuries are related to **fight wounds, chronic flea or mite infestation,** and **self-trauma in pendulous-eared dogs. Treatment** involves suturing of fresh wounds or partial resection of necrotic tissues as well as treatment of the primary cause.

    c. Neoplastic diseases

        (1) In **white cats, squamous cell carcinoma** occurs on the tips of the ears and is associated with solar dermatitis. **Treatment** involves wide surgical excision to prevent recurrence.

        (2) In **dogs, mast cell tumors, basal cell carcinoma,** and **histiocytoma** are treated by resection.

B. **External ear canal.** Surgical procedures performed on the external ear canal include procedures performed on the vertical portion alone, or in combination with the horizontal portion.

    1. Surgical procedures performed on the **vertical portion** or the external ear canal include resection of the lateral wall and ablation of the canal.

    a. Lateral wall resection (Zepp procedure)

        (1) Indications

            (a) Lateral wall resection is indicated frequently for the treatment of **chronic otitis externa** that is unresponsive to medical therapy.

                (i) Predisposing factors for otitis externa include a combination of one or more factors: primary skin disease, foreign bodies, parasites *(Otodectes)*, anatomic characteristics (e.g., floppy ears, excessive hair), excessive moisture, and secondary bacterial invaders *(Staphylococcus, Proteus, Pseudomonas)*.

                (ii) Ventilation of the canal helps resolve chronic inflammation, and provides access for topical medication.

            (b) Lateral wall resection is also frequently indicated for the **removal of neoplastic or hyperplastic lesions** of the lateral aspect of the vertical canal. Abnormal proliferative tissue from the lateral wall can be submitted for histologic evaluation and diagnosis.

        (2) Procedure (Figure 14–2)

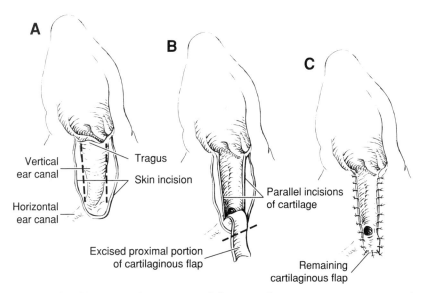

FIGURE 14–2. Lateral wall resection for treatment of chronic and recurrent otitis externa. *(A)* The skin, subcutaneous tissue, and cartilage are resected from the tragus to a level below the horizontal portion of the ear canal. *(B)* A ventral flap of the cartilage is attached distally. *(C)* The skin is sutured to the epithelium of the lateral wall to permanently expose the external ear canal.

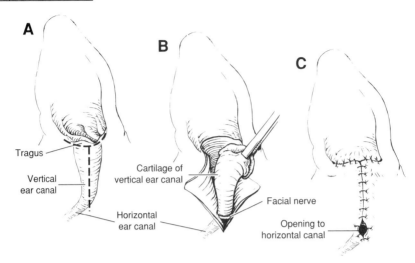

FIGURE 14–3. Ablation of the vertical canal for removal of hyperplastic lesions. (*A*) A T-shaped skin incision is made from the tragus to a point ventral to the horizontal ear canal. (*B*) The entire vertical canal is resected. (*C*) A permanent stoma is created for the horizontal canal.

        (a) Skin, subcutaneous tissue, and cartilage are resected from the tragus to a level below the horizontal portion of the canal.

        (b) A **ventral flap** or **"running board"** of cartilage is attached distally, and the skin is sutured to the epithelium of the lateral wall to create permanent exposure of the external ear canal.

    (3) Prognosis for recovery is good if predisposing factors are eliminated, there are no proliferative or occlusive lesions in the horizontal canal, and otitis media is not present.

  b. Ablation of the vertical canal is used for irreversible hyperplastic or neoplastic lesions of the lateral and medial walls of the vertical canal (e.g., ceruminous gland carcinoma or adenoma).

    (1) Procedure (Figure 14–3). The entire vertical canal is resected during ablation, and a **permanent stoma** is created for the horizontal canal. This type of surgery should not be performed in patients with lesions of the horizontal canal.

    (2) Ablation causes less postoperative discomfort and fewer complications than lateral wall resection.

2. The surgical procedure performed on the **horizontal portion** of the external ear canal involves ablation of the horizontal canal combined with removal of the vertical canal **(total ear canal ablation).**

  a. Indications for total ear canal ablation include:

    (1) Irreversible hyperplastic lesions, chronic bacterial infections (e.g., *Proteus, Pseudomonas, Staphylococcus),* or neoplastic lesions (e.g., carcinomas, sarcomas) that cause ear canal occlusion and pain

    (2) Failed lateral wall resection

    (3) Ossified cartilages

  b. Procedure (Figure 14–4). During total ear canal ablation, the vertical and horizontal portions of the canal are removed following careful perichondrial dissection.

    (1) All diseased **tissue remnants must be removed** to prevent recurrence and fistulation from infection or neoplasia.

    (2) The **facial nerve** located ventrally to the horizontal canal must be avoided to prevent postoperative facial paralysis or paresis (e.g., ipsilateral drooping lips or eyelids, decreased corneal or palpebral reflexes).

    (3) A **temporary drain** (e.g., a Penrose drain or rubber tubing for inflow/outflow) is placed in the deep subcutaneous tissues to reduce infection and accumulation of exudate.

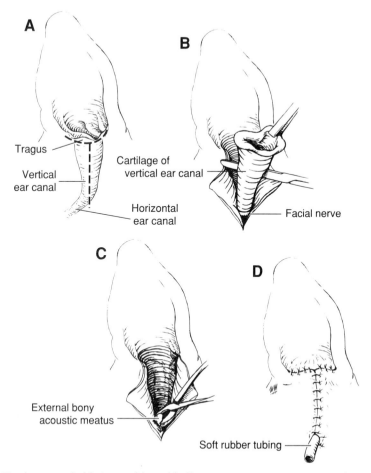

FIGURE 14–4. Total ear canal ablation and lateral bulla osteotomy. In most cases, total ear canal ablation is combined with bulla osteotomy. (*A*) A T-shaped skin incision is made. (*B*) The entire vertical ear canal is resected. (*C*) The entire horizontal ear canal is resected. (*D*) Soft rubber tubing is placed deep in the sub-cutaneous tissue and temporarily secured dorsal to the external bony acoustic meatus to reduce infection and accumulation of exudate.

    c. Prognosis following surgery is fair because of the technical demands of the procedure and complications such as recurrence of infection, nerve damage, and untreated middle ear infection. Total external ear canal ablation will reduce hearing (if present preoperatively), although sound may still be conducted through the bones of the skull.

C. **Tympanic bulla**

    1. Indications. Bulla osteotomy is indicated for **otitis media** resulting from chronic inflammatory, infectious, or neoplastic lesions.
      a. Lateral bulla osteotomy is frequently performed in combination with total ear canal ablation in animals with chronic otitis externa and media.
      b. Ventral bulla osteotomy is useful for diagnosis and treatment of bacterial infection *(Staphylococcus, Pseudomonas),* inflammatory polyps in cats, and carcinomas of the bulla.

    2. Procedure. In both surgeries, excessive dissection of the dorsomedian aspect of the bulla is avoided to prevent damage to the auditory ossicles and inner ear structures.
      a. Lateral bulla osteotomy is performed following removal of the external ear canal (see Figure 14–4).

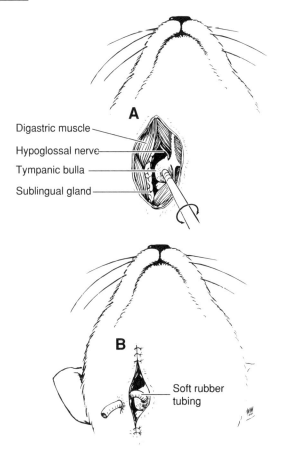

Digastric muscle
Hypoglossal nerve
Tympanic bulla
Sublingual gland

Soft rubber
tubing

FIGURE 14–5. Ventral bulla osteotomy for treatment of bacterial otitis media. (*A*) The bulla is penetrated with a Heinmann pin or bone trephine. (*B*) Soft rubber tubing is inserted to facilitate drainage.

     (1) The contents of the bulla are collected for histologic diagnosis and microbiologic testing prior to curettage and flushing of the cavity.
     (2) A drain placed within the bulla and exiting ventrally below the skin incision is useful for reducing infection and promoting healing.
  b. Ventral bulla osteotomy (Figure 14–5)
     (1) A **paramedian ventral cervical approach** is used to isolate the ventral aspect of the bulla.
       (a) The bulla is penetrated with a Heinmann pin or bone trephine.
       (b) The hypoglossal nerve and the lingual and carotid arteries should be avoided.
     (2) Tissue retrieval, curettage, and drainage are similar to the procedures performed in the lateral bulla osteotomy approach.
     (3) Care must be taken to avoid **damage to the sympathetic nerve supply** associated with the bone septum of the **feline bulla,** although both compartments need to be exposed and drained.
     (4) Resection of the base of **inflammation polyps** permits easy removal of lesions emerging through the external acoustic meatus or through the eustachian tube into the nasopharynx.

 3. Prognosis is good following removal of noninfectious or nonneoplastic lesions.
  a. Complications from surgical trauma include Horner's syndrome and inner ear disease (head tilt, ataxia, circling).
  b. Other complications include recurrence of infection or neoplasia.

SELECTED READINGS

Beckman SL, Henry WB, Cechner P: Total ear canal ablation combining bulla osteotomy and curettage in dogs with chronic otitis externa and media. *J Am Vet Med Assoc* 196:84–90, 1990.

Bojrab MJ: *Current Techniques of Small Animal Surgery,* 3rd ed. Philadelphia, Lea & Febiger, 1990, pp 133–150.

Gourley IM, Gregory CR: *Atlas of Small Animal Surgery.* Philadelphia, JB Lippincott, 1992, pp 3.1–3.7

Henderson RA, Horne RD: The pinna. In *Textbook of Small Animal Surgery,* 2nd ed. Edited by Slatter D. Philadelphia, WB Saunders, 1993, pp 1545–1576.

Siemering BH: Resection of the vertical canal for treatment of chronic otitis externa. *J Am Anim Hosp Assoc* 16:753–758, 1980.

Smeak DD: Surgery of the external ear canal and pinna. In *Saunders Manual of Small Animal Practice.* Edited by Birchard S and Sherding RG. Philadelphia, WB Saunders, 1994, pp 380–388.

Trevor PB and Martin RM: Tympanic bulla osteotomy for treatment of middle-ear disease in cats: 19 cases (1984–1991). *J Am Vet Med Assoc* 202:123–128, 1993.

Chapter 15

Spleen

Joseph Harari

I. ANATOMY

A. **Location.** The spleen is situated in the upper left quadrant of the abdomen, parallel to the greater curvature of the stomach. It is considerably longer than it is wide, and it has an irregular shape and firm consistency. In a contracted state, it is completely hidden by the caudal border of the rib cage. In medium-sized dogs, the spleen weighs approximately 50 g. In cats, the spleen varies in weight from 5–30 g.

B. **Structure.** The spleen consists of parenchyma (red and white pulps), an outer capsule rich in elastic and smooth muscle fibers, and a large, fibromuscular trabecula.

1. The **red pulp** is comprised of arterial capillaries, venules, and a reticulum filled with blood and macrophages.
   a. In **dogs,** the venous sinuses are closed, thus requiring blood cells to squeeze past adjacent endothelial cells and sometimes causing cellular fragmentation.
   b. In **cats,** the venous vessels are lined by endothelial cells that are pulled apart to create apertures, which permit cellular movement without deformation or destruction.

2. The **white pulp** consists of diffuse and nodular lymphoid tissue.

3. Between the red and white pulps is a **marginal zone** composed of vascular elements.

C. **Vasculature**

1. **Splenic artery.** The main blood supply is carried by the splenic artery, a branch of the celiac artery. It travels along the left limb of the pancreas below the stomach and divides into branches that penetrate the capsule at the hilus.

2. The **venous pathway** through the capsule parallels the arterial flow. Venous flow from the splenic vein and pancreas empties into the portal vein and, subsequently, into the liver.

II. FUNCTIONS.
Although not essential for life, the spleen has numerous functions including storage, filtration, immunologic response, and hematopoiesis.

A. **Storage.** Approximately 33% of the body's platelets and 10% of the total erythrocyte mass are contained in the spleen. Contraction of the spleen as a result of catecholamines raises the packed red cell volume in circulation, whereas barbiturates or sedatives promote splenic congestion.

B. **Filtration.** The most important function of the red pulp is removal of old or abnormal red blood cells.

1. **Selective filtration** occurs as fragile cells are trapped and fragmented during passage of blood through the trabecular network of the red pulp.

2. **Macrophages** lining the trabeculae remove abnormal blood cells and red blood cells with immunoglobulin G (IgG) or complement (e.g., C3b) on their surfaces. The blood eventually returns to the circulation by movement through the endothelial walls of the venous sinuses.

C. **Immunologic response.** The splenic parenchyma responds to blood-borne bacteria and circulating antigens.

    1. **Removal of bacteria and particulate antigens.** Bacteria and particulate antigens are removed by macrophages in the red pulp and marginal zone of the spleen.

    2. **Antibody production.** Antigenic stimulation of B lymphocytes in the white pulp results in specific immunoglobulin M (IgM) antibody production.

D. **Hematopoiesis** occurs in the spleen during fetal development and postnatally at times of increased erythrocyte demands.

III. SURGICAL PROCEDURES

A. **Biopsy.** Either percutaneous biopsy or intraoperative sampling during celiotomy can be performed.

    1. **Percutaneous biopsy** is useful in determining the cause of splenomegaly, although major complications such as hemorrhage, visceral perforation, tumor seeding, or abdominal sepsis can occur. **Ultrasonographic-guided fine-needle aspiration** performed on a sedated patient is technically easy, provides diagnostic information, and reduces the risk of morbidity or mortality.

    2. **Intraoperative biopsy** may be performed via an incision, a punch, or needle aspiration. Hemorrhage following incision or punch biopsy can be controlled with a combination of mattress sutures, absorbable hemostatic sponges, and digital pressure.

B. **Partial splenectomy** permits splenic functions to be retained, diseased tissue to be removed, and a histologic diagnosis to be obtained. Several techniques based on instrumentation and tissue handling have been described.

    1. **Digital compression.** The splenic pulp is compressed digitally and the flattened tissue is divided between forceps. A continuous suture pattern can be used to close the cut surface.

    2. **Through-and-through simple interrupted sutures** can be used to control hemorrhage or to isolate a lesion. The tissue is transected distal to the suture material. The cut surface is then oversewn with a continuous suture pattern.

    3. **Automatic stapling** devices can be used in a fashion similar to sutures.

    4. An **ultrasonic cutting device** and a **carbon dioxide laser** have also been used in performing a partial splenectomy.

C. **Total splenectomy** is performed following a ventral midline celiotomy. The abdominal incision must be large enough to permit gentle manipulation and removal of enlarged splenic tissue. Intrasplenic injection of epinephrine to reduce splenic size is not recommended because of the risk of cardiac dysrhythmia in gas-anesthetized patients.

    1. **Vascular ligation** with suture material or metallic vascular clamps can be performed at the hilus or at the level of the splenic artery, short gastric vessels, and left gastroepiploic artery distal to the vascular supply to the left limb of the pancreas.

    2. Following removal of the spleen, **hemostasis** of ligated vessels must be confirmed; and in cases involving neoplasia or sepsis, regional lymph nodes and the liver must be examined for evidence of metastasis.

    3. **Implantation** of splenic tissue into the omentum following complete splenectomy has been described, and may be useful in retaining splenic function in patients with splenic torsion or trauma.

D. **Postoperative complications** of splenic surgery include:

1. Hemorrhage and, rarely, ischemic necrosis of pancreatic or remaining splenic tissue

2. Exacerbation of blood-borne parasitemia (e.g., hemobartonellosis, babesiosis)

3. Reduced tolerance to hemorrhagic shock and strenuous exercise

4. Rapid ventricular tachycardia and low intraoperative arterial blood pressure in dogs undergoing splenectomy for tumors, torsion, and immune disorders

IV. CONDITIONS TREATED BY SURGERY

A. **Neoplasia** of the spleen is a common disorder of dogs and cats.

1. **Clinical signs** of splenic neoplasia include anemia, splenomegaly, nucleated erythro-cytes, hemoperitoneum, lethargy, and anorexia.

2. **Dogs.** Older large dogs, especially German shepherds, are most frequently affected.
   a. **Hemangiosarcoma** is the most frequent neoplasm of the canine spleen. The com-bined prevalence of all other splenic neoplasms (lymphosarcoma, leiomyosar-coma) is similar to that of hemangiosarcoma alone.
   b. **Treatment** of hemangiosarcoma by total splenectomy in dogs is palliative. The median survival time ranges from 2–6 months. Increased survival times following surgery and chemotherapy have not been reported.

3. **Cats**
   a. **Mastocytoma and lymphosarcoma** are the most common tumors of the spleen in cats. Disseminated disease is more frequent than solitary splenic lesions, thus lim-iting the usefulness of splenectomy for these conditions.
   b. **Treatment.** In cats with mast cell tumors limited to the spleen, splenectomy may increase the duration of survival. In cats with lymphosarcoma, a combination chemotherapy protocol (cyclophosphamide, vincristine, and prednisone) may be preferable to surgical treatment.

B. **Benign splenic lesions,** such as hemangioma, hematoma, and nodular hyperplasia, occur frequently. These lesions may be grossly indistinguishable from hemangiosarcoma. Long-term prognosis following splenectomy is excellent for dogs and cats with these con-ditions.

C. **Splenic torsion** is caused by twisting of the splenic pedicle and can occur in association with gastric dilation/volvulus or, less frequently, as a singular entity. Continued arterial flow and venous outflow obstruction produce **acute cardiovascular collapse** and **gastro-intestinal disturbances.** Thrombosis of splenic vessels causes **parenchymal ischemia and necrosis. Disseminated intravascular coagulation (DIC)** is an untoward sequela of the condition; therefore, surgical manipulation of hilar vessels should be minimized.

1. **Acute form**
   a. **Clinical signs** are progressive physical deterioration, cardiovascular shock, spleno-megaly, and abdominal pain.
   b. **Treatment** includes prompt fluid resuscitation, intravenous glucocorticoid ther-apy, and splenectomy following patient stabilization.

2. **Chronic form**
   a. **Clinical signs** include vague abdominal pain, splenomegaly, and recurrent gastro-intestinal upset. The patient may be anemic, neutrophilic, and hemoglobinuric.
   b. **Treatment.** An exploratory celiotomy may be required for diagnosis, and a total splenectomy should be performed.

D. **Splenic trauma** related to falls, motor vehicle accidents, or gunshot injuries can occur, although surgical intervention for hemostasis is rarely performed. Lacerations or tears usually produce slow, self-limiting hemorrhage.

    1. **Clinical signs.** In animals with acute, severe, and progressive blood loss, clinical signs include deterioration, hemoperitoneum, and possibly anemia.

    2. **Treatment.** Surgical treatment consists of vascular, parenchymal, or capsular suturing; partial splenectomy for irreparable tears; or capsular capping with synthetic mesh or omentum.

E. **Immune-mediated hematologic disorders** (e.g., thrombocytopenia, hemolytic anemia) are associated with splenic production of autoantibodies and destruction of platelets and red blood cells. These conditions may be primary or secondary to drugs, toxins, or other diseases and usually affect mature dogs.

    1. **Clinical signs** include pallor, splenomegaly, petechiae, and ecchymoses.

    2. **Treatment** includes total splenectomy in cases refractory to glucocorticoid or immunosuppressive drugs.

    3. **Prognosis** is guarded because of continued or recurrent hepatic and bone marrow phagocytosis and autoantibody production.

SELECTED READINGS

Bjorling DE: Spleen. In *Current Techniques in Small Animal Surgery,* 3rd ed. Edited by Bojrab MJ. Philadelphia, Lea & Febiger, 1990, pp 544–548.

Hosgood G and Bone DL: Splenectomy in the dog by ligation of the splenic and short gastric arteries. *Vet Surg* 18:110–113, 1989.

Hurley RE and Stone MS: Isolated torsion of the splenic pedicle in a dog. *J Am Anim Hosp Assoc* 30:119–122, 1994.

Lipowitz AJ and Blue J: Spleen. In *Textbook of Small Animal Surgery,* 2nd ed. Edited by Slatter D. Philadelphia, WB Saunders, 1993, pp 948–961.

Spangler WL and Culbertson MR: Prevalence, type, and importance of splenic diseases in dogs: 1480 cases (1985–1989). *J Am Vet Med Assoc* 200:829–834, 1992.

Spangler WL and Culbertson MR: Prevalence and type of splenic diseases in cats: 455 cases (1985–1991). *J Am Vet Med Assoc* 201:773–776, 1992.

PART III

ORTHOPEDIC SURGERY

Chapter 16

Long Bones

Joseph Harari

 ANATOMY

A. **Gross anatomy** (Figure 16–1)

1. The **epiphysis** is the articular end of the bone. It comprises compact and cancellous (woven, spongy) bone covered by hyaline cartilage.

2. The **physis** is the **growth plate** of long bones. It consists of five zones (see Figure 16–1).

3. The **metaphysis** comprises cancellous bone and a cortex of dense, compact bone.

4. The **diaphysis (shaft)** comprises compact, cortical bone and a medullary cavity.
   a. The **periosteum** (connective tissue) covers the cortex.
      (1) **Vascular elements** penetrate the periosteum at the nutrient foramen to supply the medullary cavity. Periosteal vascular supply and cellular elements are important in bone growth and fracture healing. **Haversian canals** (vascular channels) in the cortical bone run parallel to the long axis of the bone.
      (2) **Periosteal collagen fibers (Sharpey's fibers)** attach muscles, ligaments, and tendons to cortical bone.
   b. The **endosteum** is the internal connective tissue lining of cortical bone.

B. **Microscopic anatomy**

1. The **bone matrix** is composed primarily of collagen, glycoproteins, and hydroxyapatite crystals, which are responsible for the hardness of bone.

2. **Cells**
   a. **Osteoblasts** are located on the surface of bone tissue and are responsible for synthesis of the bone matrix.
   b. **Osteocytes** are mature cells found within the mineralized bone matrix that help maintain the bone matrix.
   c. **Osteoclasts** are located on the surface of mineralized bone and are active in bone resorption. They are often admixed with osteoblasts and osteocytes.

 BONE DEVELOPMENT

A. **Endochondral ossification.** Long bones develop by **osseous replacement of cartilaginous tissue.**

1. The **primary center of ossification** is the area in the central portion of the diaphysis where ossification begins.

2. The **secondary center of ossification** develops in the epiphysis to produce **longitudinal bone growth.**
   a. **Traumatic or hereditary disturbances of the physis (growth plate)** produce skeletal dysplasias (i.e., abnormal bone length, size, and shape).
      (1) Physeal injuries tend to occur in immature animals because of the weakness of the physis as compared with the joint capsule and adjacent ligaments. The **hypertrophic zone** is mechanically weak because of the large cell-to-matrix ratio in this region (see Figure 16–1).
      (2) A **Salter-Harris classification scheme** (Figure 16–2) based on the radiographic appearance of the fracture is useful for categorization of experimental animal or clinical human lesions, although it may not be an accurate indicator of

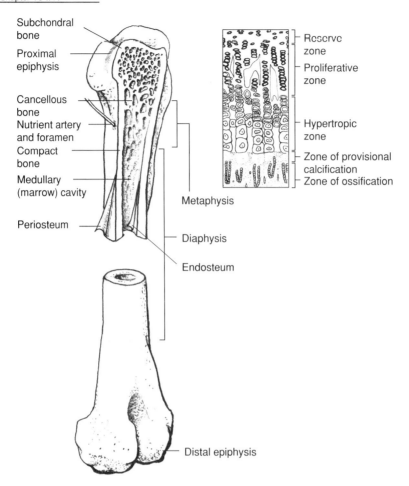

FIGURE 16–1. Anatomic subdivisions of a long bone and the histologic appearance of the physis (*inset*).

physeal injury at the cellular level or a predictor of prognosis in clinical veterinary patients. In general, **prognosis for continued growth** is enhanced by preservation of the epiphyseal blood supply and cells in the proliferative zone.

  b. **Normal closure of the growth plate** and **fusion of the epiphysis and metaphysis** occur in most long bones by 12 months of age.

B. **Intramembranous ossification** of the periosteum by osteoblasts is responsible for increasing the **diameter** of long bones. This process involves direct production of bone instead of cartilaginous replacement.

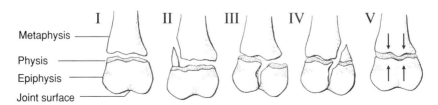

FIGURE 16–2. Salter-Harris classification of physeal injuries. Type I and II injuries occur frequently in the distal femoral physis. Note that type III and IV injuries are intra-articular fractures. Type V injuries are crush injuries.

III. BONE HEALING PROCESSES

A. **Primary fracture healing** is characterized by direct formation of bone under conditions of rigid stability and a minimal gap between the fractured ends.

1. **Mechanism.** Osteoclast resorption is followed by osteoblastic osteoid deposition and formation of a haversian system of canals surrounded by bone.

2. **Radiographic appearance.** Primary bone union is characterized radiographically by absence of a periosteal callus, disappearance of a fracture line, and continuity of the medullary cavity across the previous fracture site.

B. **Secondary bone healing** is associated with motion and gaps at the fracture site, even after stabilization of the fracture. Secondary bone healing involves the metamorphosis of granulation tissue into normal bone and is divided into inflammatory, repair, and remodelling phases.

1. The **immediate post-trauma inflammatory phase** consists of tissue damage, hemorrhage, vascular invasion, and cellular infiltration.

2. The **repair phase**, which lasts days to weeks, is characterized by differentiation of pluripotential mesenchymal cells to form a **fibrocartilaginous callus,** which unites the bone fragments. Local environmental conditions influence callus characteristics.
   a. When vascularity is poor and interfragmentary motion is present, fibrous union occurs. The greater the amount of interfragmentary motion, the larger the callus.
   b. When vascularity is abundant and interfragmentary motion is limited, osteoblasts proliferate and bone union occurs.

3. The **remodelling phase**, which lasts months to years, involves bone production and resorption of the endosteal and periosteal callus according to stresses and strains placed on the bone (Wolff's law).

C. **Abnormal bone healing**. Factors that contribute to abnormal healing include inadequate fracture stabilization, decreased osteogenesis at the fracture site, vascular impairment in osseous and soft tissue structures, and chronic infection.

1. **Delayed union** is prolongation of fracture healing, which can be demonstrated radiographically and clinically.
   a. Although **rates of union** have been described for fractures stabilized with pins and plates, variability of fractures, the severity of injury, and the health and age of the animal affect the rate of healing.
   b. **Treatment options** for delayed union include replacing the implant to increase stability, cancellous bone grafting to enhance fracture healing, infection control, and physical therapy.

2. **Malunion** is nonanatomic fracture healing resulting in cosmetic or functional defects.
   a. **Angular limb deformities** secondary to malalignment of fragment ends are most common. When the fragment ends are malaligned, the joints proximal and distal to the fracture are not in a normal anatomic or parallel relationship to each other.
   b. **Treatment** includes corrective osteotomy and stabilization with a bone plate or external fixator to realign joints and the limb axis.

3. **Nonunion** is the complete cessation of fracture healing leading to the formation of a pseudoarthrosis.
   a. **Types.** Nonunions can be biologically **active (hypertrophic)** or **inactive**. Radiographically, active nonunions are characterized by incomplete callus formation across a persistent fracture gap, whereas inactive nonunions show no callus formation and sclerosis of the bone ends.
   b. **Treatment** is based on the underlying cause.
      (1) **Active nonunions** require rigid stabilization using a compression plate or external skeletal fixation to convert the fibrous union to osseous consolidation.
      (2) **Inactive nonunions** require stabilization, compression, cancellous bone grafting, and rechannelization of the medullary canal to promote osteosynthesis.

IV. AIDS TO BONE HEALING

A. **Implants**. Selection of the proper implant (or combination of implants) is based on the type of fracture (see V A 1), the signalment of the animal, the technical expertise of the surgeon, the costs of the surgery and equipment, and the quality of postoperative care.

1. **Intramedullary pinning**
   a. **Indications**. Intramedullary pins are used to realign long bone fragments in simple or complex fractures.
   b. **Advantages**. Pins are readily available and **easy to place and remove**. A single intramedullary pin stabilizes the fracture(s) against bending forces. When three or more pins are used to fill the intramedullary cavity (**stack pinning**), the bone may also **resist rotation forces** and **shear forces** (Figure 16–3).
   c. **Disadvantages**. Variation in bone size and shape often limits the ability of pins to provide fracture stability. Pins protruding from bone (e.g., proximal femur) cause soft tissue irritation.
   d. **Equipment**
      (1) **Double-pointed trochar Steinmann pins** and **Kirschner wires** are used most frequently, especially in young animals. Kirschner wires, which are actually small pins, are used as intramedullary pins in small bones, and as components of auxiliary fixation devices (e.g., tension bands).
      (2) **Rush pins** are specialized, hooked, single-pointed pins. They are often used in pairs to stabilize metaphyseal fractures because of their ability to provide three-point fixation under tension (see Figure 16–6B).
      (3) A **pin chuck** is used to insert the pin, and **pin cutters** are necessary to trim the wires.

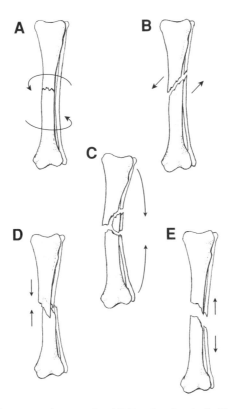

FIGURE 16–3. Distractive forces at a fracture site. (*A*) Rotation (torsion). (*B*) Shear. (*C*) Bending and fragmentation. (*D*) Compression. (*E*) Tension.

e. **Application**
    (1) Approach. An open or closed approach may be used to insert the pin into the medullary cavity to reduce the fracture and maintain stability.
    (2) Stabilization. In general, the pin or pins should fill 75% of the diaphyseal medullary cavity. Ancillary devices (e.g., cerclage wire, external fixation devices) are usually necessary to promote fracture healing by stabilizing fragments or major bone segments.
    (3) Removal. Intramedullary pins are usually removed after bone union has occurred (i.e., after approximately 1–3 months).
f. **Complications.** Inappropriate use can cause abnormal bone union, soft tissue injury, and limb dysfunction.

2. **Bone plating**
  a. **Indications.** A bone plate and screws are used to realign and stabilize bone fragments in simple or comminuted long or flat bone fractures.
  b. **Advantages.** Because bone plates can stabilize fractures by apposing (compressing) the bone, they provide a **quick return of limb function.** Bone plating **effectively counteracts all distractive fracture forces** and screws are used to appose small bone fragments.
  c. **Disadvantages**
    (1) Specialized training and equipment are required.
    (2) Extensive soft tissue dissection is necessary to permit plate application.
    (3) Second surgeries may be needed to remove broken plates, which can cause irritation, or excessively stiff plates, which can cause thinning of the underlying bone (a reaction known as **osteopenia** or **stress protection**).
  d. **Equipment**
    (1) Plates come in various shapes (e.g., straight, T-shaped, L-shaped, reconstruction) and sizes (e.g., large, mini, small, broad, narrow). Selection of a plate is based on the location of the fracture and the size and age of the animal.
    (2) Screws are used to anchor the plates. Occasionally, screws are used alone to stabilize long bone fractures involving traction physes or condylar fractures of the femur and humerus (see V A 3 a).
      (a) Screws may have cortical or cancellous threads and may be partially or completely threaded.
      (b) Selection of a screw is based on the size of the plate and where the screw will be placed in the bone.
  e. **Application**
    (1) Approach. An **extensive open approach** is used to isolate the bone shaft.
    (2) Plate application. The plate is usually applied to the **tension side** of the bone (i.e., the concave or distractive side).
      (a) Plates are contoured with bending irons or a press to approximate the shape and curvature of the bone.
      (b) Bone screws (at least three) are placed through the bone plate on either side of the fracture to provide maximum stability. Applying screws in a **lag** fashion (i.e., so that the threads of the screw only engage the far cortex) permits compression of the fragments.
    (3) Removal. Bone plates are removed from the long bones if they break and produce soft tissue irritation, are associated with infection, or produce osteopenia.

3. **Wiring**
  a. **Indications.** Orthopedic wires are used to encircle (**cerclage**) or penetrate (**hemicerclage**) the bone and provide fragmentary apposition. Wires are always used in conjunction with other implants (e.g., pins, bone plates).
  b. **Advantages.** Wires are **affordable** and **easily applied.**
  c. **Disadvantages.** Wires **require ancillary fixation** to provide fracture stability against bending and compression forces.
  d. **Equipment**
    (1) Orthopedic wire is available in a variety of gauges; selection is based on the size of the affected bone.
    (2) Wire tighteners are used to secure the wire to the bone with a twist or loop knot, and **wire cutters** are used to trim excessive lengths.

   e. Application
     (1) Approach. An open approach is necessary to isolate the segment of bone to be stabilized.
     (2) Wiring. Wires are placed across the fracture line, directly on the bone (to minimize soft tissue compromise).
       (a) Simple interrupted or **figure-eight** configurations are often used. In general, at least two cerclage wires are necessary per fracture to provide stability.
       (b) In **tension band fixation,** two Kirschner wires and a figure-eight flexible wire are placed across a fracture or osteotomy site to neutralize distractive forces.
     (3) Removal. Wires are rarely removed unless they cause soft tissue irritation or loosen and impede fracture healing.
   f. Complications. Fixation failure is most commonly associated with technical error (e.g., inappropriate application or selection of wire).

4. External skeletal fixation (see Figure 16–5 A–C)
   a. Indications. Percutaneous pins and external connecting bars and clamps are extremely useful for stabilizing long bone fractures (simple or comminuted, open or closed) in all ages and sizes of animals.
   b. Advantages
     (1) The **equipment is affordable, reusable,** and **adaptable** to various fractures.
     (2) Closed or limited open reduction **preserves bone and soft tissue vascularity** and **limits the incidence of surgical infection.**
     (3) The implant **does not interfere with treatment of extensive open wounds.**
     (4) Staged disassembly of the fixator stimulates **physiologic bone healing.**
   c. Disadvantages
     (1) Extensive postoperative patient care is required to reduce morbidity.
     (2) Externally applied devices **may be functionally and cosmetically unappealing to owners.**
   d. Equipment
     (1) Percutaneous pins are trochar-pointed and may be smooth or threaded to increase fracture stability. Pins are connected externally by **pin clamps** or grippers to **connecting bars.** Alternatively, percutaneous pins may be connected to **acrylic compounds.**
     (2) Hand chucks or **low-speed power drills** are used to place the pins in the bone.
     (3) Pin cutters are used to trim excessive pin length, and the pin clamps are tightened with **wrenches.**
   e. Application
     (1) Approach. A closed or limited open approach is used to realign major bone fragments as completely as possible. Functional anatomic realignment to preserve parallelism of the joints proximal and distal to the fractures is the goal with external fixation.
     (2) Pin placement. Pins are placed into the bone percutaneously, taking care to avoid muscle groups and the major neurovascular elements.
     (3) Fracture stabilization. External clamps are tightened or acrylic material is allowed to harden around the pins to stabilize the fracture.
     (4) Removal. Pins are sequentially removed as the bone heals during the postoperative period.
   f. Complications
     (1) Improper placement and care of pins can lead to **pin tract sepsis** or **delayed healing.**
     (2) Excessive postoperative patient activity can lead to **premature failure of the external fixator.**

B. **Bone grafts.** Cancellous and cortical bone grafts are used to enhance healing during fracture repair, arthrodesis, abnormal unions, and limb-sparing procedures (i.e., following tumor resection).

   1. Fresh, autogenous cancellous bone is used most frequently to provide osteoblasts for

osteogenesis, to serve as a trellis for incoming capillaries and osteoprogenitor cells (**osteoconduction**), and to stimulate via secretion of bone morphogenic protein host mesenchymal cells to differentiate into cartilage- and bone-forming cells (**osteoinduction**).

  a. **Harvesting.** Cancellous bone is harvested aseptically with a bone curette from the medullary cavity of the proximal aspect of the humerus, tibia or femur, or wing of the ilium.

  b. **Grafting.** Graft material is wrapped in blood-soaked sponges until delivery to the recipient bed, just prior to soft tissue closure and following lavage of the operative site.

2. **Cortical allografts** are used primarily to provide strength and mechanical support following fracture repair, limb lengthening procedures, or *en bloc* bone resection for neoplasia.

  a. **Harvesting.** Cortical allografts are harvested from donors of the same species. Harvested bone can be stored for up to 12 months in a bone bank.

   (1) **Freeze-drying and freezing.** Aseptic harvesting techniques of the long bones (humerus, radius, femur, or tibia) are necessary when freeze-drying or freezing is the preservation method of choice. Freeze-drying and freezing alter the biomechanical strength of the graft and are ineffective against bacterial pathogens; therefore, sterile technique during harvesting is important.

   (2) **Chemical preservation.** Aseptic harvesting procedures are not imperative when bone is preserved with ethylene oxide. Ethylene oxide does not greatly alter the osteoinductive and biomechanical properties of the graft, but concerns have been expressed regarding the safety of ethylene oxide sterilization in humans.

  b. **Grafting.** Because postoperative infection is a serious concern, cortical graft implantation requires strict aseptic conditions. Rigid internal fixation with a bone plate and screws and autogenous cancellous bone are used to enhance incorporation of the new bone.

3. **Other graft materials**

  a. **Nonbiologic grafts** (e.g., **hydroxyapatite, tricalcium phosphate ceramics, plaster of Paris**) have been used for osteoconduction and to extend autogenous cancellous grafts.

  b. **Heat-processed biological materials** (e.g., **coral, calf bone**) have been used for osteoconduction and reconstruction of bone defects.

V. CONDITIONS TREATED BY SURGERY

A. Fractures

1. **Introduction**

  a. **Causes of fractures**

   (1) **Trauma**

    (a) **Direct fractures** are those resulting from vehicles, firearms, falls, or fights.

    (b) **Indirect fractures** can result from excessive traumatic muscular contraction, which produces **avulsion of bone prominences** such as the tibial tuberosity or the calcaneal process.

   (2) **Pathology.** Fractures can occur as a result of underlying bone diease (e.g., neoplasia, infection).

  b. **Characteristics of fractures**

   (1) **Open versus closed**

    (a) **Open fractures** involve communication between the external environment and the bone. The degree of communication and associated soft tissue and bone injury are graded as **I (mild), II (moderate),** or **III (severe).**

    (b) **Closed fractures** do not penetrate the skin.

   (2) **Incomplete versus complete**

     (a) **Incomplete (greenstick) fractures** are characterized by a break in one side of the bone. **Fissures** are cracks in the cortex of one bone side.

     (b) **Complete fractures** involve a break through all of the bone surfaces and the medullary cavity.

        (i) A **transverse fracture** is a break perpendicular to the long axis of the bone that is caused by tension distractive forces.

        (ii) An **oblique fracture** is a break at an angle to the long axis of the bone that is caused by a compression force.

        (iii) A **spiral fracture** is a break that curves diagonally along the long axis of the bone; rotational forces are the usual cause.

        (iv) A **compression fracture** is a break that causes collapse and shortening of the bone.

   (3) Clinically, fracture patterns are often a result of a combination of destabilizing forces.

   (4) Fractures may be **single (simple), comminuted** (i.e., three or more fragments connected by fracture lines), or **multiple** (i.e., **segmental;** the fragments are not connected).

2. Scapular fractures occur infrequently because of the protection and support of the bone by medial and lateral musculature and the mobile nature of the scapula's proximal muscular attachments to the thoracic wall.

  a. Diagnosis. Obtaining the proper positioning necessary for radiographic evaluation is difficult.

  b. Preoperative considerations. In severely injured animals, brachial plexus nerve function, thoracic wall integrity, and cardiopulmonary status should be evaluated.

  c. Treatment

    (1) Minimally displaced fractures of the body, neck, or spine of the scapula can be treated with supportive external bandages (e.g., a **spica splint**).

    (2) Severely displaced fractures can be stabilized by **wire** or **plate fixation.**

    (3) Acromion and **supraglenoid tubercle fractures** are stabilized with a **tension band technique** using **wires** or a **bone screw.**

    (4) Neck and **glenoid cavity fractures** that affect the **scapulohumeral joint** are stabilized with a **small bone plate** or **Kirschner wires.**

3. Humeral fractures. Because of the proximity of the radial nerve, forelimb sensory and motor functions should be evaluated following trauma to the bone.

  a. Proximal fractures. Fracture-separation of the proximal humeral physis in young animals can be stabilized with **Kirschner wires** or **small pins** to realign the bone and shoulder joint (Figure 16–4A). **Partially threaded screws** can be used in animals with minimal growth potential.

  b. Shaft fractures

    (1) Characteristics

      (a) The majority of humeral fractures involve the **middle and distal portions** of the diaphysis.

      (b) Fractures of the diaphysis are **associated with considerable bone displacement** because of muscular contraction.

      (c) Diaphyseal fractures may be **simple or comminuted, open or closed,** and **transverse, oblique,** or **spiral.** Open fractures, which may result from vehicular or firearm trauma, are usually associated with severe soft tissue damage.

    (2) Treatment

      (a) A large **intramedullary pin** seated proximally in the greater tubercle and distally in the medial aspect of the humeral condyle can be used with cerclage and Kirschner wires, external skeletal fixation (Figure 16–4B), or transcortical screws placed into the pin (interlocking nails).

      (b) A **bone plate and screws** can be applied to the cranial (tension side), lateral, or medial aspect of the humeral shaft (Figure 16-4C) to **achieve precise anatomic alignment** and **maximum stability.**

      (c) Open, contaminated, or severely comminuted fractures may require stabilization via **external skeletal fixation.** External fixation preserves the vascularity necessary for healing and permits small fragment incorporation to serve as *in situ* corticocancellous grafting.

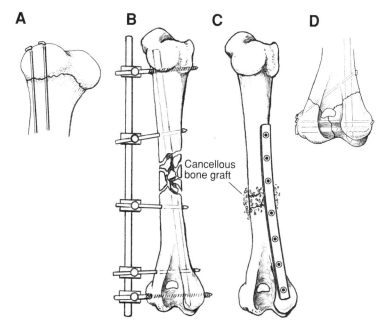

FIGURE 16–4. Fractures of the humerus. (*A*) A proximal humeral physeal fracture is stabilized with two large Kirschner wires or small intramedullary pins. (*B*) A highly comminuted humeral fracture is stabilized with an intramedullary pin and a unilateral (type I) external fixator applied to the lateral aspect of the bone. The proximal fixator pin is a positive profile threaded pin. (*C*) A comminuted midshaft fracture is stabilized with a bone plate applied to the medial aspect of the bone. Autogenous cancellous bone grafting has been used to enhance fracture healing. (*D*) A bicondylar (Y) fracture is stabilized with a transcondylar lag screw and Kirschner wire, a medial intramedullary pin, and a large lateral Kirschner wire.

  (i) Soft tissue débridement, wound drainage, and antibiotic therapy based on bacterial culture and antimicrobial sensitivity testing help control infection.
  (ii) Unilateral double bar frames or modified connecting bars across the cranial aspect of the bone can provide stability during the healing process.
 c. **Distal fractures. Supracondylar and condylar fractures** require open reduction to maintain articular cartilage alignment and elbow joint function. Cocker spaniels frequently have humeral condylar fractures, possibly because of a genetic predisposition for incomplete condylar ossification.
  (1) Supracondylar fractures can be stabilized with intramedullary pins, double Rush pins, or a bone plate applied to the caudomedial aspect of the condyle.
  (2) Unicondylar fractures occur more frequently along the lateral aspect of the bone than medially because of the smaller bone mass and greater weight-bearing status. A lateral approach permits stabilization with a transcondylar lag screw and epicondylar pin. If properly repaired, the prognosis is very good despite the articular nature of the fracture.
  (3) Intercondylar (T or Y) fractures require rigid and precise articular surface stabilization using a transcondylar lag screw and a lateral Kirschner wire along with a medial epicondylar pin or a bone plate (Figure 16–4D). A transolecranon osteotomy is performed to obtain exposure of the bone fragments and visualization of articular surfaces.
4. **Radial** and **ulnar fractures** occur frequently and are associated with significant clinical complications (e.g., elbow and carpal joint dysfunction, deformities resulting from abnormal bone union and growth).
 a. **Proximal fractures** include fractures of the olecranon, Monteggia fractures (i.e., dislocation of the radial head and fracture of the proximal ulna), and fracture-sep-

aration of the proximal radial physes. All of these lesions occur less frequently than fractures of the radial and ulnar shafts.

   (1) Olecranon fractures are stabilized with Kirschner wires and figure-eight tension band wiring or ulnar plating to counteract the distracting forces of the triceps muscles.

   (2) Monteggia fractures require suturing of the disrupted annular ligament between the radius and ulna; stabilization of the ulnar fracture with bone screws, a plate, or intramedullary pins and hemicerclage wires; and transfixation of the radius and ulna by bone screws or hemicerclage wires.

   (3) Radial physeal injuries are stabilized with Kirschner wires.

b. Shaft fractures can be open or closed, simple or comminuted, and transverse or oblique. Because the radius is the major weight-bearing bone of the forearm, ulnar fractures usually do not require fixation.

   (1) Greenstick fractures or **complete, stable fractures** can be treated with full cylinder casts, especially in young animals.

   (2) Closed or **open contaminated fractures** (comminuted, transverse, or oblique) can be stabilized with external fixators (Figure 16–5 A–C).

   (a) Applying distal traction to the paw during surgical preparation of the limb helps realign bone fragments.

   (b) Closed reduction, percutaneous application of pelvic reduction forceps, and a limited open approach to obtain cortical congruity are useful in reducing iatrogenic infection and avascular bone fragments.

   (c) Open, contaminated fractures should be stabilized and wound débridement and drainage should be performed. Delayed wound closure and cancellous bone grafting can be performed 5–7 days following the initial surgery.

   (3) Closed unstable fractures can be rigidly and anatomically reconstructed by applying a bone plate and screws along the craniomedial aspect of the radius (Figure 16–5D).

   (a) Plating provides quick limb restoration of function and is useful in patients with multiple limb injuries.

   (b) During open repair and bone plating, autogenous cancellous bone grafting is used to enhance bone healing.

   (4) Fractures of the mid or distal aspects of the radial shaft in toy or miniature dog breeds are associated with a high rate of nonunion. Contributing factors include a paucity of extraosseous soft tissue vascular supply, reduced bone marrow relative to cortical bone, and unstable fixation resulting from limited bone mass.

   (a) Small T-plates and autogenous cancellous grafting provide stabilization and osteogenic tissue.

   (b) Closed repair and external fixation provide stabilization without compromise of perosseous vascular tissue.

c. Distal fractures

   (1) Trauma to the distal ulnar physis occurs commonly.

   (a) Pathogenesis. Premature closure of the growth plate results in lateral deviation (carpus valgus) and external rotation of the carpus and cranial bowing of the radius as a result of the constrictive effect of the ulna on radial growth. Elbow joint subluxation resulting from a shortened ulna can also occur.

   (b) Treatment

   (i) In **young animals** with significant growth potential remaining, a **partial ulnar ostectomy** is performed to relieve the restraining effect of the bone on the radius.

   (ii) In **mature animals,** an **ulnar osteotomy** and corrective **radial osteotomy** are performed to realign the elbow and carpal joints along a more normal antebrachium axis. **External fixation** or **bone plating** is used to stabilize the radial osteotomy.

   (2) Trauma to the distal radial physis can result in asymmetric or symmetric closure of the growth plate.

   (a) Asymmetric closure most frequently affects the caudolateral aspect of the physis and causes carpus valgus.

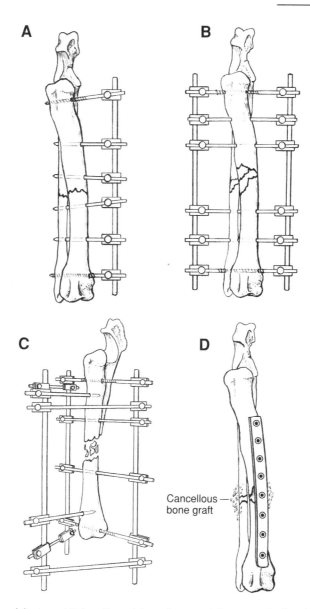

FIGURE 16–5. External fixators. (*A*) A unilateral (type I) external fixator applied to the craniomedial aspect of the radius. The most proximal and distal pins have raised threads; placement through the ulna aids in fracture stabilization. (*B*) A bilateral (type II) external fixator used to stabilize a comminuted, closed fracture of the radius and ulna. (*C*) A bilateral, biplanar (type III) external fixator is used to stabilize a comminuted, open fracture of the radius and ulna with major bone deficits. (*D*) Repair of a comminuted, closed fracture of the radius and ulna with a bone plate and screws. A cancellous bone graft has been used to aid healing.

       (i) In **young animals,** the closed aspect of the physis is resected and a fat graft is placed in the defect to permit continued radial growth.

     (ii) In **mature animals,** the angular deformity is treated with a corrective radial osteotomy similar to treatment for a closed distal ulnar physis.

  (b) **Symmetric closure** of the distal radial physis causes shortening of the radius, widening of the radiocarpal joint space, incongruity of the elbow joint, medial deviation of the carpus varus, and fragmentation of the medial coronoid process of the ulna.

       (i) In **young animals,** surgical treatment options include segmental radial ostectomy with fat replacement and external support; transverse radial osteotomy followed by distraction and bone plating; or osteotomy and continued distraction using an external fixator.

(ii) In **mature animals,** a spreading osteotomy and stabilization with a bone plate or external fixator can be used to realign the elbow joint. With mild radial shortening, a proximal ulnar ostectomy and stabilization with a single intramedullary pin can be performed to permit proximal migration of the radius and ulna; the ulnar defect has to be greater in length than the humeroradial incongruity.

(3) **Medial** or **lateral styloid fractures** cause collateral ligament insufficiency and carpal joint laxity. Open repair using Kirschner wires and figure-eight tension band wiring is useful for maintaining radiocarpal joint stability.

5. **Metacarpal fractures** usually require internal support with intramedullary pins, wires, or small plates if more than two bones are involved or fractures occur in the weight-bearing digits (i.e., numbers 3 and 4). Ancillary external support with palmar splints aids in the healing process.

6. **Phalangeal fractures** are usually treated by external support with palmar splints. Internal repair with wires or digital amputations (for nonhealing fractures) can also be performed.

7. **Femoral fractures** occur quite frequently in small animals. Surgical intervention is required to prevent displacement resulting from considerable muscle contraction and bone fragmentation. Hindlimb function depends on proper realignment of the bone segments, the quadriceps muscle axis, the patella, and normal ranges of motion in the coxofemoral and stifle joints.

a. **Proximal fractures**

(1) **Capital physeal fractures** and **dislocation** are stabilized with retrograde placement of Kirschner wires or a bone screw. Normograde application of small bone screws seated below the femoral head surface has also been described. Frequently, radiographic evidence of bone resorption occurs 3–6 weeks after surgery and may not be associated with clinical disease.

(2) **Femoral neck fractures**

(a) Stabilization can be achieved using a bone screw and Kirschner wire applied from a position distal to the greater trochanter. In cats and small dogs, multiple Kirschner wires are used to prevent rotational instability.

(b) Femoral head and neck excision is an option for chronic, comminuted, or irreparable fractures of the neck or head.

(3) **Avulsion fractures** of the greater trochanter in young animals are stabilized with Kirschner wires and figure-eight tension band wiring to neutralize the distractive forces of the gluteal muscles.

(4) **Subtrochanteric fractures**, which may be comminuted and involve the greater trochanter or femoral neck, are highly unstable. Fixation usually requires bone screws and placement of a plate along the lateral aspect of the bone in medium or large dogs, and multiple intramedullary pins and hemicerclage wiring in small dogs and cats.

b. **Shaft fractures** are usually simple or comminuted; transverse, oblique, or spiral; and closed (due to the surrounding musculature). Open repair involves stabilization using single or multiple intramedullary pins combined with wires or external fixation, or a bone plate and screws applied to the lateral (tension) surface of the bone (Figure 16–6).

(1) **External fixators** are applied unilaterally to the shaft and can be modified (connected proximally to an intramedullary pin, double lateral bars, or a curved connecting bar placed cranial to the thigh) to improve stability, although percutaneous intermuscular insertions in thigh muscles may limit postoperative patient mobility.

(a) Complications associated with intramedullary pinning include trauma to the sciatic nerve proximally and pin insertion into the stifle joint distally.

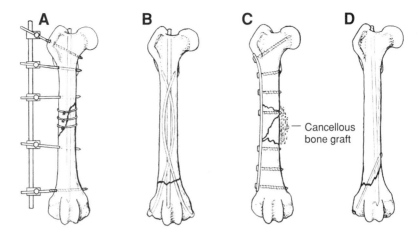

FIGURE 16–6. Fractures of the femur. (*A*) A long oblique fracture is stabilized with cerclage wires, an intramedullary pin, and a unilateral (type I) external fixator. (*B*) A supracondylar fracture is stabilized with dynamic intramedullary cross pins used in a manner similar to Rush pins. (*C*) A comminuted fracture is stabilized with a bone plate. Autogenous cancellous bone is placed in the fracture site to aid in healing. (*D*) A Salter-Harris type II fracture of the distal femoral physis is stabilized with a medially directed intramedullary pin and a large lateral Kirschner wire.

   (b) Transcortical screws may be applied through an intramedullary pin to provide interlocking stabilization.

   (2) Bone plating provides rigid stability and quick return of limb function, which is necessary to reduce morbidity in large, active dogs; dogs with multiple limb problems; or young dogs with severe bone and soft tissue injury that are likely to develop quadriceps fibrosis and extensor rigidity. In cats, thinner cuttable plates have been applied to the femur in a stacked fashion for stabilization of highly comminuted fractures.

   (3) Autogenous cancellous bone grafting is useful for osteogenesis and enhanced bone healing, especially for mature dogs or comminuted lesions.

 c. **Distal fractures**

   (1) Supracondylar fractures occur infrequently and are stabilized with cross and intramedullary pinning techniques (see Figure 16–6) or lateral plating, if enough bone is present distally to permit application of at least two screws.

   (2) Physeal fractures (most frequently Salter-Harris type I or II) affect the joint and require pinning, wiring, or the application of transcondylar screws (see Figure 18-18). The **goals of surgery** are rigid stability, establishment of articular cartilage congruency, and delicate tissue handling to preserve stifle joint function.

 8. Tibial and fibular fractures are frequently open injuries and the result of vehicular or firearm trauma.

 a. **Proximal fractures**

   (1) Avulsion of the tibial tubercle. Kirschner wires and figure-eight wiring are used to counteract distraction by the patellar tendon.

   (2) Physeal injuries are stabilized with multiple Kirschner wires placed peripherally to avoid interference with joint motion.

 b. **Shaft fractures.** The majority of injuries to the tibia and fibula involve the middle and distal diaphyses. Fractures of the fibula are rarely repaired because of its small size and lack of weight-bearing function.

   (1) Characteristics. Middle and distal shaft fractures can be open or closed; simple or comminuted; and transverse, oblique, or segmental.

   (2) Treatments for repair of tibial fractures include external coaptation (casts), external fixation, intramedullary pins and wiring, or bone plating (Figure 16–7).

     (a) Stable, minimally displaced, or **incomplete fractures,** especially in young animals, can be treated with a cast applied proximally to the stifle joint and distally to the digits. The full cylinder cast resists bending forces.

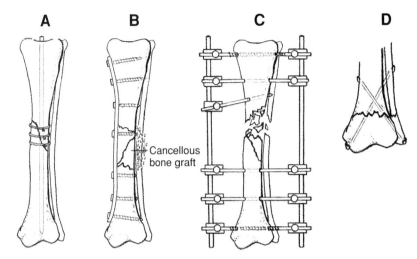

A   **B**   **C**   **D**

Cancellous
bone graft

FIGURE 16–7. Fractures of the tibia. (*A*) A long oblique fracture stabilized with an intramedullary pin and cerclage wires. (*B*) A segmental fracture repaired with a medially applied bone plate, screws, and cancellous bone grafting. (*C*) A highly comminuted fracture stabilized with a bilateral (type II) external fixator. (*D*) A distal tibial physeal fracture stabilized by two large Kirschner wires applied in a cross-pin manner.

      (b) Closed oblique fractures can be treated with intramedullary pinning and wiring. An intramedullary pin is applied normograde from a position medial to the patellar tendon into the proximal shaft to maintain stifle joint function and bone realignment.

      (c) Transverse fractures can be treated with an intramedullary pin combined with a unilateral fixator for rotational stability.

      (d) Highly unstable fractures in large animals with multiple limb injuries can be treated with bone plating and cancellous grafting. The plate is placed on the medial aspect of the bone (compression side); care should be taken to preserve the medial saphenous neurovascular bundle.

      (e) Open contaminated or comminuted fractures are frequently treated with bilateral or unilateral–biplanar fixators applied in a closed manner.

   c. Distal fractures can produce physeal fracture separation in young animals or malleolar fractures in adults.

      (1) Physeal injuries can be treated with external support if the animals are small and minimum displacement has occurred. In other cases, cross-pinning with Kirschner wires or small intramedullary pins is useful (see Figure 16–7).

      (2) Malleolar fractures require pinning and tension band wiring to preserve medial and lateral stabilities of the joint.

B.   **Developmental conditions**

   1. Hypertrophic osteodystrophy affects immature large and giant breeds of dogs. The cause of the condition is unknown.

     a. Clinical signs include recurrent pyrexia, inappetence, lameness, and metaphyseal swelling of the long bones in all four limbs.

     b. Diagnosis is by physical examination and radiographic findings, which include flared, irregular metaphyses, a radiolucent line below the physes, and periosteal soft tissue swelling.

     c. Treatment is supportive and consists of anti-inflammatory, analgesic medication; fluid and nutritional support; and avoidance of dietary mineral and vitamin supplementation.

     d. Prognosis is good for animals that are not severely affected. Permanent bone deformations may occur, although they may not be clinically significant.

   2. Osteochondromatosis is a proliferative disease of bone and cartilage that affects young dogs and cats.

     a. Etiology. Abnormal development of the periphery of the growth plate produces exostoses perpendicular to the long axis of the bone.

   b. **Clinical signs** of limb pain are mild unless adjacent soft tissue structures are compressed during phases of active bone growth.
   c. **Diagnosis** is by **radiography**, which reveals multiple radiopaque bone densities along the long bones, ribs, and vertebrae. **Biopsy** is also useful and reveals normal bone capped with hyaline cartilage.
   d. **Treatment.** Surgical resection is only necessary for compressive lesions. Animals should be neutered because of the heritable nature of the condition.
   e. **Prognosis** in dogs is good; in cats, progressive growth of the lesions following skeletal maturity and malignant transformation portend a poor outcome.

3. **Osteochondrosis** is a disturbance of endochondral ossification that affects rapidly growing medium- and large-sized dogs, more frequently males than females (see also Chapter 18 IV A).
   a. **Pathophysiology and characteristic lesions.** As a result of a failure of cartilage cells to differentiate, vascular penetration, chondroclastic activity, and subsequent resorption of cartilage cease. The remaining cartilage continues to thicken and weakens in response to stress or trauma because diffusion and metabolism of nutrients from synovial fluid are disturbed. Cartilage weakness and necrosis lead to fissures and **cartilage flaps (osteochondritis dissecans, OCD).**
      (1) **OCD** can be bilateral and is seen on the humeral head, medial humeral condyle, lateral femoral condyle, and medial ridge of the talus.
      (2) **Ununited anconeal process (UAP)** and **fragmented medial coronoid process (FMCP) of the ulna** (see Chapter 18 IV B 2) are considered manifestations of osteochondrosis by some veterinarians. Others attribute the association of OCD, FMCP, and UAP to articular incongruity; in general, most clinicians regard the three diseases within the framework of elbow dysplasia.
   b. **Clinical signs**, which usually become apparent when the animal reaches 4–12 months of age, are related to the location of the lesion and include limb lameness and joint swelling.
   c. **Diagnosis** is based on clinical examination and radiography of affected joints (see Chapter 18 IV A; Figure 18–2).
      (1) **Radiography** reveals flattening of subchondral bone, joint effusion, osteochondral joint fragments, and osteophyte formation.
      (2) **Arthrography** using aqueous iodinated solutions is useful for delineating dissecting cartilage lesions and flaps.
      (3) **Arthrocentesis** may reveal slight elevations in fluid volume and white blood cell count.
   d. **Treatment**
      (1) **Surgical treatment**
         (a) Resection of cartilage flaps or removal of osteochondral fragments (joint mice) and curettage or drilling (forage) of subchondral bone to stimulate bleeding and fibrocartilage formation in the articular defect is the most frequently used approach. If a dog has concurrent bilateral disease, both limbs can be operated on at the same time, or the procedure can be staged over a 4–6-week period.
         (b) Reattachment of flaps using tissue adhesive or small pins has also been attempted.
      (2) **Medical treatment.** Operative and nonoperative patients with osteochondroses may benefit from nonsteroidal anti-inflammatory medications or joint fluid modifiers (e.g., glycosaminoglycans, hyaluronic acid), although definitive clinical data regarding these therapies are still lacking.
   e. **Prognosis** is variable and depends on the location of the lesion (see Chapter 18 IV A).

4. **Panosteitis** is a spontaneously occurring self-limiting disease of young, large- or giant-breed dogs. The condition is characterized by medullary adipose cellular degeneration and osteoid production by stromal cells lining vascular sinusoids.
   a. **Clinical signs** include pyrexia; recurrent, shifting limb lameness; and pain evident on palpation of long bones.
   b. **Diagnosis** is by clinical signs, signalment, and radiography, which reveals in-

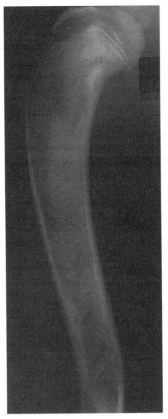

FIGURE 16–8. Panosteitis of the humerus in an 8-month-old German shepherd. Note the mottled, increased densities within the medullary cavity and the irregular endosteal surface.

creased multifocal densities of the medullary cavities and roughened endosteal surfaces of the long bones (Figure 16–8).

   c. **Treatment** consists of medication with anti-inflammatory agents, although many animals recover without the need for therapy. High-calorie diets and mineral supplementation should be avoided.

   d. **Prognosis** for recovery is excellent once animals reach maturity and the cyclical nature of the disease is passed.

  5. Retained ulnar cartilage cores affect the distal ulnar metaphysis in giant-breed dogs.

   a. **Etiology and pathophysiology.** The cause of the condition is unknown, although the pathophysiology involves accumulation of hypertrophied cartilage cells with a failure of matrix calcification (osteochondrosis).

   b. **Clinical signs** may be inapparent. Forelimb deviation (carpus valgus) and cranial bowing of the radius may result from ulnar restriction of radial growth, loss of lateral carpal support, or both.

   c. **Diagnosis** is based on the radiographic appearance of a central, radiolucent, longitudinal cone in the distal ulnar metaphysis with sclerotic margins.

   d. **Treatment** consists of an **ulnar ostectomy** in young dogs with moderate deformity or corrective **radial** and **ulnar ostectomies** in mature animals with deformity. The aim of surgery is to reduce the constrictive effects of the ulna on radial growth and function [see V A 4 c (1) (b) (i)].

   e. **Prognosis** is good for animals with mild or moderate deformations.

  6. Legg-Calvé-Perthes disease (aseptic necrosis of the femoral head) affects young, miniature- and small-breed dogs.

   a. **Etiology and pathogenesis.** The cause of the condition is unknown. Ischemic bone necrosis and repeated pressure cause collapse and deformation of the femoral head and neck.

b. **Clinical signs** include hindlimb lameness, muscle atrophy, and a reduced range of motion in affected hip joints.

c. **Diagnosis** is by signalment, clinical signs, and radiographic evidence of increased joint space width (the result of collapse and thickening of the femoral head and neck). Irregular density of the femoral epiphyseal and metaphyseal regions is also seen.

d. **Treatment** is **femoral head and neck excision** followed by physical therapy and the administration of nonsteroidal anti-inflammatory drugs to encourage return of limb function (see Chapter 18).

e. **Prognosis** for recovery is good.

C. **Osteomyelitis** is inflammation of the medullary cavity, cortex, and periosteum of the bone.

1. **Etiology**

a. Osteomyelitis is most frequently associated with **bacterial infection** (e.g., by *Staphylococcus intermedius, Escherichia coli, Streptococcus, Proteus, Pasteurella, Pseudomonas,* or *Bacteroides*). Sources of bacterial invasion include open, traumatic injuries, prolonged surgical procedures, extension from adjacent tissue, or systemic illness (bacteremia). Implant-associated biofilm or cement may protect bacteria, leading to a deep-seated ("cryptic") infection.

b. **Fungal agents** such as *Blastomyces dermatitidis, Histoplasma capsulatum, Cryptococcus neoformans,* and *Aspergillus fumigatus* are less frequently implicated; these fungi are only found in certain parts of the United States.

2. **Pathophysiology.** The pathophysiology of osteomyelitis is based on **bacterial invasion, vascular stasis, focal accumulation of inflammatory cells, release of degradative enzymes,** and subsequent bone **necrosis.** Abscessation may produce dead segments of bone **(sequestrum)** surrounded by reactive, vascular bone **(involucrum)** attempting to wall off the infection.

3. **Clinical signs** may reflect acute or chronic diseases.

a. **Acute osteomyelitis.** Initial signs include focal pain, swelling, excessive tissue warmth, and lameness. Depression, anorexia, and a persistent fever (greater than 104°F) may occur. Seepage (serosanguineous to purulent) may be seen at the surgical incision or traumatic wound.

b. **Chronic osteomyelitis.** Persistent lameness, muscle atrophy, pain at the surgery site, and multiple draining tracts are seen. Periodic episodes of depression, anorexia, and pyrexia may occur.

4. **Diagnosis** of osteomyelitis is by clinical signs and history, radiography, and microbial evaluation of infected tissues. Hematologic tests may reveal leukocytosis or anemia resulting from chronic inflammation.

a. **Radiographic examinations** may reveal soft tissue swelling within the first 10 days, whereas bone changes such as lysis, irregular periosteal reaction, and loose implants develop later (Figure 16–9). A sequestrum may appear as radiodense bone surrounded by a zone of lucency and sclerotic reactive bone.

(1) **Fistulography** can be performed to outline the location and source of fistulous tracts.

(2) **Nuclear scintigraphy** may demonstrate excessive uptake of the radioisotope because of acute inflammation early in the course of disease.

b. **Deep, fine-needle aspiration** or **biopsy** is extremely valuable in confirming the diagnosis. Bacterial culture (aerobic and anaerobic) and antimicrobial sensitivity testing of the sample are useful for establishing appropriate therapy. In patients with systemic illness, serial blood cultures should also be obtained.

5. **Treatment**

a. **Antibiotic treatment.** Long-term therapy (4–6 weeks) with antibiotics is necessary.

(1) **Agents.** Antibiotics commonly used against bacterial osteomyelitis include

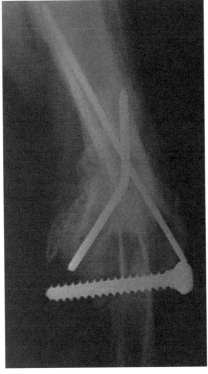

FIGURE 16–9. Chronic osteomyelitis in a 5-year-old cocker spaniel 4 weeks following repair of humeral condylar and epicondylar fractures. An irregular periosteal reaction, bone lysis, and implant failure are evident.

cephalosporins, fluoroquinolones, clindamycin, cloxacillin, and amoxicillin–clavulanate.

    (2) **Administration.** Local sustained delivery of antibiotics via antimicrobial-impregnated polymethyl methacrylate beads may be a clinical option in chronic, deep-seated infections; this delivery form also reduces the undesirable systemic effects of drugs such as gentamicin (e.g., nephrotoxicity).

  b. **Surgical treatment** involves removal of dead bone, necrotic soft tissue, and loose implants; lavage and drainage of abscessed tissue; and fracture stabilization. In chronic cases with significant sequestrum formation, delayed cancellous grafting and wound closure can be performed following débridement and development of healthy granulation tissue in the wound.

D. Neoplasia

  1. General considerations

    a. Diagnosis

      (1) A **thorough clinical history** and **examination** are necessary to rule out systemic disease, multiple limb lesions, and traumatic, non-neoplastic disorders.

      (2) **Radiography** of the affected limb is necessary to delineate the tumor for biopsy and treatment, and to predict prognosis.

        (a) Survey radiography or nuclear scintigraphy can determine multiple site involvement.

        (b) Radiography of the thorax can detect metastasis. Posttreatment radiographic examinations of the thorax may be performed on a routine basis, depending on the tumor type, treatments, and clinical signs of the animal.

      (3) **Biopsy.** Multiple samples of the affected tissue should be taken using a Mi-

chele bone trephine or Jamshidi needle to confirm the diagnosis. Radiography of the bone following biopsy assists in histologic evaluation of tissues.

(4) **Fine-needle aspiration.** Cytology of fine-needle aspirates from draining lymph nodes is performed to assist in tumor staging if lymphadenopathy is present.

(5) **Laboratory studies.** Blood work, serum biochemistries, urinalysis, and an electrocardiogram (ECG) are useful for evaluating patient health prior to operative procedures and chemotherapy.

b. **Surgical procedures**

(1) **Single limb amputation.** In many cases, single limb amputation can successfully alleviate pain, reduce the tumor burden, and improve the quality of life.

(a) **Forelimb amputations** can be performed at the mid-diaphysis of the humerus (for a lesion below the elbow joint), through the shoulder joint (this approach is technically difficult and leaves an obvious bone appendage), or by complete excision of the scapula and limb.

(b) **Hindlimb amputations** can be performed at the level of the mid-diaphysis of the femur or through the coxofemoral joint. The former approach is technically easier than disarticulation and leaves a protective stump over the male genitalia.

(c) **Technical considerations** include dissection through normal tissue and away from the tumor, control of hemorrhage by separate ligation of major arteries and veins, sharp dissection of nerves under tension, muscular reapposition to protect bone ends, and use of Penrose drains to reduce dead space.

(d) **Postoperative considerations.** Bandages are used on a short-term basis to control swelling. Analgesics are used to control postoperative discomfort.

(2) **Limb-sparing procedures** based on *en bloc* resection of affected bone (e.g., the radius) can be performed instead of amputation to preserve limb function, but adjuvant chemotherapy and radiation are required.

(a) **Minimal bone involvement** (less than 50% of the bone) **is required** to permit cortical allografting and rigid internal fixation with a bone plate and screws.

(b) **Extensive postoperative follow-up is necessary** to detect signs of infection, local recurrence, or severe metastatic thoracic disease.

2. **Osteosarcoma** is the most common feline and canine bone tumor. It frequently affects the metaphysis (distal radius, proximal humerus, distal femur, and proximal tibia) of large, old dogs and cats.

a. **Clinical signs** include an acute and persistent lameness following a mild traumatic episode and pain during palpation of the affected long bone.

b. **Diagnosis**

(1) **Radiography** reveals a focal osteoproliferative and osteolytic lesion (Figure 16–10) with a periosteal reaction. Soft tissue swelling and an adjacent bone reaction are also evident.

(2) **Histologic evaluation** of bone biopsy samples taken at the center of the lesion and angling toward the periphery is imperative to rule out osteomyelitis or other primary or secondary bone tumors. The histologic appearance of the tumor ranges from malignant cells with marked fibrogenesis and scant osteoid formation to samples containing malignant stroma and neoplastic osteoid.

c. **Treatment options** include limb amputation, a limb-sparing procedure, chemotherapy with doxorubicin or cisplatin, radiation, or combinations thereof.

(1) **Amputation alone.** Ninety percent of dogs die from metastatic pulmonary disease; a median survival time of 4–6 months is reported. In cats, the median survival time is 4 years.

(2) **Amputation combined with chemotherapy** has resulted in a 1-year survival rate of nearly 40% and a median survival time of 10 months in dogs.

(3) **Amputation combined with radiation and chemotherapy** has produced a 1-year survival rate of 35% and a median survival time of 8 months in dogs.

(4) **Limb-sparing combined with chemotherapy** has produced a 1-year survival rate of 45% and a median survival time of 11 months in dogs.

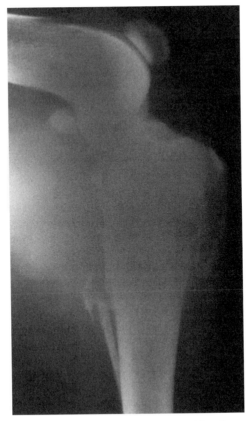

FIGURE 16–10. Osteosarcoma of the proximal tibia in a 10-year-old Doberman pinscher. A mixed proliferative and lytic bone response and soft tissue swelling are evident.

    d. Prognosis
       (1) Dogs. The prognosis for dogs with appendicular osteosarcoma is poor despite
          advances in diagnosis, surgical techniques, and chemotherapy. Most animals
          die from pulmonary metastasis within 1 year of any treatment.
       (2) Cats. In cats, the prognosis for long-term recovery is good following single
          limb amputation.
  3. Chondrosarcoma is the second most common type of primary bone tumor in dogs.
    Medium- to large-breed, middle-aged dogs are most frequently affected; chondrosar-
    coma is uncommon in cats. Flat bones (e.g., the skull, ribs) are more frequently af-
    fected than long bones.
    a. Clinical signs are related to tumor sites and include chronic lameness and
       swelling.
    b. Diagnosis. Radiographic signs are similar to those of osteosarcoma (i.e., bone
       lysis and proliferation). Histologic evaluation of biopsy specimens shows neoplas-
       tic cartilage cells with a chondroid ground substance located in bone.
    c. Treatment usually involves **limb amputation.** Chondrosarcomas tend to be resis-
       tant to radiation and chemotherapy.
    d. Prognosis is fair; the lesion is slow-growing and localized, and metastasis is infre-
       quent. Following amputation, a median survival time of 1.5 years is reported.
  4. Fibrosarcoma occurs infrequently in dogs and cats.
    a. Clinical signs. Fibrosarcoma has clinical characteristics similar to those of chon-
       drosarcoma and osteosarcoma.
    b. Diagnosis. Histologic characteristics include interlacing bundles of neoplastic fi-
       broblasts located within a collagenous matrix. Fibrosarcoma may be misdi-

agnosed as osteosarcoma or chondrosarcoma because of the morphologic hetero-geneity of these tumors.

   c. **Treatment options** include limb amputation, limb-sparing procedures, and chemo-therapy.

   d. **Prognosis** is guarded and based on the degree of cellular differentiation. In general, metastasis occurs more frequently with fibrosarcomas than chondrosarcomas but less frequently than with osteosarcomas.

5. **Hemangiosarcoma** most frequently affects the proximal humerus and femur in older dogs, particularly German shepherds. It is rare in cats.

   a. **Clinical signs** may reflect the location of the tumor. Signs of systemic disease (e.g., anemia, splenomegaly, cardiac disease) are common because of the disseminated nature of the tumor.

   b. **Diagnosis**

     (1) **Radiography** reveals extensive intramedullary osteolysis.

     (2) **Biopsy** reveals numerous vascular channels lined with endothelial cells, hemorrhage, and thrombosis.

     (3) **Ultrasonographic evaluations** of the spleen, liver, and heart are useful.

   c. **Treatment options** include **amputation** and **chemotherapy** with **doxorubicin and cyclophosphamide.**

   d. **Prognosis** is poor because of systemic metastasis.

6. **Squamous cell carcinoma** can affect the digits of cats and dogs, especially large breeds with dark coats. Tumors arise from the subungual epithelium and produce tissue necrosis and bone lysis. Treatment is by **amputation** of the affected digits and prognosis is fair.

7. **Multiple myeloma**, a neoplastic proliferation of plasma cell clones within the bone marrow, occurs infrequently in dogs and is rare in cats. It is a multicentric tumor that affects flat bones, vertebrae, and long bones.

   a. **Diagnosis.** Multiple myeloma is characterized radiographically by mottled osteolytic ("punched-out") lesions.

   b. **Treatment** involves **combination chemotherapy** (with **melphalan** and **prednisone**) and the prognosis is good.

8. **Periosteal (juxtacortical) osteosarcoma** arises from the outer periosteal covering of long and flat bones in dogs and cats. **Amputation** or **wide surgical excision** may provide a good long-term prognosis.

9. **Metastatic neoplastic conditions** that affect long bones include lymphosarcoma and adenocarcinoma from mammary, prostatic, or lung tissues. Surgical and medical **treatments are aimed at the source of disease.**

E. **Bone cysts** occur infrequently in dogs and cats and may be simple, benign cysts lined by a membrane and filled with fluid, or osteolytic spaces filled with vascular elements (aneurysmal bone cysts). Treatments include **curettage** and **cancellous bone grafting.**

F. **Hypertrophic osteopathy** is a diffuse periosteal proliferative condition of long bones that affects dogs and, rarely, cats.

1. **Etiology.** Hypertrophic osteopathy is associated with neoplastic or infectious masses in the thoracic or abdominal cavity, which inexplicably stimulate peripheral periosteal vascularization.

2. **Clinical signs** include diffuse long bone pain, lameness, and reluctance to move.

3. **Diagnosis** is by clinical signs and a history of thoracic or abdominal masses. Radiography reveals long bone periosteal reaction in all four limbs that progresses in a distal to proximal direction.

4. **Treatment** includes **surgical resection of the inciting thoracic or abdominal masses,** and analgesics to reduce periosteal discomfort. **Unilateral intrathoracic vagotomy** to block the suspected nervous reflex associated with increased peripheral vascular flow has also been advocated for cases involving non-resectable masses.

5. Prognosis is fair but depends on identification and treatment of the underlying cause of disease.

G. **Bone infarction** is an uncommon clinical entity in small animals.

1. **Etiology.** Vascular impairment of the bone is suspected to be associated with neoplasia, infection, or lipid abnormalities.

2. **Diagnosis** is by radiography; an irregular radiopaque density within the medullary cavity is characteristic.

3. **Treatment** is aimed at correcting the underlying disease.

VI. **NUTRITIONAL AND METABOLIC BONE DISORDERS.** Although these conditions are not treated surgically, animals with these conditions are often referred to surgeons.

A. **Nutritional secondary hyperparathyroidism** is seen in young animals fed an unsupplemented all-meat or grain diet.

1. **Pathogenesis.** The unsupplemented diet produces deficiencies in calcium and vitamin D. In response to the hypocalcemia, the parathyroid gland produces excessive amounts of parathyroid hormone (PTH), which stimulates bone resorption and the transfer of calcium into the circulation.

2. **Clinical signs** include lameness, long bone deformities, and spontaneous fractures.

3. **Diagnosis**
   a. Laboratory analysis reveals increased serum phosphorus, alkaline phosphatase, and PTH levels.
   b. Radiography reveals evidence of systemic bone resorption, fractures, and increased linear metaphyseal densities.

4. **Treatment** is by dietary improvement (i.e., complete rations, calcium supplementation) and restriction of activity to prevent additional bone damage and allow fracture healing.

5. **Prognosis** for recovery is good in the absence of severe skeletal deformation.

B. **Renal secondary hyperparathyroidism** is seen in young animals with congenital renal insufficiency or old animals with chronic renal failure.

1. **Pathogenesis.** Impaired renal phosphorus excretion and failure to convert vitamin D to its active form result in hypocalcemia and subsequent PTH release (i.e., bone resorption).

2. **Clinical signs** include polydipsia, polyuria, vomiting, diarrhea, weight loss, and anorexia as a result of uremia and bone resorption, primarily in the skull and jaw.

3. **Diagnosis** is based on clinical signs, laboratory findings of renal failure, and radiographic evidence of demineralization, pathologic fractures, and periodontal lucencies in the skull and mandible.

4. **Treatment.** Measures are taken to treat the renal failure (e.g., fluid therapy, peritoneal dialysis, renal transplantation).

5. **Prognosis** is guarded and based on the severity of the renal disease and the response to therapy.

C. **Rickets** and **osteomalacia** are rare conditions caused by vitamin D deficiency in young and mature animals, respectively.

1. **Pathogenesis.** In immature animals, the absence of vitamin D prevents conversion of growth plate cartilage into bone, whereas in mature animals, bone osteoclastic resorption is impaired.

2. **Clinical signs** include lameness, bone deformation, and pathologic fractures.

3. **Diagnosis**
   a. Laboratory studies reveal hypocalcemia, hyperphosphatemia, and increased serum alkaline phosphatase levels.
   b. Radiography reveals widened, irregular growth plates and metaphyseal cupping in young animals and reduced bone density in mature animals.

4. **Treatment**. The animal is fed a nutritionally complete diet, supplemented initially with vitamin D.

5. **Prognosis** for functional recovery is good if severe and chronic skeletal deformations have not occurred.

D. **Hypervitaminosis A** has been described in cats fed predominantly whole liver and milk diets, causing confluent exostoses of the long bones and cervicothoracic vertebrae.

1. **Clinical signs** include lameness, muscle atrophy, and cervical pain.

2. **Diagnosis**. Laboratory studies reveal elevated serum vitamin A levels. Radiography reveals evidence of vertebral and joint fusion along with long bone exostoses.

3. **Treatment** is based on dietary modification, including cessation of the liver diet, and upright feedings. Analgesics may reduce musculoskeletal pain.

4. **Prognosis** is guarded because the bone lesions are irreversible.

E. **Mucopolysaccharidosis** is a group of primary metabolic disorders caused by deficits in glycosaminoglycan metabolism. Siamese cats, Plott hounds, and dachshunds are most often affected.

1. **Clinical signs** include facial dysmorphia, abnormal gait, joint pain, diffuse neurologic deficits, and ocular and respiratory discharge.

2. **Diagnosis.** Laboratory studies reveal glycosaminoglycans in the urine and abnormal granular material in neutrophils. Radiography reveals vertebral and joint fusion, pectus excavatum, and bilateral coxofemoral luxation.

3. **Treatment** is supportive in terms of alleviating discomfort.

4. **Prognosis** for recovery is poor.

SELECTED READINGS

Ablin L, Berg J, Schelling SH: Fibrosarcomas of the appendicular skeleton. *J Am Anim Hosp Assoc* 27:303–309, 1991.

Avon D, Palmer R, Johnson A: Biologic strategies and a balanced concept for repair of highly comminuted long bone fractures. *Comp Cont Educ Pract* 17:35–49, 1995.

Berg J, Weinstein MJ, Schelling SH: Treatment of dogs with osteosarcoma by administration of cisplatin after amputation or limb-sparing surgery: 22 cases (1987–1990). *J Am Vet Med Assoc* 200:2005–2008, 1992.

Bojrab MJ: *Current Techniques in Small Animal Surgery*, 3rd ed. Philadelphia, Lea & Febiger, 1990, pp 756–769, 783–801, 682–693, 722–727.

Bojrab MJ (ed): *Disease Mechanisms in Small Animal Surgery*, 2nd ed. Philadelphia, Lea & Febiger, 1993, pp 644–648, 663–684, 689–700.

Brinker WO, Piermattei DL, Flo GF: *Handbook of Small Animal Orthopedics and Fracture Management*, 2nd ed. Philadelphia, WB Saunders, 1990, pp 105–139, 140–209.

Durall I, Diaz MC, Morales I: Interlocking nail stabilization of humeral fractures. *Vet Comp Ortho Traum* 7:3–8, 1994.

Gentry SJ, Taylor RA, Dee JF: The use of veterinary cuttable plates: 21 cases. *J Am Anim Hosp Assoc* 29:455–459, 1993.

Harari J (ed): *Surgical Complications and Wound Healing in the Small Animal Practice.* Philadelphia, WB Saunders, 1993, pp 203–252.

Johnson JM, Johnson AL: Histological appearance of naturally occurring canine physeal fractures. *Vet Surg* 23:81–86, 1994.

Johnson KA: Osteomyelitis in dogs and cats. *J Am Vet Med Assoc* 205:1882–1887, 1994.

Johnson KA, Watson ADJ, Page R: Skeletal diseases. In *Textbook of Veterinary Internal Medicine*, 4th ed. Edited by Ettinger SJ and Feldman EC. Philadelphia, WB Saunders, pp 2077–2103, 1994.

Leighton RL: *Small Animal Orthopedics.* London, Mosby-Year Book Europe Ltd, pp 2.2–4.9.

Michellin-Little DJ, DeYoung DJ, Ferris KK: Incomplete ossification of the humeral condyle in spaniels. *Vet Surg* 23:475–487, 1994.

O'Brien MG, Straw RC, Withrow SJ: Recent advances in the treatment of canine appendicular osteosarcoma. *Comp Contin Educ Pract* 15:939–946, 1994.

Popovitch CA, Weinstein MJ, Goldschmidt MH: Chondrosarcoma: a retrospective study of 97 dogs (1987–1990). *J Am Anim Hosp Assoc* 30:81–85, 1994.

Sherding RG: *The Cat: Diseases and Clinical Management*, 2nd ed. New York, Churchill Livingstone, 1994, pp 1599–1710.

Slatter D (ed): *Textbook of Small Animal Surgery*, 2nd ed. Philadelphia, WB Saunders, 1993, pp 1703–1709, 1716–1728, 1736–1768, 1805–1816, 1866–1877.

Waters DJ, Breur GJ, Toombs JP: Treatment of common forelimb fractures in miniature and toy breed dogs. *J Am Anim Hosp Assoc* 29:442–448, 1993.

Chapter 17

Pelvis

Joseph Harari

I. **ANATOMY** (Figure 17–1). Because of the **structure** and **location** of the pelvis, most fractures are **closed injuries** that **involve multiple bones or joints** and, frequently, severe **soft tissue trauma.**

A. **Concomitant orthopedic lesions**

1. **Within the pelvic girdle.** With multiple hemipelvic fractures, reduction and stabilization of the cranial segments (i.e., the sacroiliac or iliac segments) helps reduce other fragments (i.e., in the pubis, caudal acetabulum, or ischium).

2. **Outside the pelvic girdle.** Sacral body fractures, coccygeal vertebrae fractures, coxofemoral luxation, and femoral fractures are often seen in conjunction with pelvic fractures.

B. **Associated soft tissue injuries** include urinary bladder or urethral rupture, lumbosacral trunk or sciatic nerve damage, traumatic myocarditis, diaphragmatic hernia, pneumothorax, and regional soft tissue hemorrhage. Sciatic neurapraxia is usually self-limiting and recovery occurs within 2–3 weeks of the injury.

II. **PELVIC FRACTURES.** Approximately 20% of all fractures in dogs and cats involve the pelvis. Vehicular trauma and falls from great heights are the most common causes.

A. **Patient evaluation.** Because of the high incidence of associated injuries, the animal should be carefully assessed prior to treatment of the pelvic fracture.

1. **Essential diagnostic tests** include physical examination, a complete blood count (CBC), a chemistry profile and urinalysis, thoracic and abdominal radiography, electrocardiography, urinary catheterization, and abdominal paracentesis.

2. **Ancillary evaluations** include abdominal ultrasonography, cystography, computed tomography, magnetic resonance imaging, and exploratory celiotomy.

B. **Patient stabilization**

1. **Treatment of severe soft tissue injuries** (e.g., ruptured urinary bladder, diaphragmatic hernia, myocarditis) **may be required before orthopedic repairs can be pursued.**

2. Animals often require **fluid resuscitation** and **glucocorticoids** for hypovolemic shock and **analgesic therapy** to reduce discomfort.

C. **Selection of treatment.** Factors influencing the choice of therapy include the location and severity of the lesions and the owner's finances. Evaluations that can help determine the course of therapy include gait analysis (to reveal lameness), palpation of the iliac crest (to reveal sacroiliac instability), palpation of the hip joint (to reveal crepitation), gentle rectal palpation (to reveal displaced bone segments), and multiple radiographs of the pelvis.

1. **Indications for surgical stabilization** of pelvic fractures include the following:
   a. **Inadequate hindlimb weight-bearing capability** as a result of unstable sacroiliac separation, iliac fractures, or acetabular fractures
   b. **Medial displacement of bone fragments,** which can compromise the pelvic canal

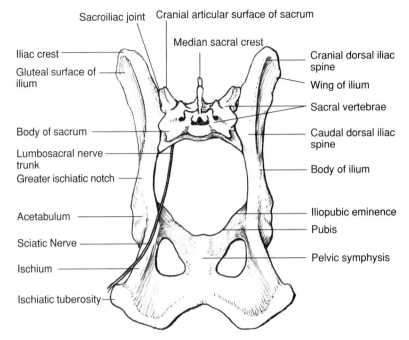

Iliac crest

Gluteal surface of ilium

Body of sacrum

Lumbosacral nerve trunk

Greater ischiatic notch

Acetabulum

Sciatic Nerve

Ischium

Ischiatic tuberosity

Sacroiliac joint   Cranial articular surface of sacrum

Median sacral crest

Cranial dorsal iliac spine

Wing of ilium

Sacral vertebrae

Caudal dorsal iliac spine

Body of ilium

Iliopubic eminence

Pubis

Pelvic symphysis

FIGURE 17–1. Caudodorsal view of the basic anatomy of the pelvis and sacral vertebrae.

c. **Cranioventral displacement of the pubis** and **tearing of the prepubic tendon,** which can lead to caudal abdominal visceral herniation
d. **Ischiatic tubercle avulsion,** which can cause hindlimb lameness

2. **Indications for conservative therapy. Cage rest for 4–8 weeks** is often appropriate for ambulatory animals with **minimally displaced sacroiliac luxations,** or those with **caudal acetabular, ischial,** or **pubic fractures.**

D. General surgical considerations

1. Pelvic fractures **tend to heal quickly** (i.e., within 6–10 weeks) because of the **abundant cancellous bone** content of the pelvic girdle (i.e., ilium, acetabulum) and the supportive **periosseous muscle mass,** which provides an abundant blood supply to the fracture.

2. **Implants** (e.g., plates, screws, and pins) are not routinely removed following bone healing because of the degree of surgical invasiveness necessary for a second surgery and an absence of clinical problems associated with leaving the implant in place.

3. **Healed, collapsed fractures of the pelvis** that cause urinary or bowel compromise **may require pelvic symphyseal osteotomy, distraction,** and **insertion of a cortical bone or a synthetic (polyethylene, polyester mesh) graft** to increase the pelvic diameter.

E. Types of fractures

1. **Sacroiliac joint luxation**
   a. **Technique.** Most displacements occur in a cranial direction and require open reduction and stabilization with screws or pins. Anatomic reduction and adequate stabilization are important for clinical recovery and require identification of the sacral body to permit seating of implants and ensure avoidance of the vertebral canal.
      (1) A **dorsolateral or ventrolateral approach** is used to reflect the gluteal muscles from the ilium and permit visualization and palpation of the sacroiliac joint.
      (2) **Reduction.** The iliac wing is grasped with bone-holding forceps and traction is applied in a caudal direction.

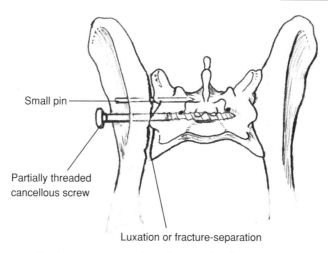

Small pin

Partially threaded
cancellous screw

Luxation or fracture-separation

FIGURE 17–2. Two-point fixation and compression of a sacroiliac luxation, using a partially threaded bone screw and pin.

(3) **Stabilization. Screws or pins** are **placed across the ilium** and **into the body of the sacrum** (Figure 17–2).
 (a) Implants should penetrate to a point that is equal to at least 60% of the width of the sacrum (based on the ventrodorsal radiographic view) to provide maximum stability.
 (b) **Transilial bolt.** In overweight animals with severely unstable fractures, bilateral luxations, or impaction of the sacrum, a partially threaded Steinmann pin is placed transversely through both iliac wings, dorsal to the lumbar vertebrae. A nut is placed on the threaded portion of the Steinmann pin, and the smooth end is bent over to stabilize both ilia.
 b. **Prognosis.** For animals without severe neurologic deficits, the prognosis for recovery is excellent following a 2–4-week period of convalescence.
 2. **Iliac fractures** are usually oblique with medial displacement and narrowing of the pelvic canal by the caudal segment of bone.
 a. **Technique**
 (1) A **lateral approach** is used and the gluteal muscles are periosteally elevated from the bone.
 (2) **Reduction of the caudal fragment** often requires leverage, traction, and rotation using bone-holding forceps.
 (3) **Stabilization** is most commonly achieved with a **contoured bone plate and screws** (Figure 17–3) or **lag screw fixation** across the fracture. The plate is usually applied to the caudal ilial segment and then secured to the cranial frag-

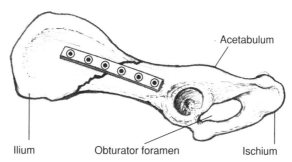

Acetabulum

Ilium Obturator foramen Ischium

FIGURE 17–3. Stabilization of an oblique ilial fracture with a laterally applied neutralization plate and screws (lateral view).

ment, leveraging the medially displaced distal fragment laterally. Alternatively, **intramedullary pins** can be placed within the ilium or **pins and wires** can be placed across the fracture in small dogs or cats.

    b. Prognosis. For animals without neurologic deficits, the prognosis is excellent following a 2–4-week period of convalescence.

3. Acetabular fractures

    a. Treatment options. The cranial two-thirds of the acetabulum is involved in weight-bearing.

        (1) Stabilization is recommended for fractures involving any portion of the articular surface, even those not directly related to weight-bearing, because of the risk of developing degenerative arthritis.

        (2) Cage rest and slings. Some surgeons prefer to treat minimally displaced caudal acetabular fragments with cage rest or the application of non–weight-bearing slings to the affected limb. Subsequent development of arthritis and lameness can be treated with anti-inflammatory medication or femoral head and neck resection.

    b. Surgical techniques

        (1) Approaches

            (a) A **dorsal approach** to the hip joint **via trochanteric osteotomy** is performed to adequately visualize the acetabulum. A dorsal approach is indicated for fractures in the cranial two-thirds of the bone.

                (i) The skin and underlying tissues are incised along the cranial aspect of the greater trochanter.

                (ii) Following transection of the superficial gluteal insertion below the trochanter, the greater trochanter is osteotomized and reflected proximally to reveal the acetabulum and sciatic nerve. Care should be taken to protect the sciatic nerve.

                (iii) Following stabilization of the fracture, the trochanteric osteotomy needs to be stabilized using a tension band technique [see Chapter 16 IV A 3 e (2) (b)].

            (b) A **caudal approach,** which requires **transection of the external rotator muscles** of the hip, is useful for treatment of caudal acetabular fractures.

                (i) Dissection is similar to that used for the dorsal approach.

                (ii) The femur is rotated internally and the insertions of the internal obturator and gemelli muscles are transected (instead of performing a trochanteric osteotomy).

                (iii) The muscles are reflected dorsally and used to protect the sciatic nerve as the caudal acetabulum is exposed.

            (c) For fractures of the ilium and acetabulum, a **combination lateral** and **dorsal approach** (to the ilium and acetabulum, respectively) permits exposure of the hemipelvis.

        (2) Stabilization is via **acetabular plates** and **screws** (Figure 17–4). In racing greyhounds, non-displaced ''Y'' stress fractures of the acetabulum occur; dorsal acetabular plating is required to prevent malunion. **Intramedullary pin and wir-**

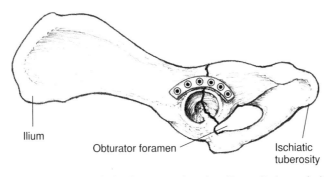

Ilium   Obturator foramen   Ischiatic tuberosity

FIGURE 17–4. Stabilization of an acetabular fracture with a dorsally applied acetabular plate and screws.

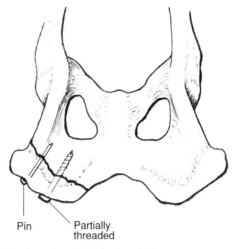

Pin   Partially
         threaded

FIGURE 17–5. Tension band fixation of an ischial tubercle fracture using a partially threaded bone screw and pin.

ing techniques are reserved for the repair of small bone fragments in light-weight animals.

(3) **Femoral head and neck excision** is indicated for **highly comminuted, irreparable fractures with loss of the medial buttress** of the acetabular wall. Caudal acetabular segments that are severely displaced medially and cranially may need to be realigned to prevent trochanteric contact pain and loss of extension following femoral head and neck excision.

c. **Prognosis.** In most animals, prognosis is good following stabilization and reestablishment of acetabular articular congruity. **Long-term complications** (e.g., sciatic nerve injury, degenerative osteoarthritis, lameness following femoral head and neck resection) can occur.

4. **Ischial fractures**
    a. Ischial fractures are usually associated with iliac or acetabular fractures. Primary repair of these bones produces nearly normal realignment of ischial segments; therefore, surgery to repair the ischial fragment is infrequently performed.
    b. **Fracture and avulsion of the ischiatic tubercle** that causes hindlimb lameness should be repaired with screws or pins and wires in a **tension band technique** (Figure 17–5).

5. **Pubic fractures**
    a. As with ischial fractures, isolated pubic fractures occur infrequently; pubic fragments associated with other pelvic bone fractures are reduced during other primary repairs or are left *in situ* to heal.
    b. **Cranioventral displacement of the pubis**, which can lead to abdominal herniation, requires wiring of the bone fragments and suturing of the prepubic tendon or the abdominal muscular sheaths.

SELECTED READINGS
Betts CW: Pelvic fractures. In Slatter D (ed): *Textbook of Small Animal Surgery*, 2nd ed. Philadelphia, WB Saunders, 1993, pp 1769–1785.

Bojrab MJ: *Current Techniques in Small Animal Surgery*, 3rd ed. Philadelphia, Lea & Febiger, 1990, pp 649–661.

Bookbinder PF, Flanders JA: Characteristics of pelvic fracture in the cat. *Vet Comp Ortho Traum* 5:122–127, 1992.

Brinker WD, Piermattei DL, Flo GL: *Handbook of Small Animal Orthopedics and Fracture Treatment*, 2nd ed. Philadelphia, WB Saunders, 1990, pp 76–104.

Butterworth SJ, Gribben S, Skerry TM: Conservative and surgical treatment of canine acetabular fractures: a review of 34 cases. *J Sm Anim Pract* 139–143, 1994.

Houlton J, Dyce J: Management of pelvic fractures in the dog and cat. *Waltham Focus* 4: 17–25, 1994.

Hulse DA: Pelvic fractures, conservative and surgical management. *Vet Med Rep* 2:267–278, 1990.

Payne JT: Selecting a method for managing pelvic fractures in dogs and cats. *Vet Med* 88: 969–973, 1993.

Verstraete FJM, Lambrechts NE: Diagnosis of soft tissue injuries associated with pelvic fractures. *Comp Contin Educ Pract* 14:921–930, 1993.

Chapter 18

Joints

Spencer A. Johnston

I. INTRODUCTION

A. **Classification.** A **joint** is a junction between two or more bones. The amount of movement occurring between the bones is variable and depends on the specific anatomy of the joint.

1. A **fibrous joint,** or **synarthrosis,** is an immovable joint with adjoining bone ends separated by a thin membrane (e.g., cranial sutures).

2. A **cartilaginous joint,** or **amphiarthrosis,** has a fibrocartilage pad between the bone surfaces and allows limited movement between bones (e.g., vertebrae, pubic symphysis).

3. A **synovial joint,** or **diarthrosis,** has adjacent bone ends covered with hyaline cartilage. The bones are joined by ligaments and a fibrous capsule lined by a synovial membrane. The major motion joints of the body (e.g., elbow, stifle, hip) are synovial joints, and are those most commonly associated with injury. All joints discussed in this chapter are synovial joints.

B. **Synovial joint anatomy**

1. **Hyaline cartilage** is made up primarily of water, collagen (predominantly type II), proteoglycans, and ground substance.
   a. Hyaline cartilage is unique in that it allows smooth, nearly frictionless movement and absorbs shock. Its **viscoelasticity** results from the high water content and structure of cartilage. Like a wet sponge, hyaline cartilage weeps fluid when compressed. Collagen gives the tissue resiliency and the ability to resist force.
   b. Cartilage is avascular and receives nutrition from the synovial fluid. Cartilage has a poor capacity for repair following injury; therefore, damage to this tissue is usually permanent.

2. The **joint capsule** of synovial joints is composed of a thin inner layer (the intima) and an outer fibrous layer. The intima, or synovial membrane, is a vascular tissue that lines the joint cavity and contains cells that produce synovial fluid. The outer fibrous layer helps to stabilize the joint. Inflammation of the synovial membrane can occur with injury; mild inflammation may occur with degenerative joint disease (DJD) [see II A 3]. Fibrous thickening of the joint capsule occurs with chronic DJD and joint instability.

3. **Synovial fluid** is an ultrafiltrate of plasma that contains hyaluronic acid, proteoglycans, protein, white blood cells, and other biochemical mediators. The main function of synovial fluid is to lubricate the joint and provide nutrition for cartilage.
   a. Synovial fluid is normally clear and viscous, has relatively few cells (of which more than 90% are mononuclear cells), and is present in low volumes (approximately 0.5 ml per joint).
   b. The quality of synovial fluid deteriorates with joint injury and inflammation. For this reason, synovial fluid analysis is valuable when diagnosing joint disease (Table 18–1).

4. **Ligaments** are dense bands of collagen that connect bones across a joint. They differ from tendons, which connect muscle to bone. Ligaments are flexible tissues that are relatively inelastic.

TABLE 18–1. Common Synovial Fluid Findings Indicative of Disease

Synovial Fluid Characteristic	Normal Joint	Noninflammatory		Inflammatory			
		Degenerative Joint Disease	Hemarthrosis	Rheumatoid Arthritis	Lupus Arthropathy	Neoplastic Joint Disease	Septic Arthritis
Color	C	PY	R	YBT	YBT	YBT	CCS
Turbidity	Clear	Slight	Marked	Moderate	Moderate	Moderate	Marked
Viscosity	Normal	Normal	Reduced	Reduced	Reduced	Reduced	Reduced
Mucin clot	Good	Good	Fair	Poor	Fair	Good	Poor
RBCs	None	Few	Many	Moderate	Moderate	Moderate	Moderate
WBCs $\times 10^3/\mu l$	0.25–3	1–5	3–10	8–38	4.4–371	3–10	40–267
% PMN cells	0–6	0–12	60–75	20–80	15–95	15–75	90–99
% Mononuclear cells	94–100	88–100	25–40	20–80	5–85	25–85	1–10
Ragocytes	–	–	–	–	+	–	–
LE cells	–	–	–	–	+	–	–
Neoplastic cells	–	–	–	–	–	+	–
Microorganisms	–	–	–	–	–	–	+
SF glucose (% of blood glucose)	100	80–100	100	50–80	50–80	50–80	< 50

C = colorless; PY = pale yellow; R = red; YBT = yellow to blood-tinged; CCS = cream-colored to sanguineous.
RBCs = red blood cells; WBCs = white blood cells; PMN = polymorphonuclear; LE = lupus erythematosus; SF = synovial fluid.
 – = absent; + = present.
(Adapted from Toombs JP, Widmer WR: Bone, joint, and periskeletal swelling or enlargement. In *Small Animal Medical Diagnosis,* 2nd ed. Edited by Lorenz MD, Cornelius LM. Philadelphia, JP Lippincott, 1993, p 409.)

II. **NONINFLAMMATORY JOINT DISEASE** is characterized by a paucity of inflammatory cells (neutrophils and macrophages) in the synovial fluid. Noninflammatory joint disease includes DJD and hemarthrosis.

 A. **DJD** is an inclusive term that includes congenital, developmental, and acquired diseases.

1. **Pathophysiology.** DJD is characterized by progressive deterioration of articular cartilage and formation of new bone at joint surfaces and margins. Deterioration results from abnormal stresses (i.e., trauma) on normal cartilage or normal stress on abnormal cartilage leading to the release of inflammatory mediators from synoviocytes and chondrocytes. These mediators cause enzymatic degradation of the cartilage. Pathologic changes include cartilage degeneration, synovial effusion, bone remodeling, low-grade synovitis, and periarticular fibrosis.

2. **Clinical presentation.** Signs associated with DJD are variable and tend to progress from intermittent mild lameness to constant, severe lameness. Signs of lameness include shortened stride, decreased joint motion, decreased weight bearing, and shifting of weight to other limbs. Signs tend to worsen after exercise and during wet and cold weather.

3. **Diagnosis**
   a. **Physical examination** reveals variable joint pain, periarticular swelling, joint effusion, crepitus, and decreased range of motion. In chronic cases, the fibrous joint capsule is enlarged.
   b. **Radiographic changes** tend to be progressive, and include periarticular swelling and joint effusion, joint space narrowing due to loss of articular cartilage, subchondral bony sclerosis, osteophyte production, and, in severe cases, bony remodeling.

4. **Treatment**
   a. **Nonsurgical treatment** may be adequate for the management of DJD, depending on the cause. Medical and nonmedical approaches can be utilized.
      (1) **Nonmedical**
         (a) **Controlled exercise** on soft surfaces is of benefit to patients suffering from

DJD. Swimming or whirlpool therapy provides musculoskeletal stimulation without traumatic concussive forces across joint surfaces.

(b) **Weight control.** While obesity alone does not cause degenerative joint disease, excess weight does cause extra stress on joints and can further injure an abnormal joint.

(c) **Therapeutic heat and cold** relaxes tissues and decreases activity of sensory nerve endings.

(2) **Medical therapy** includes local and systemic therapy to modify the degradative processes associated with DJD.

(a) **Nonsteroidal anti-inflammatory drugs (NSAIDs).** The most commonly used NSAIDs are aspirin and phenylbutazone. These drugs decrease prostaglandin synthesis by damaged synovial cells and chondrocytes, reducing inflammation and pain.

(i) Other NSAIDs (e.g., ibuprofen, naproxen) are available as prescription and nonprescription drugs. These drugs should be used with great caution, however. The metabolism of these drugs by human beings is different from that by dogs, and **extrapolation of the human dose to veterinary patients can be fatal**.

(ii) The most common side effects of NSAIDs are gastrointestinal irritation and bleeding. Clinical signs include vomiting, hematemesis, melena, and anemia. NSAIDs should not be given to patients with renal disease because prostaglandin inhibition can alter renal hemodynamics.

(b) **Corticosteroids** are potent inhibitors of the inflammatory process. They also inhibit prostaglandin synthesis. Chronic administration may hasten degeneration of cartilage and has negative systemic effects as well, the most notable being depression of the hypothalamic–pituitary–adrenal axis.

(c) **Joint fluid modifiers** include polysulfated glycosaminoglycan (PSGAG) and hyaluronic acid (sodium hyaluronate).

(i) **PSGAG** is believed to work by increasing the production of hyaluronic acid and decreasing the activity of degradative enzymes (such as neutral metalloproteinases and lysosomal enzymes) within the joint environment. Although this drug has been demonstrated to be beneficial in experimentally induced arthritis, clinical data are insufficient to recommend routine use at this time. Furthermore, experimental data suggest a potentially greater benefit if given early in the course of disease before degenerative changes are established.

(ii) **Sodium hyaluronate** is administered by intra-articular injection. The exact mechanism of action is unknown, but sodium hyaluronate is suspected to inhibit inflammatory cell migration, phagocytosis, and prostaglandin synthesis. Although hyaluronan has been demonstrated to reduce biochemical and morphological changes in experimentally induced arthritis of the canine stifle, clinical data regarding its use are lacking.

b. **Surgical treatment.** If nonoperative management fails to control the progression of DJD, surgical intervention may be necessary to preserve limb function or normal activity levels. If a primary cause of joint degeneration, such as a torn cranial cruciate ligament, is identified, then specific surgical treatment is aimed at the underlying lesion.

(1) **Arthrodesis,** the surgical union of two adjoining bones, is performed to eliminate joint pain and improve limb function. Joints that are relatively straight, such as the carpus, are arthrodesed more successfully than joints with a large natural angle, such as the elbow or stifle. The principal techniques of joint fusion include cartilage débridement, rigid stability using pins, screws, a bone plate, or an external fixator, and autogenous cancellous bone grafting to enhance bone union. External splints such as casts are often used to provide postoperative stability and enhance joint fusion.

(2) **Joint replacement (arthroplasty)** is an excellent method of treating the degen-

erate joint and maintaining optimum joint and limb functions. Unfortunately, only total hip replacement is commonly performed in veterinary medicine.

(3) **Joint excision** or **excision arthroplasty** can be performed in selected cases. Relief is provided by eliminating the source of pain (i.e., abnormal articulation and joint capsule). Limb function, however, is biomechanically altered. The best known example is the femoral head and neck ostectomy performed for DJD or other injuries of the coxofemoral joint [see IV B 1 e (2) (c)].

(4) **Amputation.** In cases of severe limb injury or deformity affecting the joints, the most effective treatment may be amputation. In these animals, single limb amputation offers excellent recovery from disease and return to near-normal activity. Careful consideration must be given to the status of the joints of the remaining limbs when choosing this option.

B. **Hemarthrosis**

1. **Trauma.** Treatment of hemarthrosis associated with trauma is directed toward the specific injury.

2. **Coagulopathy.** Hemarthrosis associated with a coagulopathy is usually the result of a clotting factor deficiency; treatment is directed at the underlying condition.

III. **INFLAMMATORY JOINT DISEASE** is characterized by moderate to severe inflammation of the synovium and increased numbers of inflammatory cells (polymorphonuclear neutrophils and macrophages) within the synovial fluid. It is usually associated with an infectious, neoplastic, or immune-mediated cause.

A. **Immune-mediated arthritis**

1. **Classification**
   a. **Erosive arthritis** is associated with the destruction of articular cartilage and subchondral bone. Examples include rheumatoid arthritis, erosive polyarthritis of greyhounds, and feline chronic progressive polyarthritis.
   b. **Nonerosive arthritis** is also characterized by inflammation, but with no radiographic or histopathologic evidence of joint destruction. The most common examples are idiopathic nondeforming arthritis and systemic lupus erythematosus (SLE). Nonerosive arthropathies associated with various concurrent conditions (e.g., bacterial endocarditis, discospondylitis, neoplasia, enteropathy, drug administration) occur infrequently.

2. **Signalment**
   a. **Erosive.** Rheumatoid arthritis typically affects small dogs at any age.
   b. **Nonerosive.** The most common forms of nonerosive disease typically occur in larger dogs of any age.

3. **Clinical presentation.** Signs for erosive and nonerosive arthropathy are similar. Although both forms can result in joint instability, erosive disease tends to cause more severe deformity and progressive clinical signs than nonerosive disease.
   a. Immune-mediated arthropathies usually involve multiple joints, and most frequently involve the small distal joints, such as the carpus, tarsus, and interphalangeal joints.
   b. Local signs such as pain, joint effusion, soft tissue swelling, and local hyperthermia may be noted.
   c. Systemic signs, such as fever, malaise, anorexia, and generalized muscle pain may accompany the lameness.
   d. Waxing and waning of clinical signs is very common for both erosive and nonerosive forms.

4. **Diagnosis** is by physical examination, radiographs, arthrocentesis, and serologic testing.

a. **Radiographic imaging**
  (1) **Erosive arthropathy.** Animals typically demonstrate collapse of the joint space, destruction of subchondral bone, and periarticular swelling.
  (2) **Nonerosive arthropathy** is characterized by periarticular swelling and joint effusion, but not joint collapse or subchondral bone lesions.
b. **Laboratory testing**
  (1) **Arthrocentesis** reveals synovial fluid that characteristically lacks viscosity (a string less than 2.5 cm in length forms when a drop of fluid is placed between two fingers or between the needle and the slide). Nucleated cell counts are increased, with the majority of cells being neutrophils (see Table 18–1).
  (2) **Serologic testing** is performed in cases of suspected immune-mediated disease, but is generally unrewarding because most animals are rheumatoid factor (RF)- and antinuclear antibody (ANA)-negative. Only 25% of dogs with rheumatoid arthritis test positive for RF. Most animals with immune-mediated arthritis are ANA-negative, although most dogs with SLE are ANA-positive.
  (3) **Microbial culture.** In cases of inflammatory arthritis, synovial fluid culture is indicated to rule out an infectious etiology (see III C 1). Analysis of synovial fluid cytology alone, although helpful, usually cannot completely rule out infection.
  (4) **Histopathologic changes** noted on synovial or articular cartilage biopsy can be valuable in distinguishing erosive from nonerosive disease.
    (a) Erosive disease is associated with synovial hypertrophy and plasmacytic, lymphocytic infiltration of synovial tissue, along with articular cartilage erosion at the joint margins.
    (b) Nonerosive arthritis is associated with a milder synovitis. Polymorphonuclear neutrophils are elevated, but destruction of bone or cartilage is absent.
c. **Diagnostic criteria.** Criteria for diagnosis of rheumatoid arthritis and SLE have been established. However, clinical features of erosive and nonerosive disease overlap considerably. Immune-mediated arthritis frequently can be defined only as erosive or nonerosive.

5. **Treatment** of these conditions entails interrupting the process of inflammation. Drugs commonly used include corticosteroids, chrysotherapy (gold salts), or cytotoxic drugs, such as cyclophosphamide, azathioprine, or methotrexate. These drugs may be used alone or in combination. NSAID therapy is usually ineffective.

6. **Prognosis.** As with human beings, treatment for immune-mediated arthritis can be unrewarding, with continued progression of the disease. The prognosis for nonerosive disease is better than for erosive disease. Approximately 50% of nonerosive animals can eventually be weaned from therapy, whereas nearly all animals with erosive disease require lifelong therapy and may worsen despite therapy.

B. **Arthritis associated with neoplasia**

1. **Overview**
  a. **Clinical presentation.** Neoplastic processes involving the joint are relatively uncommon. Pain and lameness of variable duration are typical presenting complaints.
  b. **Diagnosis**
    (1) **Physical examination** frequently reveals an inflamed, painful, swollen joint.
    (2) **Radiographs** may demonstrate only soft tissue swelling, or may reveal lysis of adjoining bone ends.
    (3) **Differential diagnosis.** The main differential diagnoses for lysis of adjoining bone ends are infection and rheumatoid (erosive) arthritis.

2. **Synovial cell sarcoma** is the most common malignant tumor involving the joints. The tumor arises from primitive mesenchymal cells outside of the synovial membrane. Metastasis is detected at the time of diagnosis in approximately 25% of patients. **Amputation** is the therapy of choice, and most animals survive 3 or more years.

3. **Osteosarcoma.** Primary bone neoplasia typically does not cross the joint. However, because of its location in the metaphyseal region, osteosarcoma may interfere with normal joint function and result in periarticular swelling. The carpal, shoulder, and stifle joints are most commonly affected. Treatment may include **chemotherapy, amputation,** or **limb salvage** procedures.

C. **Infectious arthritis**

1. **Bacterial arthritis** is the most common type of infectious arthritis.
   a. **Etiology**
      (1) **Hematogenous seeding** of the joints occurs infrequently in small animals.
         (a) Hematogenous seeding may be associated with umbilical infection or retropharyngeal lymph node abscessation in young animals.
         (b) In mature dogs, hematogenous seeding can be associated with urogenital tract, skin, oral, respiratory, or cardiac infections (e.g., endocarditis).
      (2) **Penetrating trauma.** Bacterial arthritis can also occur following surgery, intra-articular injection, or accidental wounding.
   b. **Clinical signs** of bacterial arthritis include acute onset of pain and lameness—both of which may be severe—along with warmth and joint effusion detected on palpation. Systemic signs may be vague, and include malaise, fever, and anorexia. If hematogenous spread is the cause of the arthritis, signs may be specific to the body system involved.
   c. **Diagnosis**
      (1) **Radiographic imaging.** Early in the disease course, joint distention and swelling may be the only radiographic changes, while subchondral lucency and DJD are detected in chronic cases (those lasting more than 3 weeks).
      (2) **Laboratory testing.** Confirmation of septic arthritis is performed by arthrocentesis and bacterial culture.
         (a) **Arthrocentesis** demonstrates large numbers of inflammatory cells ($> 40,000/mm^3$ with $> 90\%$ neutrophils) that may be degenerate, and possibly bacteria. A Gram stain may be helpful for preliminary bacterial identification. The synovial fluid is usually cloudy, has decreased viscosity, and may have a gross purulent appearance with or without blood.
         (b) **Bacterial culture.** It may be difficult to successfully culture bacteria from the synovial fluid of a septic joint because of a propensity for bacteria to adhere to the synovial membrane. Bacterial culture is best performed by placing synovial fluid in blood culture media in a $1:9$ fluid-to-culture media ratio, or by obtaining a synovial biopsy for culture. Direct swabbing of synovial fluid frequently results in no growth of bacteria, even in joints known to be septic.
            (i) *Staphylococcus, Streptococcus,* and coliforms are the most common bacteria isolated.
            (ii) If no penetrating injury has occurred, serial blood cultures may help to identify the organism.
   d. **Immediate treatment is imperative** because of the articular destruction that results from degradative enzymes released by bacteria, neutrophils, and damaged chondrocytes. Appropriate **intravenous antibiotic therapy** is instituted. Irrigation of the joint by **needle arthrocentesis** or **surgical débridement and joint lavage** are also recommended.

2. **Other causes of infectious arthritis**
   a. **Rickettsial diseases. Rocky mountain spotted fever** and **ehrlichiosis** are rickettsial diseases transmitted by ticks. The diagnosis is based on clinical signs, clinical laboratory changes including thrombocytopenia, serologic testing, and response to therapy (e.g., tetracycline, doxycycline, or chloramphenicol). If arthropathy is associated, synovial fluid analysis reveals an elevated white blood cell count and an increased percentage of neutrophils.
   b. **Spirochetal disease. Lyme borreliosis** is caused by the spirochetal organism *Borrelia burgdorferi,* for which hard ticks are the primary vector. The disease is characterized by acute or chronic fever, anorexia, lethargy, stiffness, and recurrent, in-

termittent joint pain. Synovial fluid has elevated leukocyte counts (approximately 40,000/mm^3) with 80% neutrophils. Diagnosis is based on clinical signs, synovial fluid analysis, serology or isolation of the organism, and response to therapy (tetracycline).

IV. CONGENITAL AND DEVELOPMENTAL JOINT DISORDERS

A. **Osteochondrosis** is a disturbance of the normal process of endochondral ossification. **Osteochondritis dissecans** (OCD) is a form of osteochondrosis that develops when the hyaline cartilage fractures vertically, forming a cartilage flap and allowing communication of synovial fluid with underlying subchondral bone (see Chapter 16 V B 3). It most frequently affects the shoulder, elbow, stifle, and tarsus. OCD lesions are usually treated by surgical excision of the cartilage flap and curettage of the subchondral bone to stimulate bleeding and fibrocartilage filling of the bone defect.

1. **Shoulder.** Osteochondrosis is most frequently recognized in the shoulder joint.
   a. **Diagnosis**
      (1) **Physical examination** reveals pain on flexion or extension of the joint.
      (2) **Radiographic confirmation.** A radiolucent region is visible on the caudal border of the humeral head (Figure 18–1).
   b. **Prognosis** for return to function following surgical treatment [see Chapter 16 V B 3 d (1)] is excellent.
2. **Elbow.** Osteochondrosis of the elbow occurs on the medial aspect of the humeral condyle. It is frequently associated with a **fragmented medial coronoid process (FMCP) of the ulna** (see IV B 2 a).
   a. **Diagnosis**
      (1) **Radiographic confirmation** of a radiolucent defect may be difficult. The craniocaudal view is usually most valuable, but radiographs may only demon-

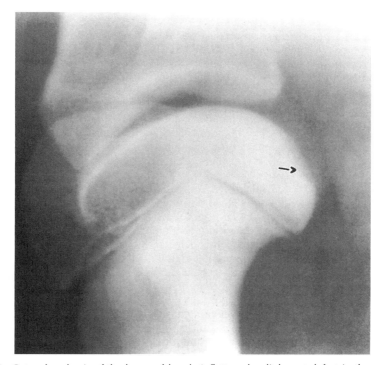

FIGURE 18–1. Osteochondrosis of the humeral head. A flattened radiolucent defect in the subchondral bone is visible *(arrow)*.

strate osteoarthritic changes of the radial head, medial humeral condyle, coronoid process, and anconeal region.

(2) **Exploratory surgery** is often necessary to confirm the presence of an OCD lesion.

b. **Prognosis** is fair following surgical treatment if concurrent disease (e.g., FMCP) has not produced a highly degenerative joint environment.

3. **Stifle.** The medial aspect of the lateral femoral condyle is the classic location for osteochondrosis of the stifle, but the disease can occur in the medial condyle as well.

a. **Diagnosis**

(1) **Clinical signs.** Joint effusion is often present.

(2) **Radiographic confirmation** of the condition is necessary; the craniocaudal view is the most valuable. The fossa of the long digital extensor tendon, located on the lateral condyle, should not be mistaken for an OCD lesion.

b. **Prognosis** for recovery with surgical treatment is fair to good.

4. **Tarsus.** The medial trochlear ridge of the talus is the typical location of an osteochondrosis defect, except in rottweiler dogs, where the lesion is often found on the lateral trochlear ridge.

a. **Diagnosis**

(1) **Clinical signs.** Joint effusion and hyperextension of the tibiotarsal joint are common.

(2) **Radiographic confirmation** is difficult, and often requires multiple views of the tarsus, including flexed and oblique views.

b. **Prognosis.** Because some dogs exhibit little improvement with surgery, the value of surgical treatment is debatable. The long-term prognosis following surgery for OCD of the talus is guarded because of joint instability and degeneration associated with lesions of the trochlear ridges.

B. **Dysplasia**

1. **Hip dysplasia** is the most common congenital canine orthopedic abnormality.

a. **Etiology.** Hip dysplasia results from a combination of nutritional, environmental, and genetic factors. The genetic contribution is polygenic. The nutritional contribution is recognized because obesity and rapid weight gain are associated with more severe dysplasia in predisposed dogs. Environmental factors include excessive exercise and rapid growth.

b. **Predisposing factors.** Large- and giant-breed dogs are at greatest risk, although smaller dogs and cats may be affected.

c. **Clinical presentation**

(1) **Younger dogs**

(a) **Joint laxity** is the hallmark sign of the dysplastic hip in the young dog. The Ortolani and Bardens signs are used to detect laxity. Because nonsedated dogs may object to the manipulations necessary to perform these tests, the most consistent results are obtained when the patient is sedated or anesthetized.

(i) The **Ortolani sign** is detected by placing the dog on its back and forcing the femurs dorsally. The limbs are then slowly abducted. A positive Ortolani sign exists when the femoral head palpably seats into the acetabulum as the limb is abducted (Figure 18–2).

(ii) The **Bardens sign** is detected by exerting a lateral force on the femur while palpating the femoral head. Palpable lateral movement of the femoral head is considered to be a positive sign.

(b) **Other signs** recognized early (4–12 months of age) include lameness and bunny-hopping. The muscles of hind limbs may be poorly developed. Pain is elicited on flexion and extension of the coxofemoral joints.

(2) **Older dogs.** Clinical signs in mature dogs are typical of DJD.

(a) Lameness and pain are intermittent or constant.

(b) Joint laxity is absent or less marked because joint stabilization is associated with joint capsule thickening, periarticular fibrosis, and periarticular osteophyte production.

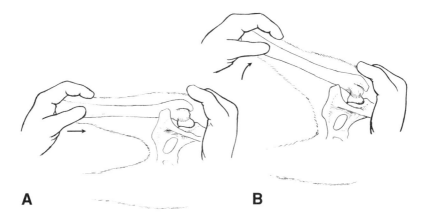

FIGURE 18–2. Ortolani sign. *(A)* Subluxation resulting from hip dysplasia may be demonstrated by pushing the stifle proximally and parallel to the femur. *(B)* Reduction of the subluxation results in a "thud" that is detected by the other hand on the greater trochanter region when the stifle is abducted. (From Brinker WO, Piermattei DL, Flo GL: *Handbook of Small Animal Orthopedics and Fracture Treatment,* 2nd ed. Philadelphia, WB Saunders, 1990, p 277.)

    (c) Range of motion is decreased.
    (d) Crepitation is more noticeable on palpation than in young animals.
    (e) The animal is usually not tolerant of strenuous manipulations of the coxofemoral joint unless sedated.
  d. **Diagnosis.** The disease is confirmed **radiographically.** Currently, standard radiographic views developed by the Orthopedic Foundation for Animals taken at 2 years of age are used to determine whether a dog is free of dysplasia.
    (1) Radiographic findings consistent with hip dysplasia include:
      (a) A shallow acetabulum, flattened femoral head, or both
      (b) Poor coverage (less than 50%) of the femoral head by the acetabulum in young animals (i.e., subluxation) (Figure 18–3)
      (c) Subchondral bone sclerosis
      (d) Femoral neck remodeling (in older dogs)
      (e) Periarticular osteophyte formation
    (2) Although generally related, the severity of radiographic changes and the degree of lameness can be widely disparate.
    (3) A dorsal acetabular rim radiographic view is used by some surgeons to evaluate candidates for triple pelvic osteotomy.
    (4) A stress-radiographic method for quantitating hip-joint laxity has recently been described. Compression and distraction are applied to the hip joints and measurements of the femoral head relative to the acetabulum are made to assess hip joint laxity.
  e. **Treatment**
    (1) **Nonsurgical** management includes exercise restriction, weight reduction, anti-inflammatory medications, and joint fluid modifiers (see II A 4 a).
    (2) **Surgical**
      (a) **Pectineal muscle** or **tendon resection** has been used to alleviate pain from abnormal concussion of the femoral head against the dorsal acetabular rim. For this procedure, a medial approach to the pectineal muscle is used, and either the muscle or tendon of origin is removed. The long-term clinical benefits of this procedure are debatable because DJD continues to progress.
      (b) **Triple pelvic osteotomy**
        (i) **Indications.** The procedure is performed in young dogs with clinical signs and subluxation, that lack secondary DJD. The value of triple pelvic osteotomy in asymptomatic dogs with joint laxity and radiographic signs is controversial.

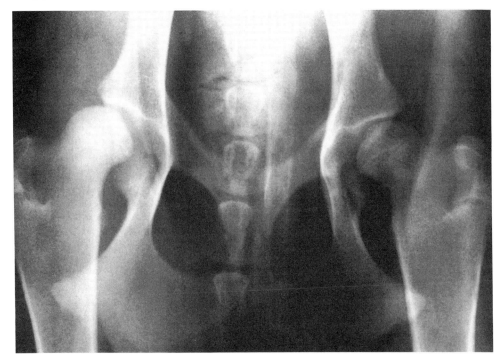

FIGURE 18–3. Bilateral hip dysplasia in a young dog. Note the inadequate seating of the femoral heads in the acetabula.

        (ii) Procedure. Cuts are made in the ilium, ischium, and pubis to allow rotation of the acetabulum so that there is greater coverage of the femoral head by the acetabulum. The ilial segment is secured in its new angled position with a bone plate. The ilial osteotomy usually heals within 6–8 weeks, but bilaterally affected dogs can undergo separate procedures 3–6 weeks apart.

    (c) Femoral head and neck ostectomy is performed as a salvage procedure to eliminate the source of pain associated with dysplasia.

        (i) Indications. Femoral head and neck ostectomy may be performed in mature or immature animals.

        (ii) Procedure. The femoral head and neck are excised using a craniolateral approach to the hip joint. The osteotomy is angled from the greater to the lesser trochanters and smoothed with a bone rasp. A pseudarthrosis is thus created based on the remaining joint capsule, fibrous scar tissue, and support of the limb by gluteal muscles.

        (iii) Prognosis. Early postoperative activity and physical therapy are associated with a good prognosis. The placement of muscle tissues interposed between the acetabulum and resected femoral neck remains controversial in improving patient outcome.

    (d) Total hip replacement with synthetic prostheses has the greatest ability to reestablish normal mechanical function of the hip. Eighty percent of animals with bilateral dysplasia regain satisfactory function following unilateral surgery.

        (i) Procedure. The diseased femoral head and neck are excised using a craniolateral approach. The acetabulum and femoral medullary canal are scraped and bone cement is used to adhere the prostheses to the bone. The cemented total hip is the most commonly used implant, although research on cementless implants is currently being performed.

(ii) **Prognosis.** Approximately 90%–95% of animals exhibit normal or near normal function following hip replacement. Strict surgical asepsis and careful postoperative care are integral to the success of this procedure.

2. **Elbow dysplasia** is a term that describes generalized incongruence of the elbow associated with FMCP of the ulna, ununited anconeal process (UAP), or osteochondrosis of the medial humoral condyle. These conditions may exist singularly or in combination.

  a. **FMCP** results from abnormal development or abnormal forces applied to the region.

    (1) **Predisposing factors.** This disease is most frequently recognized in large-breed dogs, especially Labrador retrievers. It can occur in dogs of any age, but usually manifests at 6 months of age or older.

    (2) **Clinical presentation.** It is characterized by mild to moderate lameness that worsens with exercise. Physical examination may reveal swelling of the medial aspect of the joint and pain on palpation in this region.

    (3) **Diagnosis.** Radiographic confirmation is often difficult and may require oblique views of the elbow joint or computed tomography. Often the only radiographic evidence is periarticular osteophyte production in the region of the anconeal process, medial epicondyle, or radial head (Figure 18–4). Surgical exploration is often used to confirm the disease.

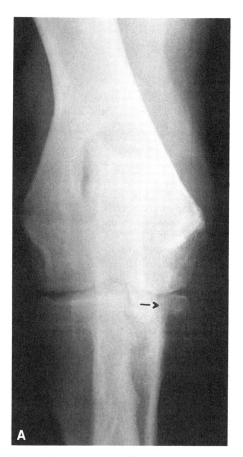
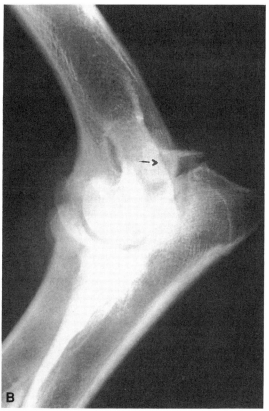

FIGURE 18–4. A canine elbow joint with fragmented medial coronoid process (FMCP) and ununited anconeal process (UAP) of the ulna. *(A)* Craniocaudal view shows periarticular osteophyte formation *(arrow)* along the medial border of the radius. *(B)* Lateral to medial projection shows the UAP *(arrow)* and periarticular osteophytosis along the cranial border of the radius.

(4) **Treatment** by surgical excision of the fragmented coronoid process through a medial approach is recommended.
(5) **Prognosis.** Surgery usually results in improvement of clinical signs but not normality, because degenerative changes may progress.

b. **UAP**
(1) **Predisposing factors.** UAP typically occurs in large-breed dogs, such as German shepherds. Small, chondrodystrophic breeds such as basset hounds may also be affected.
(2) **Diagnosis.**
(a) Lameness is usually intermittent and exacerbated by exercise. Joint effusion is usually present.
(b) The diagnosis is confirmed radiographically when an open anconeal physis is identified in an animal 20 weeks of age or older (see Figure 18-4B). Because the growth plate of the anconeal process does not normally close before 20 weeks of age, diagnosis cannot be confirmed until this time.
(3) **Treatment.** Surgical excision of the anconeal process is most frequently performed. Surgical stabilization with a bone screw can be attempted, but requires anatomic alignment and reduction, which may not be possible in many cases.
(4) **Prognosis.** Surgical excision provides good functional recovery, although arthritis may progress. The presence of DJD prior to surgery worsens the prognosis.

C. **Legg-Calvé-Perthes disease** (aseptic necrosis of the femoral head) is discussed in Chapter 16 V B 6.

D. **Congenital luxation**

1. **Patellar luxation** occurs when the patella does not articulate with the trochlear groove, but is located laterally or medially to its proper location. **Medial luxation** typically occurs in small-breed dogs, and **lateral luxation** in large-breed dogs, although any dog can have a medial or lateral luxation.
a. **Pathophysiology.** Patellar luxation rarely occurs as an isolated event, and is more appropriately thought of as being associated with deformity of the entire hindlimb.
(1) Abnormalities associated with **medial patellar luxation** include coxa vara, lateral bowing of the femur and internal rotation of the proximal tibia, a shallow trochlear groove, bowing of the tibia, and hypoplasia of the medial femoral condyle (Figure 18–5).
(2) For congenital **lateral luxations,** bone rotations and bowing are reversed (i.e., coxa valga, medial bowing of the femur, external rotation of the proximal tibia, and hypoplasia of the lateral femoral condyle).
b. **Classification.** A grading system of I to IV is used to describe severity of patellar luxation.
(1) **Grade I:** The patella can be forced out of the trochlear groove but returns to the groove when the external force is removed. Deformity and lameness are minimal.
(2) **Grade II:** The patella freely moves in and out of the trochlear groove. An infrequent "skipping" lameness occurs when the patella luxates. Normal gait returns when the patella spontaneously repositions.
(3) **Grade III:** The patella is naturally out of the trochlear groove, but can be forced back into the normal position. Lameness occurs frequently and tends to be more constant than in grade II patients.
(4) **Grade IV:** This is the most severe deformity. The patella is out of the trochlear groove and cannot be forced back into the normal position. Lameness and hind limb deformity are severe. In a grade IV medial luxation, the tibia is rotated 90° internally in relation to the femur. The animal may be unable to walk because of a flexed hind limb position.

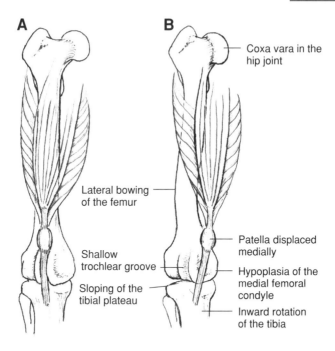

A

B

Coxa vara in the
hip joint

Lateral bowing
of the femur

Shallow
trochlear groove

Patella displaced
medially

Hypoplasia of the
medial femoral
condyle

Sloping of the
tibial plateau

Inward rotation
of the tibia

FIGURE 18–5. *(A)* Normal pelvic limb. *(B)* Bone deformities associated with congenital medial patellar luxation.

c. **Clinical presentation.** Intermittent or continuous lameness is usually the presenting clinical sign. Lameness tends to be absent or mild with grade I and worsens with higher grades of patellar luxation or concurrent cranial cruciate ligament and medial meniscal injuries.

d. **Treatment** depends on the severity and progression of disease.

(1) **Indications for surgery.** Treatment for asymptomatic dogs is controversial. If clinical signs do not exist, and patellar luxation is detected on routine examination, surgical treatment may not be warranted. Some surgeons believe that a luxating patella may predispose the dog to greater degenerative change, and therefore asymptomatic dogs should have surgery. Most surgeons, however, believe that only dogs with clinical lameness benefit from surgery.

(2) **Treatment options** involve a combination of soft tissue and orthopedic procedures to keep the patella in the trochlear groove. In general, the greater the severity of luxation, the greater the number of techniques needed.

(a) **Soft tissue techniques**

(i) **Imbrication or plication.** The joint capsule and fascia on the side opposite the luxation are tightened to provide stabilization of the patella. Large, nonabsorbable or synthetic absorbable sutures can be used in a mattress pattern.

(ii) **Release.** The joint capsule and fascia on the side of the luxation are incised to allow the patella to be pulled to the opposite side by imbrication techniques. It is not necessary to close these deep layers primarily, although the joint capsule should be sutured if possible.

(iii) **Fabellar suture.** A suture or strip of fascia lata is placed around the fabella opposite the direction of luxation and through the patellar ligament or the tibial crest. This pulls the patella and rotates the limb in the direction opposite the luxation, and helps to align the patella in the trochlear groove (Figure 18–6).

(b) **Orthopedic techniques**

(i) **Tibial crest transposition.** An osteotomy is performed and the tibial crest is moved in the direction opposite the luxation. This realigns

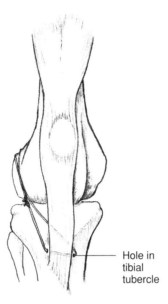

Hole in
tibial
tubercle

FIGURE 18–6. Fabellar suture technique for reducing medial patellar luxation. Nonabsorbable suture is passed from around the lateral fabella through the tibial tuberosity to externally rotate the tibia. (Redrawn and modified with permission from Brinker WO, Piermattei DL, Flo GL: *Handbook of Small Animal Orthopedics and Fracture Treatment,* 2nd ed. Philadelphia, WB Saunders, 1990, p 384.)

the tibial crest and trochlear groove so that the patella may rest within the trochlear groove.

(ii) **Trochleoplasty.** All trochleoplasty techniques deepen the trochlear groove. The simplest technique in mature animals is **trochlear sulcoplasty,** which involves using a rongeur or rasp to remove the articular cartilage and subchondral bone, deepening the trochlear groove so that the patella stays in place. A technically more demanding, but cartilage-sparing and, therefore, preferred technique, is **wedge recession trochleoplasty,** in which a V-shaped piece of bone is cut from the trochlea and then replaced after additional exposed bone is removed (Figure 18–7).

(iii) **Trochlear chondroplasty.** In immature patients, a cartilage flap can be elevated and underlying subchondral bone removed. The flap,

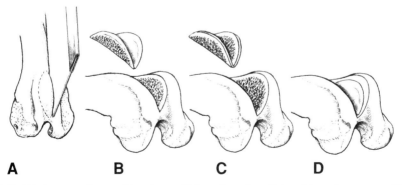

A   B   C   D

FIGURE 18–7. Wedge recession trochleoplasty. *(A)* Location of medial and lateral saw cuts. *(B)* Removal of osteochondral wedge. *(C)* Deepening of trochlear bed by removal of a second wedge. *(D)* Placement of the original osteochondral wedge (i.e., the one with the cartilage surface) into the trochlear bed. (Redrawn with permission from Boone EC, Jr., Hohn RB, Weisbrode SE: Trochlear recession wedge technique for patellar luxation: an experimental study. *J Am Anim Hosp Assoc,* 19:735, 1983.)

still attached proximally or distally, is placed back over the bone defect to provide a hyaline cartilage base for patellar articulation.

(iv) Other techniques. Corrective osteotomy, stifle arthrodesis, or amputation can be considered for grade IV luxations if the animal is unable to walk and other corrective procedures are inadequate.

Corrective osteotomy. Transverse cuts are made in the femur or the tibia or both, and the bones are rotated to align the patella in the trochlear groove. Bone stabilization is usually accomplished through internal fixation using a bone plate and screws.

Stifle arthrodesis [see II A 4 b (1)]. To compensate for a loss of bone length during cartilage and subchondral bone curettage, the stifle is fixed at an angle slightly greater (130°–150°) than the contralateral joint.

Limb amputation (see Chapter 16 V D 1 b) involves midshaft resection of the femur or disarticulation at the coxofemoral joint, using the thigh muscles for soft tissue coverage.

e. **Prognosis.** The prognosis for recovery with surgery is excellent for grades I and II, good for grade III, and poor for grade IV.

2. **Shoulder luxation.** Cranial, caudal, medial, or lateral luxation may occur. Congenital medial luxation of the shoulder is typically associated with small-breed dogs. Concurrent incongruence of the glenoid cavity and proximal humeral head is common, and therefore this malarticulation is best left untreated if the animal is pain-free and only mildly lame. Arthrodesis or excision arthroplasty of the humoral head can be performed if the animal is lame and in pain.

3. **Elbow luxation.** Congenital luxation of the elbow is typically associated with severe incongruence of the olecranon fossa and distal humerus. Surgical intervention can be attempted using a transarticular pin or external fixator, but the joint is usually incongruent and degenerate, and the prognosis is guarded.

V. TRAUMATIC CONDITIONS

A. General considerations

1. **Fractures** of the physis and articular surface can cause premature closing of the growth plate, leading to shortening of the limb and angular deviation (see Chapter 16 II A 2 a). These abnormalities stress the adjacent joints, which can cause malarticulation and DJD.

2. **Luxations** result from third-degree sprains and joint capsule disruption. Secondary DJD is also a likely complication of luxations.

3. **Sprains**
   a. **Classification.** Sprains are classified according to the degree of tissue disruption.
      (1) **First-degree** sprains involve stretching or minimal tearing of the ligament. Mild inflammation, swelling, tenderness, and pain may be present.
      (2) **Second-degree** sprains involve partial tearing of the ligament. Inflammation, swelling, tenderness, and pain are moderate in severity.
      (3) **Third-degree** sprains are complete tears of the ligament that can result in joint instability. Inflammation, swelling, tenderness, and pain are severe.
   b. **Diagnosis** can be difficult.
      (1) **Differential diagnosis.** Sprains are often diagnosed by exclusion, when fractures and other causes of lameness cannot be identified.
      (2) **Radiography.** Third-degree sprains can be diagnosed by stress radiography—an abnormal joint space is visible when angular forces are applied to the joint.
   c. **Treatment** is based on the severity of the injury.
      (1) **Conservative treatment.** First- and second-degree sprains, and stable third-de-

gree sprains, are treated with **rest** and **bandaging. NSAIDs** can be useful for reducing acute inflammation and discomfort.

(2) **Surgical treatment.** If the joint is unstable, surgical repair, either by direct suturing of the ligament or by prosthetic ligament techniques (e.g., suture support of the adjoining bone ends) may be required. Arthrodesis of the joint may be necessary in chronic and severe cases of multiple ligamentous injury.

B. **Shoulder injuries**

1. **Fractures** involving the articular surface of the scapula or proximal humerus are uncommon.
   a. **Scapula.** Articular fractures of the scapula are best treated by **internal fixation** with pins, wires, or small plates and screws [see Chapter 16 V A 2 c]. Prognosis for return to normal function is poor if articular congruency is not recovered postoperatively.
   b. **Proximal humerus.** Salter-Harris type I and II fractures of the proximal humerus can be repaired satisfactorily with either **closed reduction and immobilization** by a Velpeau sling, or by **open reduction and internal fixation** with intramedullary pins (see Chapter 16 V A 3 a).

2. **Luxations** can be either medial or lateral, but typically occur laterally and in large-breed dogs. Surgical stabilization by transposition of the biceps tendon is recommended if reduction cannot be maintained with either a Velpeau sling (for medial luxation) or a Spica bandage (for lateral luxation).

C. **Elbow injuries**

1. **Fractures**
   a. **Lateral humeral condyle fractures** are common in young dogs, and also occur occasionally in mature dogs, especially cocker spaniels.
      (1) **Types of condylar fractures**
         (a) A **Salter-Harris type IV fracture** typically occurs when the dog jumps from a surface and lands on the front limbs, transmitting excess force up the radius to shear off the lateral humeral condyle.
         (b) **T and Y fractures** involving both the medial and lateral humeral condyles also occur, and create even greater instability than lateral humeral condyle fractures.
      (2) **Surgical treatment of these fractures is imperative for satisfactory outcome** (see Chapter 16 V A 3 c). Casting, splinting, or bandaging is inadequate and results in a severely compromised joint.
      (3) **Complications.** Although infrequent, Salter-Harris type V injury of the radial and ulnar growth plates can occur as a result of the forces applied to the limb that cause distal humeral fractures. This may result in angular limb deformity (see Chapter 16 V A 4 c). Frequent examinations during convalescence to monitor for the development of this abnormality are indicated. Radiographic examination should be performed if angular limb deformity is suspected from physical examination findings.
   b. **Radial head and ulnar trochlear notch fractures** should be treated by rigid internal fixation with anatomic alignment of the articular surface. Radial head fractures are difficult to repair because of the small size of the bone fragments and the proximity of vital neurovascular structures.
   c. **Monteggia fractures** are a combination of cranial luxation of the radial head and fracture of the proximal portion of the shaft of the ulna. Treatment consists of realignment and internal fixation of the ulna and suturing of the torn radial collateral ligament [see Chapter 16 V A 4 (a) (2)].

2. **Luxation** of the elbow is nearly always lateral (i.e., lateral luxation of the ulna with respect to the humerus). The large medial epicondylar ridge of the humerus effectively prevents medial luxation. Collateral ligament damage is suspected but not always confirmed. Closed reduction and external coaptation is usually successful in acute cases. If not, open reduction and stabilization with external coaptation can be performed.

3. **Isolated collateral ligament damage** is detected by stressing the joint to open medially or laterally. These injuries usually do not require surgical intervention and heal with conservative management and temporary immobilization. Repair by reattaching an avulsed bone fragment or by employing a prosthetic ligament technique (i.e., using wire or nonabsorbable suture in a figure-of-eight pattern) can be performed.

D. Carpal injuries

1. **Fractures. Secondary degenerative change** occurs commonly with fracture of any carpal bone.
   a. **Fractures of the radial and accessory carpal bones** are rare except in the working or racing animal. The fixation method depends on the degree of comminution.
      (1) Highly comminuted fractures are usually treated with external coaptation because they lack fragments of sufficient size to hold pins or screws.
      (2) Fractures that include larger fragments can be treated with pins or screws, or external coaptation if displacement is minimal.
   b. **Fracture of the numbered carpal bones** occurs less frequently and is usually treated by splinting, fragment excision, or, infrequently, internal fixation.

2. **Hyperextension** is the most common injury, and occurs when excessive force, usually from jumping off an elevated surface, is applied to the carpus. It can occur at several levels simultaneously, including the antebrachiocarpal, the middle carpal, and the carpometacarpal joints.
   a. **Clinical presentation.** Tearing of supporting ligamentous structures of the carpus (i.e., the palmar carpal ligaments and palmar fibrocartilage) results in the plantigrade stance characteristic of this injury. The animal typically attempts to walk on the injured limb, particularly after the pain of the acute injury diminishes, although function usually does not improve with time.
   b. **Treatment. Arthrodesis** is usually necessary for these third-degree sprains. Splint or cast management is generally unsuccessful.
      (1) **Pancarpal arthrodesis** is indicated for complete disruption of the radiocarpal joint or of all carpal joints.
      (2) **Partial arthrodesis** is indicated for injuries involving the middle or distal carpal joints, and may preserve function of the antebrachiocarpal joint. It is performed by fusing the carpometacarpal and middle carpal joints.
   c. **Prognosis.** Limb function following partial or pancarpal arthrodesis is good. Complications include breakage and irritation from bone plates, necessitating implant removal.

3. **Shear injuries** to the carpus occur when the carpus is trapped between a tire and pavement and the animal is dragged for a distance. There is loss of overlying skin, muscle, and tendon, and, frequently, collateral ligaments and bone. Complete carpal luxation may occur. These wounds are usually heavily contaminated. **If the joint becomes infected, severe damage to the articular cartilage occurs.**
   a. **Treatment.** Open wound management [i.e., soft tissue débridement, lavage with polyionic solution (e.g., lactated Ringer's), and systemic antibiotics] and stabilization are necessary.
      (1) **External fixation** allows the joint to be stabilized without restricting access to the soft tissue injuries. Once soft tissue injuries are satisfactorily addressed, the joint injury can be definitively treated. In less severe cases, temporary stabilization with an external fixator or coaptation may allow the formation of sufficient scar tissue, eliminating the need for additional treatment.
      (2) **Prosthetic ligament techniques** and **arthrodesis** can be used to provide more rigid joint stabilization. Treatment is based on the amount and quality of articular cartilage remaining. If complete carpal luxation occurs, **pancarpal arthrodesis** may be necessary to salvage the limb.
   b. **Prognosis** is guarded, although many patients recover satisfactory ambulation despite the devastating appearance of the initial injury. **Amputation should not be performed routinely** in the early management of these cases. With proper wound care and external fixation, recovery is often successful.

E. **Phalangeal injuries. Interphalangeal joint luxation** is an uncommon but painful injury that can be devastating to the working dog. Treatment by open **reduction and imbrication of the joint** is recommended. Other alternatives include **arthrodesis** or **amputation** of the digit.

F. **Hip injuries**

1. **Fractures**
   a. **Acetabular fractures** are common and usually require surgical intervention (see Chapter 17 II E 3).
   b. **Fracture of the femoral head** occurs as a Salter-Harris type I fracture in young animals and is referred to as a **capital physis fracture** [see also Chapter 16 V A 7 a (1)]. This fracture is treated by open reduction and stabilization using multiple small pins or Kirschner wires (Figure 18–8) or a lag screw. Alternatively, femoral head and neck ostectomy can be performed [see IV B 1 e (2) (c)].
   c. **Femoral neck fractures** occur in mature animals. Techniques for repair are similar to those used for femoral head fractures.

2. **Luxation.** Traumatic coxofemoral luxation usually results in cranial and dorsal displacement of the femoral head in relation to the acetabulum.
   a. **Closed reduction** is performed with the animal under general anesthesia to reduce muscle tone and resistance to manipulation.
      (1) Technique
         (a) Craniodorsal luxations are reduced by externally rotating the limb and pulling caudodistally until the femoral head sets in the acetabulum. The joint is then put through a range of motion with pressure over the greater trochanter to make sure no portion of the joint capsule is between the femoral head and acetabulum.
         (b) Once reduced, positioning is confirmed radiographically.

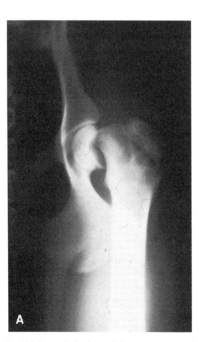
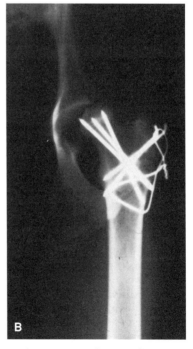

FIGURE 18–8. *(A)* A capital physeal fracture-separation and a greater trochanteric fracture. *(B)* The capital physeal fracture-separation has been reduced and stabilized with three divergent Kirschner wires. The greater trochanter fracture has been reduced and stabilized using two Kirschner wires and a tension band wire.

(c) The limb is placed in an Ehmer sling to maintain abduction, internal rotation, and flexion of the coxofemoral joint. The limb remains in the sling for 10–14 days.

(2) Success rate. Reduction is maintained in approximately 50% of dogs that are treated with closed reduction shortly after injury. Chronic cases have a poorer success rate.

b. Open reduction is performed if closed reduction fails.

(1) Techniques include capsulorrhaphy, trochanteric transposition, prosthetic capsule techniques, transacetabular or De Vita pinning, application of a flexible external fixator, and toggle pinning.

(2) Success rate. Despite open reduction, some animals fail to maintain reduction. **Femoral head and neck ostectomy and total hip replacement** are remaining options.

G. Stifle injuries

1. Ligament injuries

a. Cranial cruciate ligament injury results both from traumatic causes and from chronic degeneration of the ligament. Midsubstance tears may be complete or partial. Bone avulsion of the origin of the cranial cruciate ligament occurs infrequently.

(1) Clinical presentation. Acute onset of lameness and pain is typical. Pain usually diminishes after 3–5 days, but lameness persists for much longer. Untreated dogs may begin to bear weight 2–4 weeks after injury, if not sooner. If pain and severe lameness persist, concurrent medial meniscal injury is suspected. Partial cranial cruciate ligament injury typically results in chronic weight-bearing lameness that does not improve, and frequently worsens.

(2) Diagnosis is made by detecting abnormal cranial drawer motion during flexion and extension. Partial ligament tears are more difficult to diagnose because of the lack of cranial drawer motion. Diagnosis of these tears is typically based on a history of chronic lameness, physical examination findings of fibrous enlargement of the medial aspect of the joint (i.e., medial buttressing) and slight cranial drawer movement (usually greater in flexion than extension), and radiographic evidence of secondary DJD.

(3) Treatment. Surgical intervention is usually beneficial, particularly in active dogs weighing more than 15 kg. The goal of surgery is to reduce abnormal cranial motion and internal rotation of the tibia. A variety of techniques are available and are typically classified as intracapsular or extracapsular. Arthrotomy is performed to examine the menisci for injury. Although debate over various repair techniques has been extensive, the overall clinical success rate regardless of technique is approximately 85%.

(a) Intracapsular techniques involve passing a piece of autogenous tissue (i.e., fascia lata, patellar ligament) through the joint to biomechanically mimic the cranial cruciate ligament. The strip is secured to the lateral condyle by a bone screw and spiked washer or by suturing the strip to the periosteum. Procedures described include:

(i) Paatsama technique: Passing a fascia lata strip through a tunnel drilled in the lateral condyle and proximal tibia

(ii) Over-the-top techniques: Placing portions of the patellar tendon or combined patellar tendon and fascia lata through the joint and over the caudolateral aspect of the lateral femoral condyle

(iii) Under-and-over technique: Passing the fascia lata strip under the intermeniscal ligament into the joint and then over the lateral condyle

(iv) Brinker technique: Passing the fascia lata medially through the tibial tuberosity and then into the joint

(b) Extracapsular techniques

(i) Suture techniques involve placing monofilament suture material around the lateral fabella and through a hole drilled in the tibial crest. Variations include placing two lateral and one medial suture (modified retinacular imbrication technique), or placing sutures from the lateral fabella to the distal portion of the patellar ligament (DeAngelis technique).

(ii) **Fibular head transposition** involves advancing the fibular head cranially and securing it to the tibia with a pin and wire. Joint stabilization is provided by the taut lateral collateral ligament, which attaches to the fibular head.

(iii) **Imbrication** of the joint capsule and retinacular tissue can be performed as primary stabilization, but it is most useful in addition to intracapsular or other extracapsular techniques. Lateral advancement of the bicep femoris insertion or medial advancement of the sartorius insertion also provides soft tissue stabilization of the joint.

(4) **Damage to the medial meniscus** frequently accompanies cranial cruciate ligament injury. Medial meniscus injury is suspected if a meniscal click is palpated during physical examination, and is confirmed during arthrotomy. If the medial meniscus is damaged, **partial or complete meniscectomy** is performed. Experimentally, total meniscectomy causes greater damage to the joint. Clinically, however, the difference between partial and total meniscectomy remains controversial. The prognosis for dogs with cruciate ligament rupture and damaged menisci is generally less favorable than for those with intact menisci.

b. The **caudal cruciate ligament** is rarely injured as an isolated structure. A torn caudal cruciate ligament is frequently associated with other stifle joint injuries, such as cranial cruciate or collateral ligament rupture.

(1) **Diagnosis.** Caudal cruciate ligament injury is characterized by abnormal caudal drawer movement. Diagnosis can be hampered by difficulty in distinguishing between caudal and cranial drawer movement.

(2) **Treatment.** Surgical treatment of this injury may only be necessary after conservative management fails. Large, nonabsorbable sutures have been used between the patellar tendon and head of the fibula or caudoproximal aspect of the tibia to reduce abnormal caudal motion of the stifle joint. However, results have been equivocal.

c. **Isolated medial and lateral collateral ligament** damage occurs relatively infrequently. Collateral injury damage is frequently associated with damage to the cranial and caudal cruciate ligaments and the medial meniscus.

(1) **Diagnosis.** Damage is diagnosed on physical examination by applying lateral and medial forces to open one side of the joint.

(2) **Treatment.** Repair is performed by arthrotomy with attempted suturing of the ligament, reattachment of the avulsed fragment, or prosthetic ligament support and joint imbrication. Cruciate ligament repair and meniscectomy are also performed, if indicated.

2. **Luxation**

a. **Stifle luxation.** Damage to both medial and lateral collateral and both cruciate ligaments results in stifle luxation, a devastating injury. Repair is performed by stabilizing the individual injuries. An alternative method that has worked satisfactorily in cats and small dogs is transarticular pinning. This repair is simpler than repair of each individual injury. Regardless of treatment method, the overall prognosis is poor.

b. **Traumatic patellar luxation** occurs infrequently in large dogs. The condition is characterized by an acute onset of lameness, pain, and swelling of the stifle, usually following vigorous exercise. Surgical stabilization by closure of the tear in the joint capsule and imbrication of the surrounding retinaculum is usually successful.

3. **Fractures**

a. **Salter-Harris I and II fractures of the distal femur** occur more frequently than similar fractures of the proximal tibia. These fractures are best stabilized with

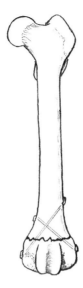

FIGURE 18–9. Static intramedullary cross-pinning for repair of a distal femoral physeal fracture using small pins or large Kirschner wires.

small Steinmann pins used as dynamic or static cross pins, Rush pins, or large Kirschner wires (Figure 18–9).

    b. Articular fractures involving the stifle are not common. Articular fractures should be treated with precise anatomic reduction and stabilization using pins, screws, plates, or a combination of these treatments.

    c. Patellar fractures are rare and should be treated by pin-and-wire stabilization if large fragments exist, or by partial patellectomy.

H. Tarsal injuries

    1. Fractures and luxations of the tarsal bones occur both in performance and nonperformance animals. Because of the small size of the bones, these injuries are difficult to treat. External coaptation is sometimes beneficial in the nonworking pet. If fragments are large, internal fixation with bone screws and Kirschner wires is usually beneficial.

        a. Fractures of the calcaneus must be stabilized with Kirschner wires or tension band wiring to neutralize the distracting forces of the common calcanean tendon.

        b. Central tarsal bone fractures in racing greyhounds require lag screw fixation.

        c. Luxation of the small tarsal bones can be treated with partial arthrodesis of the tarsus using a bone plate or pins and external support.

        d. Severe injury of the talocrural joint can be treated with pantarsal arthrodesis with a bone plate or external fixator.

    2. Fractures of the medial and lateral malleolus involve the articular surface. Joint instability results because collateral ligaments are attached to these structures. Anatomic repair is necessary to minimize secondary DJD, and is performed using small screws, pins, or pins and tension band wiring.

    3. Shear injury of the tarsus occurs with automobile trauma when the limb is caught between the tire and the road and dragged for some distance. Treatment is similar to that for carpal shear injury (see V D 3).

SELECTED READINGS
Alexander JW: Canine hip dysplasia. *Vet Clin North Am: Small Anim Pract.* Philadelphia, WB Saunders, 1992, 22(3):503–743.

Altman RD, Dean DD, Muniz OE, et al: Therapeutic treatment of canine osteoarthritis with gly-cosaminoglycan polysulfuric ester. *Arthritis Rheum* 32:1300–1307, 1989.

Bennett D, May C: Joint diseases of dogs and cats. In *Textbook of Internal Medicine,* 4th ed. Edited by Ettinger SJ and Feldman EC. Philadelphia, WB Saunders, 1994, pp 2032–2075.

Brinker WO, Piermattei DL, Flo GL: *Handbook of Small Animal Orthopedics and Fracture Treatment.* 2nd ed. Philadelphia, WB Saunders, 1990.

Gilson SD, Piermattei DL, Schwartz PD: Treatment of humeroulnar subluxation with a dynamic proximal ulnar osteotomy. *Vet Surg* 18:114–122, 1989.

Huber ML, Bill RL: The use of polysulfate glycosaminoglycan in dogs. *Comp Contin Educ* 16:501–505, 1994.

Johnson JM, Johnson AL, Eurell JC: Histological appearance of naturally occurring canine phy-seal fractures. *Vet Surg* 23:81–86, 1994.

Korvick DL, Johnson AL, Schaeffer DJ: Surgeons' preferences in treating cranial cruciate liga-ment ruptures in dogs. *J Am Vet Med Assoc* 205:1318–1324, 1994.

Lipowitz AJ: Degenerative joint disease. In *Textbook of Small Animal Surgery,* 2nd ed. Edited by Slatter D. Philadelphia, WB Saunders, 1993, pp 1921–1984.

Manley PA: The hip joint. In *Textbook of Small Animal Surgery,* 2nd ed. Edited by Slatter D. Philadelphia, WB Saunders, 1993, pp 1786–1805.

Moore GA: Degenerative joint disease. Pharmacology and therapeutics of treatment. *Vet Med Rep* 2:89–96, 1990.

Roush JK: Stifle surgery. *Vet Clin North Am: Small Anim Pract.* Philadelphia, WB Saunders, 1993, 23(4):691–914.

Schiavinato A, Lini E, Guidolin D, et al: Intraarticular sodium hyaluronate injections in the Pond-Nuki experimental model of osteoarthritis in dogs: II. Morphological findings. *Clin Or-thop* 241:286–299, 1989.

Smith GK, Biery DN, Gregor TP: New concepts of coxofemoral joint stability and the develop-ment of a clinical stress radiographic method for quantitating hip joint laxity in the dog. *J Am Vet Med Assoc* 196:59–70, 1990.

Todhunter RJ, Lust G: Polysulfate glycosaminoglycan in the treatment of osteoarthritis. *J Am Vet Med Assoc* 204:1245–1251, 1994.

Vail DM, Powers BE, Getzy DM, et al: Evaluation of prognostic factors for dogs with synovial sarcoma: 36 cases (1986–1991). *J Am Vet Med Assoc* 205:1300–1307, 1994.

Chapter 19

Skull

Alan J. Schulman

I. ANATOMY

A. **Bones** (Figure 19–1). The skull bones (i.e., those of the cranium, face, mandible, and maxilla) consist of compact, dense bone and spongy bone (diploë).

B. **Cavities.** The skull may be divided into a number of cavities. For example:

   1. The **cranial cavity** contains the brain.
      a. The roof of the cranial cavity is the **calvaria,** which is formed by the parietal and frontal bones. The base is formed by sphenoid bones rostrally and the basioccipital bone caudally. The caudal wall is formed by the occipital bone, and the rostral wall is formed by the cribriform plate of the ethmoid bone. The lateral walls are formed by the temporal, parietal, and frontal bones.
      b. Because the brain is enclosed within the rigid confines of the skull, there is a limit to which any of the intracranial constituents (i.e., the brain parenchyma, cerebrospinal fluid, and vascular system) may expand before causing an increase in **intracranial pressure.**

   2. The **nasal cavity** contains the facial portion of the respiratory tract.

   3. The **paranasal sinuses** include the maxillary, frontal, and sphenoid sinuses.

C. **Vasculature**

   1. **Arterial supply.** The carotid artery and its branches supply the head. The vascular supply to the brain is divided into rostral and caudal circulations.
      a. The **rostral circulation** is derived from the external carotid artery.
      b. The **caudal circulation** is derived from the basilar artery, which originates from the vertebral artery.
      c. The **arterial circle of the brain** (the **circle of Willis**) is found at the base of the brain; it is formed by branches of the internal carotid and basilar arteries.

   2. **Venous drainage.** Blood from the brain drains into the dorsal sinuses and is transported to the maxillary, internal jugular, and vertebral veins, as well as the vertebral venous plexus. The main channel for return of venous blood from the head is the external jugular vein.

II. GENERAL CONSIDERATIONS

A. **Advances in skull surgery.** Precise diagnostic tools (e.g., radiography, magnetic resonance imaging, computed tomography, nuclear imaging) have allowed numerous advances in skull surgery. Advances in anesthetic and surgical techniques have reduced patient morbidity and mortality.

B. **Goals of surgical intervention**

   1. The primary objective of **cranial surgery** is to prevent or reverse damage to neural tissue. Neurologic damage occurring immediately after trauma is potentially reversible if treatment is immediate and appropriate.

   2. The major objectives of **mandibular and maxillary fracture repair** are accurate rees-

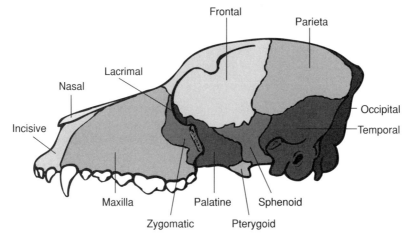

FIGURE 19–1. Bones of the skull, lateral aspect. The zygomatic arch and mandible have been removed. (Redrawn with permission from Evans HE: *Miller's Anatomy of the Dog*, 3rd ed. Philadelphia, WB Saunders, 1993, p 114.)

tablishment of dental occlusion, restoration of masticatory function, and reversal of respiratory obstruction, oronasal communication, or both.

III. CONDITIONS OF THE SKULL TREATED BY SURGERY

A. Trauma

1. **Preoperative considerations**
   a. **Examination.** It is usually safe to assume that an animal with a skull fracture has been subjected to severe head trauma. Although a client may be concerned with the immediate external appearance of the animal, a complete physical examination is necessary to evaluate potentially life-threatening injuries affecting other body systems.
      (1) The **cardiopulmonary, urologic, gastrointestinal,** and **musculoskeletal systems** should be evaluated, triaged, and treated accordingly.
      (2) Palpation and visual **examination of the affected area** is necessary to determine the degree of damage. Thorough evaluation of the oral cavity and skull, using imaging techniques if necessary, is best performed after the animal is stabilized and can be safely anesthetized (see III A 1 b).
   b. **Stabilization.** In the absence of neurologic deterioration, anesthesia and surgical intervention should be delayed until the animal is stable. Considerations unique to intracranial surgery (e.g., reducing intracranial pressure) are discussed in Chapter 21 I A–C.
      (1) **Ensuring adequate ventilation.** A patent airway is of paramount concern.
         (a) The mouth and upper airway should be inspected for foreign bodies or other causes of obstruction.
         (b) Thoracic radiography, auscultation, and blood gas analysis can also be used to assess the adequacy of ventilation.
      (2) **Ensuring adequate tissue perfusion.** Once adequate ventilation has been established, the circulatory status should be assessed.
         (a) The quality of the pulse should be evaluated and the blood pressure measured. However, young, otherwise healthy animals can maintain normal or near normal pulse and blood pressure parameters despite continuing hemorrhage until a point when irreversible shock develops as compensa-

tory mechanisms fail. At this point, initiation of aggressive support measures may be too late.
- **(b)** Peripheral perfusion can be assessed using transcutaneous oximetry.
- **(c)** The circulating blood volume should be assessed, based on urine output and central venous pressure, and maintained as necessary.
  - **(i)** Infusion of small volumes of hypertonic saline and colloids provides cardiovascular support without worsening brain edema and increasing intracranial pressure.
  - **(ii)** Hemorrhage must be controlled.
- **c. Anesthesia**
  - **(1)** In animals with fractures causing dental malocclusion, an endotracheal tube may hinder jaw manipulation and prevent evaluation of the occlusion during fracture repair. In these animals, tracheal intubation is accomplished via pharyngostomy or tracheostomy.
  - **(2)** Anesthesia protocols for intracranial surgery are discussed in Chapter 21 I C.

2. Basic principles of skull and jaw fracture repair
- **a. Standard aseptic preparation** of the surgical site is performed and the endotracheal tube cuff is inflated to prevent aspiration of blood or lavage fluid. Gauze sponges can be placed in the oropharynx to help prevent aspiration from the nasal and oral cavities.
- **b. Antibiotic therapy.** Because oral cavity fractures are open and contaminated, broad-spectrum bactericidal antibiotics are administered preoperatively to prevent brain infection, which can have devastating effects.
- **c. Thorough débridement of nonviable tissues** and removal of foreign material should be performed.
- **d. Additional trauma should be avoided** [e.g., to the central nervous system (CNS), teeth, or soft tissue].
- **e. Stable fixation** should be used to neutralize distracting forces on the fracture line.
- **f. Postoperative care**
  - **(1) Extraoral fractures.** Symptoms of CNS disease and airflow obstruction (in cases involving the bones encasing the nasal turbinates) must be managed.
  - **(2) Oral cavity fractures.** Postoperative care involves feeding of soft foods (except when the repair involves forced occlusion, which entails a liquid diet or parenteral nutrition) and prevention of self-induced trauma to the fracture repair. Initial antibiotic treatment should be followed by the administration of a specific agent (based on the results of bacterial culture and sensitivity testing of samples obtained during surgery).

3. Fractures of the lower jaw are relatively common in dogs and cats, accounting for approximately 3% and 15% of all fractures, respectively. Mandibular symphyseal fractures predominate in cats, whereas fractures in the premolar region predominate in dogs (Figure 19–2).
- **a. Fracture-separation of the mandibular symphysis**
  - **(1) Circumferential wiring** (Figure 19–3) is the most commonly used method of mandibular symphyseal fracture-separation repair. Approximately 4 weeks of fixation are necessary to allow sufficient healing.
  - **(2) Interfragmentary transmandibular pins** or **lag screw fixation** may be indicated for additional stabilization in large animals or if significant tissue loss or damage is present.
- **b. Fractures of the mandibular body (horizontal ramus).** A wide variety of fractures occur in this region and usually affect the alveoli and teeth. Teeth in the fracture site may affect bone healing: If the teeth are fractured, luxated, or infected, they are usually removed unless they contribute to fracture stability.
  - **(1)** A **tape muzzle** may work well when temporary jaw fracture stabilization is required, or as an adjunct to internal fixation. Tape muzzles may also be used as the primary method of repair in minimally displaced stable fractures.
    - **(a)** An intact contralateral mandible acts as a splint to help stabilization.
    - **(b)** A 0.5- to 1.5-cm gap between the upper and lower incisors should be

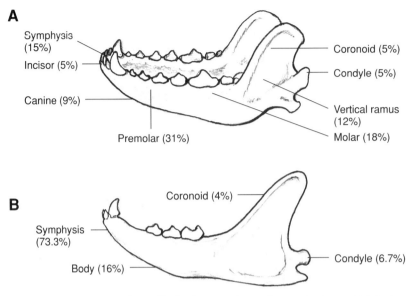

FIGURE 19–2. Common locations of mandibular fractures in (*A*) dogs and (*B*) cats. [(*A*) Redrawn and modified with permission from Umphlet RC, Johnson AL: Mandibular fractures in the dog: a retrospective study of 157 cases. *Vet Surg* 19(4):273, 1990. (*B*) Redrawn and modified with permission from Umphlet RC, Johnson AL: Mandibular fractures in the cat: a retrospective study. *Vet Surg* 17(6):334, 1988.]

provided to allow prehension of food. Alternatively, the mouth may be taped shut if extraoral alimentary feeding techniques are employed.

   (c) Common problems with tape support include intolerance, contact dermatitis, and prolonged healing times.

(2) **Interarcade fixation** may be more effective for treating rostral fractures in cats and brachycephalic dogs than application of a tape muzzle.

   (a) Bilateral loops of wire are passed between the mandible and maxilla to maintain dental occlusion (Figure 19–4A).

   (b) Alternatively, special pins can be placed on the buccal surfaces of all four canine teeth and joined with wire or acrylic.

(3) **Intraoral acrylic splints** are an easy, relatively noninvasive means of fixation recommended for fractures rostral to the first molar.

   (a) Once the fracture is reduced and proper occlusion reestablished, the

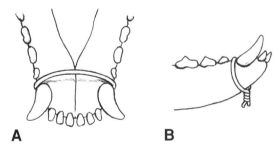

FIGURE 19–3. Circumferential wiring technique for simple symphyseal fracture separations. (*A*) A hypodermic needle is used to pass a single, 18- to 22-gauge stainless steel wire beneath the mandibular mucosa and caudal to the canine teeth, encircling the mandible. (*B*) The wire ends are twisted together to provide reduction. If the canine teeth diverge, the wire may be twisted in a figure-of-eight pattern around the canine teeth, tightened, and, in some cases, covered with intraoral acrylic (not shown). (Redrawn with permission from Nunamaker DM: Fractures and dislocations of the mandible. In *Textbook of Small Animal Orthopedics.* Edited by Newton CD, Nunamaker DM. Philadelphia, JB Lippincott, 1985, p 302.)

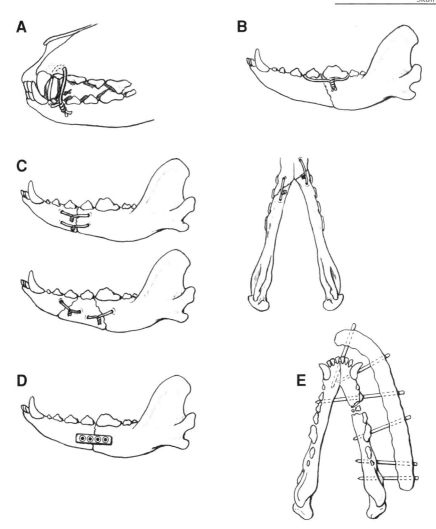

FIGURE 19–4. Repair of fractures of the mandibular body. (*A*) Interarcade fixation is effective for treating rostral fractures in cats and brachycephalic dogs. Bilateral wire loops are passed through holes in the mandible and maxilla. The loops are tightened enough to maintain occlusion; enough space is left between the teeth to permit prehension of liquids and soft foods. (Redrawn with permission from Egger EL: Skull and mandibular fractures. In Slatter D: *Textbook of Small Animal Surgery*, 2nd ed. Philadelphia, WB Saunders, 1993, p 1912.) (*B*) Interdental wiring technique. The wire is passed around the bases of the teeth adjacent to the fracture. Alternatively, the wire may be passed through holes drilled between the roots of the adjacent teeth (not shown). (Redrawn with permission from Brinker WO, Piermattei DL, Flo GL: Fractures and dislocations of the upper and lower jaw. In *Handbook of Small Animal Orthopedics and Fracture Management*. Philadelphia, WB Saunders, 1983, p 186.) (*C*) Interfragmentary wiring technique. Interfragmentary wiring is most successful when the opposite mandible is intact, at least two wires are placed across the fracture site, the wires are oriented at right angles to the fracture line, and the wires are passed so that they avoid tooth roots. (Redrawn with permission from Brinker WO, Piermattei DL, Flo GL: Fractures and dislocations of the upper and lower jaw. In *Handbook of Small Animal Orthopedics and Fracture Management*. Philadelphia, WB Saunders, 1983, p 187.) (*D*) Bone plate and screws. A small bone plate is applied across the fracture near the ventral border of the bone in order to avoid the roots of the teeth and the medullary canal of the mandible. (*E*) Application of a percutaneous skeletal fixation device to a fractured mandible. A low-speed drill is used to make holes between the tooth roots for the insertion of fixation pins through small skin incisions. The acrylic is molded around the pins and allowed to cure. Alternatively, the fracture can be reduced and temporarily stabilized with connecting clamps and bars while the acrylic is applied and allowed to harden.

splint is constructed and orthopedic wire is incorporated into the splint to allow fixation to the teeth.

(b) Complications include potential mucosal damage (because of the exothermic reaction produced while the acrylic is setting) and accumulation of food, debris, and exudate in the fracture site.

(4) **Interdental wiring** (see Figure 19–4B) works best when there is a solid, intact tooth on each side of a relatively stable fracture site. Incorporation of two teeth on each side of the fracture provides the most surgical stability.

(a) Depending on the size of the animal, 18- to 24-gauge wire is used.

(b) Overtightening the wire must be avoided to prevent distraction of the ventral mandibular border.

(5) **Interfragmentary wiring** (see Figure 19–4C). Short oblique and simple transverse fractures can be stabilized with simple interrupted cerclage wiring techniques. Interfragmentary wiring is not recommended for stabilization of highly comminuted fractures associated with bone loss, because reduction and stability are difficult to achieve.

(6) **Intramedullary pins** have been used for repair of mandibular body fractures; however, malunion and malocclusion as a result of malalignment and inadequate stability are fairly common. These complications result because of the difficulty of passing pins through dense mandibular bone. Other complications include damage to vessels, nerves, and tooth roots, as well as thermal necrosis of bone associated with power drilling.

(7) **Bone plate and screw fixation** of complex and bilateral mandibular fractures (see Figure 19–4D) provides excellent stability and anatomic reduction and allows reestablishment of dental occlusion immediately after surgery. Specialized plating equipment (e.g., reconstruction, "T," "L," or "mini" plates) provides tremendous versatility in approaching fracture repair.

(a) Theoretically, bone plates should be applied near the alveolar (dorsal) border, which is the tension side of the mandible. However, application of bone plates to this area causes gingival erosion and damage to tooth roots and neurovascular structures.

(b) Ventrolateral placement of bone plates provides accurate and rigid reduction with rapid return of function.

(8) **Percutaneous skeletal fixation devices** are excellent for the treatment of complex comminuted compound fractures associated with bone loss and severe soft tissue trauma.

(a) This technique provides rigid stability with minimal soft tissue dissection and excellent versatility.

(b) Acrylic can replace the more cumbersome bar and pin configurations associated with a metal apparatus. The acrylic is adaptable and easily contoured to treat bilateral and multiple fractures (see Figure 19–4E).

(9) **Partial mandibulectomy** [see Chapter 10 I G 2 f (2)] can be used as a salvage procedure in cases where primary fixation has failed or if extreme trauma and infection preclude reduction and stability.

(10) **Intraoral dental bonding of canine teeth** has been used to stabilize mandibular fractures and luxations in dogs and cats. A dental composite is applied to the teeth and the mouth is maintained in an open position to permit eating following surgery.

c. **Fractures of the vertical ramus and condyle**

(1) **Conservative treatment.** Fractures of the vertical ramus and condyle are often treated with **tape muzzles** and **interarcade wiring** because the surgical approach is difficult and the bone of the vertical ramus is thin and weak.

(2) **Surgical treatment. Application of a small** or **"mini" bone plate** or **interfragmentary wiring** via a lateral approach allows accurate reduction. It is important to preserve the masseter and digastricus muscles, the facial artery vein and nerve, and the parotid salivary gland and duct.

4. **Fractures of the upper jaw**
   a. **Diagnosis.** Fractures of the upper jaw are usually easily diagnosed by direct observation and palpation.
      (1) **Clinical signs.** Animals typically exhibit epistaxis, bleeding from the mouth, respiratory distress (open mouth breathing), and disfigurement with varying degrees of dental malocclusion.
      (2) **Radiography** can delineate the full extent of the injury.
   b. **Treatment**
      (1) **Premaxillary (nasal and incisive bone) fractures.** Fortunately, many premaxillary fractures have minimal displacement and heal rapidly without surgical stabilization.
         (a) **Indications for surgical treatment.** Treatment is indicated when malocclusion, oronasal communication, severe facial deformity, or airflow obstruction is present.
         (b) **Methods of treatment.** While the animal is anesthetized, the bones are realigned and occlusion is checked with the lower dental arcade. Stabilization using pins and wires is similar to that described for mandibular fractures.
      (2) **Maxillary fractures.** Like premaxillary fractures, many maxillary fractures are simple fractures without significant displacement that heal well without surgical stabilization. Because these bones have thin cortices, rigid internal fixation is difficult to achieve.
         (a) **Indications for surgical treatment**
            (i) **Multiple fractures** and **fractures with depressed fragments** require reduction, fragment elevation, and stabilization.
            (ii) In some cases, highly comminuted fractures may preclude anatomic reduction and **the value of achieving a desirable cosmetic result must be weighed against surgically induced** loss of vascularity to individual bone fragments, which can lead to **sequestration.**
         (b) **Methods of treatment.** Methods of closed reduction and fixation are similar to those employed for mandibular fractures. Because closure is important in order to prevent the development of postoperative subcutaneous emphysema, care must be taken to preserve the periosteum.
      (3) **Avulsion fractures** of alveolar bone and teeth are reduced and stabilized by driving multiple divergent Kirschner wires across the fragment into the hard palate.
         (a) Care should be taken to avoid the tooth roots.
         (b) If an avulsion fracture fragment is nonviable or missing, a number of mucosal flap techniques are available to prevent oronasal fistula formation.

5. **Fractures of the hard palate**
   a. **Diagnosis.** Animals with palatine fractures may present with minimal clinical signs unless the palatine fracture is associated with other severe fractures. In most cases, a **complete tear of the overlying mucosa** is present, making diagnosis more straightforward.
   b. **Treatment.** Interdental wiring and simple suture repair of the mucosal tissue is usually sufficient to stabilize these injuries (Figure 19–5).

6. **Fractures of the zygomatic arch**
   a. **Diagnosis.** Fractures in this region are frequently associated with periorbital soft tissue swelling, masticatory dysfunction, and pain on opening or closing the mouth.
   b. **Treatment**
      (1) **Nondisplaced fractures** do not require surgical intervention.
      (2) **Depressed fragments** may injure the globe or interfere with mastication and require elevation and stabilization.
         (a) **Interfragmentary wiring techniques** are usually sufficient for simple fractures.
         (b) In highly comminuted fractures where reconstruction cannot be achieved, **resection of the arch** may be necessary.

7. **Fractures of the occipital bone.** Although relatively uncommon, fractures of the oc-

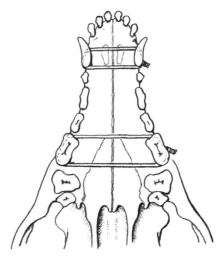

FIGURE 19–5. Interdental wiring technique for longitudinal fractures of the hard palate.

cipital condyle do occur and the potential for severe brain or brain stem injury is great. Management of these fractures is conservative **(cervical support until union is complete),** because surgical exposure is difficult and internal fixation has not resulted in consistent success rates.

8. **Fractures of the brain case**
   a. **Extracranial fractures** do not penetrate the bones of the brain case to involve the brain.
      (1) **Diagnosis.** Extracranial fractures are associated with soft tissue swelling, crepitus, deformity, and subcutaneous emphysema. Neurologic signs depend on the concussive effects of the injury.
      (2) **Treatment**
         (a) **Most extracranial fractures do not require surgery.**
         (b) **Fixation may be necessary** for cosmetic reasons (e.g., with depressed frontal sinus fractures) or if fracture fragments invade the orbit and endanger the globe. **Interfragmentary wiring techniques** or **"mini" bone plates** can be used to stabilize the fracture.
   b. **Intracranial fractures** penetrate the brain case and, potentially, the brain parenchyma. These fractures are uncommon; but when they do occur, **detection and treatment of CNS damage take precedence over fracture repair.**
      (1) **Nondisplaced linear fractures** may not require surgical intervention.
      (2) **Depression fractures.** The fragmented portion of the bone must be elevated. Burr holes are drilled adjacent to the fracture, and a curved, blunt elevator is passed through the holes to gently elevate the fracture site from underneath.
      (3) **Highly comminuted fractures** are difficult to treat. Multiple sharp fragment edges may easily tear the meninges, venous sinuses, or brain parenchyma; therefore, individual fragments must be removed to prevent further neurologic damage.

B. Neoplasia

1. **Oral neoplasia** is discussed in Chapter 10 I G 2.

2. **Craniofacial neoplasia** (e.g., **osteosarcoma, sinochondrosarcoma, osteochondrosarcoma**)
   a. **Treatment.** Tumors that do not invade the oral cavity can be treated by **craniofacial resection.**
      (1) The difficulty of these resections depends on the exact location of diseased tissues. Resection of portions of the brain case or nasofacial bones can result in surgical invasion of the nasal passages, sinuses, orbit, or intracranial vault.

        (2) Strict attention to surgical technique and anesthetic management are necessary when resecting tumors that require removal of a substantial portion of the brain case.

    b. Postoperative care

        (1) Administration of intravenous fluids and **systemic analgesics** may be necessary throughout the immediate postoperative period.

        (2) An **Elizabethan collar** may be necessary to prevent self-induced trauma to the surgical site.

C. **Temporomandibular joint abnormalities** may occur secondary to trauma or dysplasia.

  1. Craniomandibular osteopathy is a proliferative bone disease of the mandible and tympanic bullae that causes masticatory discomfort and pain.

    a. The **etiology** is unknown.

    b. Treatment

        (1) Surgical treatment does not consistently provide clinical improvement.

        (2) Medical treatment. Steroids and nonsteroidal anti-inflammatory agents are used to alleviate pain. Function is impaired in most animals, but not to the extent that they are incapable of maintaining normal nutritional status.

  2. Temporomandibular joint luxations may occur unilaterally or bilaterally as an isolated injury, or in conjunction with mandibular fractures.

    a. Diagnosis

        (1) With **unilateral luxation** and **rostral displacement** of the condyle, the mandibular canine teeth shift rostrally and away from the side of the luxation.

        (2) With **caudal displacement** of the condyle, the mandibular canine teeth shift caudally and toward the side of the luxation.

    b. Treatment

        (1) Closed reduction is usually successful and is accomplished by placing a fulcrum transversely across the back of the mouth, applying pressure to close the mouth, and manipulating the mandible to reengage the condyle with the temporal joint surface. If the joint is unstable after closed reduction, a muzzle or interdental wiring may be used to prevent reluxation.

        (2) Open reduction is indicated if closed reduction is unsuccessful. Suture imbrication of the joint capsule is used to stabilize the joint.

        (3) Condylar resection and **pseudarthrosis** (i.e., formation of a false joint supported by fibrous tissue) may be necessary in refractory cases or when significant injury to the joint has occurred.

        (4) Tethering the mandibular condyle to the zygomatic process of the temporal bone with nonabsorbable polyester sutures has been successfully used to treat cats with recurrent luxations.

  3. Intermittent open-mouth lower jaw locking

    a. Pathogenesis. Intermittent open-mouth lower jaw locking is associated with temporomandibular joint dysplasia, which causes joint subluxation. Subluxation of the diseased temporomandibular joint either laterally displaces the contralateral coronoid process or causes it to contact the ventral aspect of the adjacent zygomatic arch. This mechanical interference prevents the mouth from closing.

    b. Treatment. Excision of the rostroventral portion of the involved zygomatic arch prevents future locking episodes.

SELECTED READINGS

Bennet JW, Kapatkin AS, Maretta SM: Dental composite for the fixation of mandibular fractures and luxations in 11 cats and 6 dogs. *Vet Surg* 23:190–194, 1994.

Brinker WO, Piermattei DL, Flo GS: *Handbook of Small Animal Orthopedics and Fracture Treatment.* Philadelphia, WB Saunders, 1990, pp 230–243.

Capon TM: Traumatic temporomandibular joint luxation in a cat and treatment by condylar tethering. *Vet Comp Ortho Traum* 8:61–65, 1995.

Dewey CW, Budsberg SC, Oliver JE: Principles of head trauma management in dogs and cats—parts I & II. *Compend Contin Educ Pract Vet* 15(2):177–193, 199–220, 1993.

Dewey CW, Downs MO, Aron DN: Acute traumatic intracranial hemorrhage in dogs and cats. *Vet Comp Ortho Traum* 6:153–159, 1993.

Kirby R: Treatment of dogs and cats with severe head injuries in the first 24 hours. *Prog Vet Neurol* 5:2–74, 1994.

Lantz GC: Surgical correction of unusual temporomandibular joint conditions. *Compend Contin Educ Pract Vet* 13:1570–1576, 1991.

Slatter D: *Textbook of Small Animal Surgery*, 2nd ed. Philadelphia, WB Saunders, 1993, pp 521–530, 1910–1921, 2272–2276.

PART IV

NEUROSURGERY

Chapter 20

Introduction to Neurosurgery

Rodney S. Bagley

I. **OVERVIEW OF THE NERVOUS SYSTEM.** The nervous system can be divided into three major areas, according to function.

A. **Intracranial nervous system**

1. **Supratentorial (forebrain) structures** (i.e., the **cerebral hemispheres, basal nuclei, diencephalon,** and **rostral part of the mesencephalon**) are located rostral to the tentorium cerebelli (Figure 20–1).
   a. **Functions.** These structures are associated with **conscious functions** (e.g., movement, sensation, hearing). The diencephalon controls many **autonomic functions.**
   b. **Clinical signs produced by unilateral supratentorial lesions** include:
      (1) A contralateral menace response deficit accompanied by normal pupillary light reflex activity and normal cranial nerve VII function
      (2) Contralateral hemiparesis
      (3) Contralateral facial sensation deficit
      (4) Seizures
      (5) Behavioral abnormalities
      (6) Circling or head turning (usually toward the side of the lesion), pacing, head-pressing
      (7) Alterations in consciousness

2. **Infratentorial structures** are located caudal to the tentorium cerebelli (see Figure 20–1).
   a. **Brain stem** (i.e., the **caudal mesencephalon, pons,** and **medulla oblongata**)
      (1) **Functions.** The brain stem controls many physiologic functions (e.g., **blood pressure, respiration, body temperature, sleep**). In addition, the brain stem houses the majority of the **cranial nerve nuclei** (Table 20–1) and the **reticular formation,** which plays an important role in consciousness.
      (2) **Clinical signs produced by brain stem lesions.** Brain stem lesions may produce signs of ipsilateral hemiparesis or alterations in consciousness. Cranial nerves III through XII are most often affected.
   b. **Cerebellum**
      (1) **Function.** The cerebellum controls the rate, range, and force of movement.
      (2) **Clinical signs produced by cerebellar lesions** include ataxia, dysmetria, intention tremor, menace deficit (ipsilateral to the lesion), and pupillary abnormalities.

B. **Spinal cord.** The spinal cord is divided functionally into the **upper motor neuron (UMN) system** and the **lower motor neuron (LMN) system.** By determining which limbs are abnormal and then identifying UMN or LMN signs in the affected limbs, a lesion involving specific spinal cord segments can be localized.

1. **UMNs** are descending fibers within the white matter of the spinal cord that do not leave the central nervous system (CNS).
   a. **Function.** UMNs influence, either positively or negatively, the LMNs.
   b. **Clinical signs produced by UMN lesions** include loss of motor function, hyper- to normoreflexia, hypertonia or normotonia, and disuse muscle atrophy (mild and slow in onset).
      (1) **Paresis** implies a neurologic cause for motor dysfunction and that some degree of motor function is retained. It can occur with UMN or LMN lesions.
         (a) **Tetraparesis (quadriparesis)** is neurologic impairment of **all limbs.**
         (b) **Paraparesis** is neurologic impairment of **both pelvic limbs.**
         (c) **Hemiparesis** is neurologic impairment of a **thoracic limb and the ipsilateral pelvic limb.**

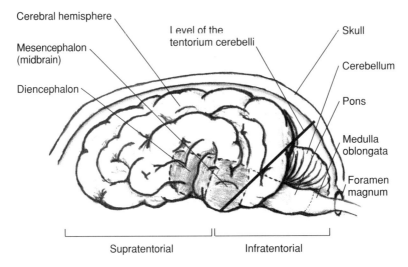

FIGURE 20–1. Classification of the intracranial structures based on their relationship to the tentorium cerebelli.

    (d) Central cord syndrome. Rarely, both thoracic limbs are more affected than the pelvic limbs. Central cord syndrome results from preferential involvement of the spinal tracts that terminate in the thoracic limbs.

  (2) Plegia implies loss of voluntary motor function. The same prefixes used to describe paresis may be applied to plegia.

 c. Localization of lesions (Figure 20–2)

  (1) If intracranial functions are normal and there are **UMN signs in all limbs,** the lesion is in the **C1–C5** spinal cord segment.

  (2) If there are **UMN signs in the pelvic limbs** only, then the lesion is in the **T3–L3** spinal cord segment.

2. LMNs exit the CNS, forming the final common pathway for performance of a function.

 a. The cell bodies of the LMNs innervating the **thoracic limbs** reside in the **cervical intumescence.** The cell bodies of the LMNs innervating the **pelvic limbs** reside in the **lumbosacral intumescence.**

TABLE 20–1. Cranial Nerves

Number	Name	Summary of Function
I	Olfactory	Olfactory
II	Optic	Vision
III	Oculomotor	Ocular movement, pupillary constriction
IV	Trochlear	Ocular movement
V	Trigeminal	Sensory to head and eye; motor to masticatory muscles
VI	Abducens	Ocular movement
VII	Facial	Motor to muscles controlling facial expression; taste; lacrimation
VIII	Vestibulocochlear	Balance; orientation in space; hearing
IX	Glossopharyngeal	Swallowing; taste
X	Vagus	Swallowing; autonomic innervation to the GI tract and heart; taste
XI	Spinal accessory	Motor to the trapezius muscle
XII	Hypoglossal	Tongue movement

GI = gastrointestinal.

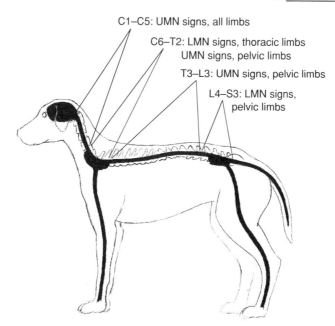

C1–C5: UMN signs, all limbs

C6–T2: LMN signs, thoracic limbs
UMN signs, pelvic limbs

T3–L3: UMN signs, pelvic limbs

L4–S3: LMN signs,
pelvic limbs

FIGURE 20–2. Functional areas of the spinal cord. It is possible to localize spinal cord lesions by identifying upper motor neuron (*UMN*) or lower motor neuron (*LMN*) signs in the limbs.

    b. Clinical signs produced by LMN lesions include paresis or plegia, hyporeflexia or areflexia, hypotonia or atonia, and neurogenic muscle atrophy (acute in onset and severe).

        (1) Note that **paresis or plegia can occur with either UMN or LMN lesions.**

        (2) Because the sympathetic nerves to the eye exit at the T1–T3 spinal cord segment, **Horner's syndrome** (i.e., **miosis, enophthalmus, ptosis, vasodilation, and prolapse of the nictitating membrane**) may be seen ipsilateral to a unilateral lesion in this area.

        (3) Because the lateral thoracic nerve responsible for the cutaneous trunci reflex is formed and exits at the C8–T1 spinal segment, **loss of cutaneous trunci movement** can occur ipsilateral to a unilateral lesion in this area.

    c. Localization of lesions (see Figure 20–2)

        (1) If a spinal cord lesion causing **LMN signs in the thoracic limbs** and **UMN signs in the pelvic limbs** is suspected, a **C6–T2** lesion is likely.

        (2) If **LMN signs** are present in the **pelvic limbs only,** a lesion in the **L4–S3** segment is suspected.

C. **Peripheral nervous system (PNS).** The PNS begins at the intervertebral foramina of the vertebrae.

    1. Histology

        a. Schwann cells. Both myelinated and unmyelinated axons can exist in a peripheral nerve; however, **all nerves myelinated by Schwann cells are members of the PNS.**

        b. Connective tissue elements

            (1) The **endoneurium** covers individual myelinated axons and groups of unmyelinated axons.

            (2) The **perineurium** encircles groups of nerve fibers (fascicles) and forms the blood–nerve barrier.

            (3) The **epineurium** is the outer connective tissue layer.

    2. Clinical signs produced by PNS lesions

        a. Lesions of the **PNS, neuromuscular junction (NMJ),** and, occasionally, **muscle** may produce LMN signs (see I B 2 b).

        b. Lesions restricted to the **NMJ** and **muscle** may cause muscle weakness without other obvious neurologic signs.

II. DIAGNOSIS OF NEUROLOGIC CONDITIONS

A. Physical and neurologic examinations permit definition and localization of the lesion.

B. Differential diagnoses. After the lesion has been localized, a list of appropriate differential diagnoses should be generated.

C. Ancillary tests
   1. **Intracranial disease**
      a. **Computed tomography** and **magnetic resonance imaging** can be used to determine the structural integrity of the CNS (Figure 20–3).
         (1) Imaging studies should be performed **prior** to cerebrospinal fluid (CSF) collection (see II C 1 b) in animals with suspected structural brain disease because

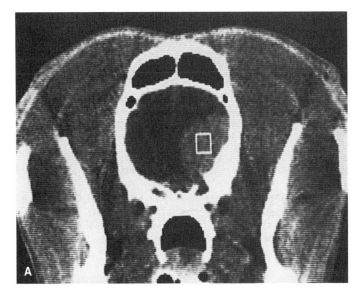

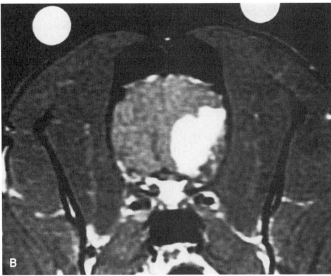

FIGURE 20–3. Images at the level of the frontal lobes of a dog with a meningioma. (*A*) Contrast-enhanced computed tomography scan. (*B*) T_1-weighted, contrast-enhanced magnetic resonance image.

CSF collection in the presence of increased intracranial pressure may cause brain herniation.

(2) If a structural brain lesion is found with advanced imaging, the risk of CSF collection may outweigh the benefits.

b. CSF analysis may be helpful for defining inflammatory processes involving the brain. Its utility, however, is often limited by lack of specificity. For example, many dogs with brain tumors have inflammatory changes detectable by CSF analysis; however, additional testing is necessary to determine the actual cause of the inflammation (e.g., tumor, infection, degeneration).

c. Electroencephalography may be helpful for evaluating nonstructural encephalopathy and localizing seizure foci. However, electroencephalography often provides no more information than that obtained by imaging studies and CSF evaluation in animals with structural brain disease.

d. Brain stem auditory evoked potential testing, often indicated for diagnosis of deafness, may provide information about brain stem integrity.

e. Angiography and **venography** are useful for evaluating cerebral arterial or venous integrity. In addition, these studies may provide information regarding the structural integrity of intracranial structures around the vessels. For example, cavernous sinus venography provides information concerning structural lesions of some cranial nerves and the pituitary.

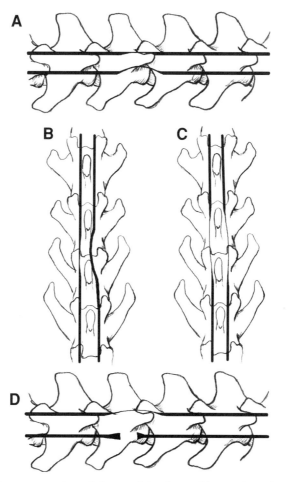

FIGURE 20–4. Schematic representation of abnormalities detected by myelography. (*A*) A ventral, extradural compressive lesion (lateral view). (*B*) A lateral, extradural compressive lesion (ventrodorsal view). (*C*) An intramedullary spinal cord lesion (ventrodorsal view). (*D*) An intradural, extramedullary lesion (lateral view).

2. Spinal cord abnormalities
   a. Radiography and **myelography** are used to determine whether a compressive or expansive lesion of the spinal cord is present.
      (1) Survey radiography may be helpful in defining vertebral abnormalities (e.g., fractures, luxations, neoplasia, diskospondylitis).
      (2) Myelography can be used to localize a spinal cord lesion and determine where the lesion is in relationship to the meninges and spinal cord parenchyma (Figure 20–4). Two radiographic views (i.e., a dorsoventral and a lateral view) are imperative for accurate diagnosis.
         (a) An extradural lesion results in axial deviation of one or both contrast columns in the dorsoventral or lateral view.
         (b) An intradural, extramedullary lesion produces the classic myelographic pattern of the "golf tee" sign when the contrast agent outlines the lesion.
         (c) An intramedullary lesion results in abaxial movement of contrast columns in both the dorsoventral and lateral views.

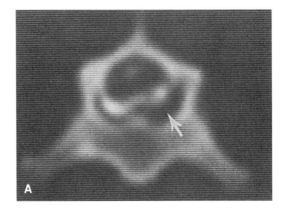

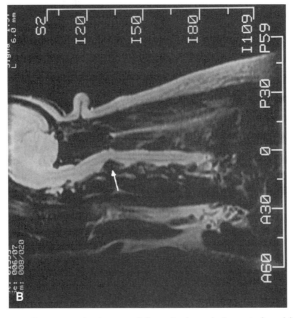

FIGURE 20–5. (*A*) Computed tomography image of the spinal cord. A ventral and lateral compressive lesion is noted (*arrow*). The final diagnosis was intervertebral disk extrusion. (*B*) Sagittal T$_2$-weighted, non–contrast-enhanced magnetic resonance image of the cervical spinal cord showing a herniated intervertebral disk at C2–C3 (*arrow*).

    b. Computed tomography and **magnetic resonance imaging** may be helpful when myelography is not definitive (Figure 20–5).

       (1) Computed tomography is most beneficial for definition of vertebral abnormalities.

       (2) Magnetic resonance imaging is most helpful for visualizing perispinal and intraspinal cord lesions.

    c. CSF analysis may be helpful for diagnosis of inflammatory lesions or neoplastic lesions.

    d. Evoked potentials (e.g., spinal cord evoked potentials, magnetic evoked potentials, somatosensory evoked potentials) may allow localization of the lesion and prediction of prognosis in selected cases.

3. PNS abnormalities

    a. Nerve conduction velocity (NCV) testing assesses the integrity of the peripheral nerves.

    b. Late potentials (F waves, H waves) provide information concerning the integrity of the proximal peripheral nerve, nerve roots, and cell bodies within the gray matter of the spinal cord.

    c. Electromyography provides evidence of muscle disease.

       (1) Fibrillation potentials and positive sharp waves are suggestive of denervation of muscle.

       (2) Single fiber electromyography and **decremental responses** can be used to assess the NMJ.

    d. Peripheral nerve or muscle biopsies are used to evaluate the morphology of these structures (see Chapter 23).

SELECTED READINGS

Braund KG: *Clinical Syndromes in Veterinary Neurology,* 2nd ed. St. Louis, Mosby, 1994.

Chrisman CL: *Problems in Small Animal Neurology,* 2nd ed. Philadelphia, Lea & Febiger, 1991.

deLahunta A: *Veterinary Neuroanatomy and Clinical Neurology,* 2nd ed. Philadelphia, WB Saunders, 1983.

Oliver JE Jr, Lorenz MD: *Handbook of Veterinary Neurology,* 2nd ed. Philadelphia, WB Saunders, 1993.

Chapter 21

Brain

Rodney S. Bagley

I. PREOPERATIVE CONSIDERATIONS

A. Preoperative evaluation

1. Preoperative evaluation of animals with suspected intracranial disease requires precise **neuroanatomical localization** of the lesion (see Chapter 20 I A, II C 1].

2. In many instances, regardless of the primary disease, intracranial disease may result in common intracranial **pathophysiologic alterations.**
   a. **Increased intracranial pressure** is common with intracranial structural disease.
      (1) **Monro-Kellie doctrine.** Within the confines of the skull, the brain parenchyma, blood, and cerebrospinal fluid (CSF) exist in equilibrium at a stable intracranial pressure. Any increase in volume of one of these intracranial components must be equally compensated for by a decrease in one or both of the other intracranial components, or the intracranial pressure will increase. A point of maximum compensation exists, after which a continual increase in intracranial volume causes dramatic elevations of the intracranial pressure.
      (2) **Effects.** With dramatic elevations of intracranial pressure, **brain function** is **altered** and **brain herniation** is common.
   b. **Cerebral edema** can be classified as vasogenic, cytotoxic, or interstitial.
      (1) **Vasogenic edema** is the result of alterations in vascular permeability (i.e., in the **blood–brain barrier**). This edema, which is often caused by brain tumors, commonly occurs in the cerebral white matter.
      (2) **Cytotoxic edema** is intracellular edema resulting from energy failure within neurons. Toxic and metabolic causes often cause this type of edema.
      (3) **Interstitial edema** within the brain is caused only by hydrocephalus.
   c. **Hemorrhage** within the brain can occur spontaneously or secondary to head trauma. Hemorrhage can be **intraparenchymal** or **subdural;** extradural hemorrhage is uncommon because the dura is normally tightly adherent to the calvaria.
   d. **Seizures** are most commonly associated with disease within the supratentorial structures.

B. Perioperative medical treatment of animals with intracranial disease is important in reducing patient morbidity and mortality.

1. **Reduction of intracranial pressure** is accomplished by administration of diuretics, corticosteroids, or hyperventilation of intubated animals.
   a. **Diuretic therapy**
      (1) **Mannitol,** an osmotic diuretic, decreases brain edema rapidly and is used in acute, life-threatening situations (1–2 g/kg intravenously). Although there may be a risk of increasing bleeding with mannitol, the occurrence of clinically significant epidural or subdural hematoma is rare, whereas edema is common.
      (2) **Furosemide,** a loop-sparing diuretic, is used to potentiate the effects of mannitol. Furosemide (0.7–1 mg/kg intravenously) is administered approximately 15 minutes after the mannitol.
   b. **Administration of corticosteroids** (e.g., methylprednisolone, dexamethasone) may lower intracranial pressure by decreasing cerebral edema. In addition, corticosteroids have anti-inflammatory effects.
   c. **Hyperventilation** decreases the arterial carbon dioxide partial pressure. The cerebral vasculature is directly responsive to arterial carbon dioxide concentrations, so decreasing the arterial carbon dioxide partial pressure causes vasoconstriction

of the cerebral vessels and decreases blood flow to the brain, ultimately decreasing the intracranial pressure.

2. **Seizure control.** Many animals with supratentorial disease experience seizures.
   a. **Diazepam** administered intravenously is used for acute termination of seizure activity.
   b. **Phenobarbital** and **potassium bromide** administered orally are most commonly used for chronic seizure control.

3. **Infection control**
   a. Cephalosporins may be administered prophylactically to decrease the incidence of brain infection.
   b. Trimethoprim–sulfa, chloramphenicol, or ampicillin may be used to treat bacterial brain infections. Chloramphenicol potentiates the effects of phenobarbital; therefore, the two should not be used concurrently.

C. **Anesthesia.** A knowledge of the effects of injectable and inhalation anesthetics on cerebral blood flow, intracranial pressure, and the autoregulatory mechanisms that maintain normal cerebral perfusion pressure is of critical importance.

1. **Fluid therapy** should be instituted to support circulation; care should be taken to avoid exacerbation of cerebral edema.

2. **Selection of protocol.** There is no single ideal anesthetic protocol for intracranial surgery; however, dissociative agents, halothane, and enflurane should be avoided. Intravenous barbiturates are recommended for induction and isoflurane and opioids are recommended for maintenance of anesthesia.

3. **Respiratory depression must be prevented.** Assisted ventilation or hyperventilation may help to lower the arterial carbon dioxide partial pressure, thus preventing cerebral vasodilation and increases in intracranial pressure.

II. INTRACRANIAL SURGERY

A. **Indications** include diagnosis and treatment of a variety of intracranial disease processes.

1. **Biopsy of brain tissue** may be necessary to definitively diagnose diffuse encephalopathy or encephalitis.

2. **Removal of masses** is accomplished via a craniotomy.

3. **Trauma.** Animals with head trauma may require intracranial surgery to remove depressed skull fragments, débride abnormal tissue, and evacuate subdural hematoma.

4. **Seizure control.** In some human patients, surgery has been used to control seizures that are poorly controlled with currently available anticonvulsant medications.
   a. **Callosotomy** (i.e., longitudinal division of the corpus callosum) eliminates a potential conduit for seizure generation.
   b. **Focal resection.** If a discrete seizure focus can be localized, surgical resection of this focus may eliminate the abnormal electrical activity causing the seizures.

5. **Placement of ventriculoperitoneal shunts** and **intracranial pressure monitoring devices** requires intracranial surgery.

B. **Procedures**

1. **Craniotomy** and **craniectomy** permit exposure of the brain. During craniotomy, a portion of the skull is removed and the resected bone is replaced following surgery. During craniectomy, the skull is not replaced, thus allowing space for the brain to swell.
   a. **Preoperative considerations.** To minimize the incidence of brain trauma during

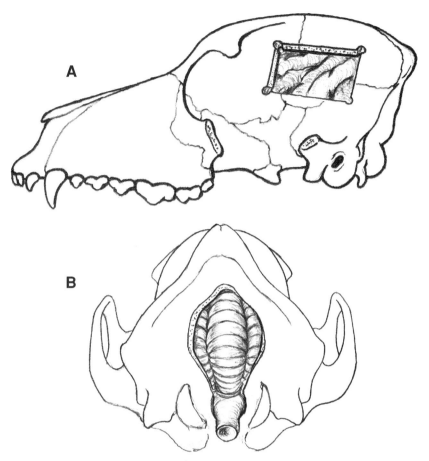

FIGURE 21–1. (*A*) Lateral rostrotentorial approach. (*B*) Caudotentorial (suboccipital) approach.

craniotomy and dural incision, attempts to decrease the intracranial pressure should be made prior to surgery.

b. **Approach.** A variety of surgical approaches to the brain have been described. Approaches to the canine brain are believed to be limited by the presence of normal vascular channels within the skull; however, as intracranial surgical techniques continue to improve, this consideration may cease to be valid.

   (1) The **lateral rostrotentorial** approach allows visualization of the lateral aspects of the ipsilateral cerebral hemisphere (Figure 21–1A). The zygomatic arch can be removed to increase ventral exposure.

   (2) A **bilateral rostrotentorial** approach exposes the dorsal aspects of the cerebral hemispheres and the dorsal sagittal sinus.

   (3) The **caudotentorial (suboccipital)** approach allows visualization of the dorsal caudal cerebellum and brain stem (Figure 21–1B).

   (4) The **transfrontal** approach is used to expose the rostral portions of the cerebrum. Because this area is approached via the frontal sinus, the postoperative infection rate increases.

   (a) A watertight dural closure may decrease the risk of brain infection associated with this approach.

   (b) An autogenous fat graft or placement of an absorbable gelatin sponge in the frontal sinus prior to closure may also decrease the risk of infection.

   (5) A **radical frontal** approach combines the lateral rostrotentorial and the transfrontal approaches.

   (6) A **ventral transsphenoidal** approach to the brain can be used for surgical removal of the pituitary.

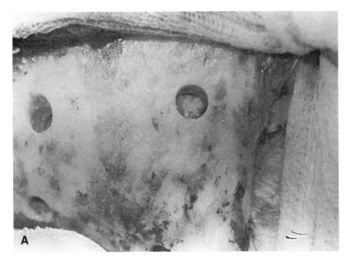

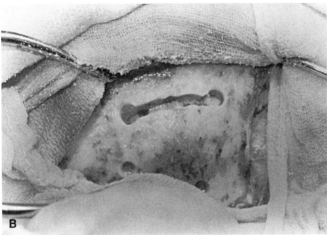

FIGURE 21–2. Exposure of the brain during a craniotomy/craniectomy. (*A*) Two burr holes are placed in the left lateral skull in preparation for a rostrotentorial craniotomy. The dura can be seen in the depth of each hole. (*B*) The burr holes are connected with a high-speed air drill.

      c. Exposure of the brain. Following periosteal dissection of the overlying musculature, a portion of the skull is removed using a high-speed air drill or craniotome. The dura is carefully incised (Figure 21–2).

      d. Resection or biopsy

        (1) Cortical lesions and biopsies

          (a) Masses can be removed by establishing a plane of dissection around the lesion. If the lesion is encapsulated, the mass can be incised, the center removed, and the capsule resected to avoid unnecessary manipulation of the brain.

          (b) Cortical biopsies are taken if an obvious lesion is not encountered or if a diffuse pathologic process is suspected.

        (2) Subcortical lesions. If a lesion is not visible on the surface of the brain, incision into the cortex may be necessary.

          (a) Ultrasound may be helpful for defining lesions below the brain surface.

          (b) The cortex is entered through a gyrus to avoid damaging the vessels that lie within the sulci of the brain. The incision through the cortex is best made with the sharp end of a Freer periosteal elevator or Penfield dissector.

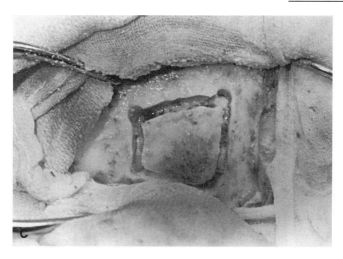

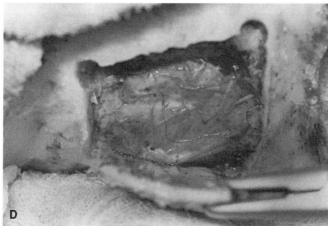

FIGURE 21–2. (*cont*) (*C*) All burr holes are connected in a similar manner to isolate the skull flap. (*D*) The free skull fragment is removed, exposing the underlying dura.

    (c) Hemorrhage is controlled with gelatin sponges and bipolar cautery. Larger vessels can be occluded with sutures (4-0 silk) or small vascular clips. In some instances, the bipolar cautery can be attached to a small metal suction device for concurrent suction and coagulation.

  e. Closure. After resection or biopsy has been performed, the exposed brain is covered with dura, a temporalis muscle–fascia graft, or absorbable gelatin sponges. Often with surgical manipulation, brain swelling occurs and skull fragments are not replaced to accommodate for this edema. The brain underlying the craniectomy site is then protected only by the temporalis muscle and fascia.

2. Ventriculoperitoneal shunting is used to treat hydrocephalus.

  a. Approach. The approach is the same as that described for craniotomy, up to the point where the temporalis muscle is removed from the skull.

  b. Exposure. Instead of removing a large portion of the skull as for a craniotomy, a small burr hole is made in the lateral dorsal aspect of the occipital region.

  c. Placement of the shunt (Figure 21–3)

    (1) The dura is incised and the ventriculoperitoneal shunt is advanced through the dura and cortex to enter the lateral ventricle at its caudal aspect. The shunt is advanced rostrally so that the tip resides in the rostral lateral ventricle.

    (2) The shunt is tunnelled subcutaneously from the cranial incision caudally to a

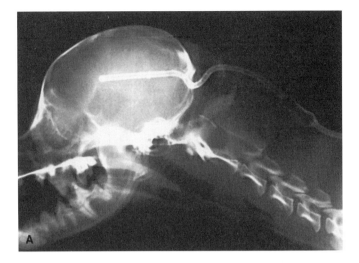

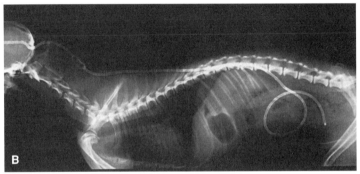

FIGURE 21–3. Lateral radiograph of a dog with a ventriculoperitoneal shunt. One end of the shunt is placed in the lateral ventricle (*A*) and the other extends into the peritoneal cavity (*B*).

small incision made behind the last rib. The peritoneal end of the shunt is advanced into the abdomen and secured with sutures.

d. **Complications of shunt placement**
   (1) **Iatrogenic brain trauma** can occur during shunt advancement.
   (2) **Hemorrhage** can result from direct laceration of intracranial vessels. Subdural hematoma may occur when too low a pressure shunt is used, causing a rapid decrease in ventricle size and leading to damage of small brain vessels.
   (3) **Occlusion** of the shunt may occur.
   (4) **Infection** can result in shunt failure.

3. **Monitoring intracranial pressure.** A device to measure intracranial pressure may be inserted into the ventricle, subdural space, or brain parenchyma. The most commonly used device is a fiberoptic cable system.
   a. Placement requires drilling a small hole in the lateral skull.
   b. The fiberoptic catheter is advanced into the brain parenchyma and secured with a cranial bolt.

C. **Postoperative care** of the animal requiring intracranial surgery involves intensive monitoring of vital signs and neurologic function. Imaging studies (e.g., computed tomography) can be performed immediately after surgery to examine the extent of lesion removal.

1. Because increases in intracranial pressure can cause bradycardia and respiratory abnormalities, **heart rate** and **respiration** should be closely monitored.

2. **Pupil size, equality,** and **responsiveness** to light should be evaluated to assess for possible brain herniation.

3. Recumbent animals should be kept on soft bedding and should be turned frequently to lessen the incidence of **decubital ulceration** and **pulmonary atelectasis. Thoracic auscultation** should be performed daily to detect early signs of **pneumonia,** which is also common in these animals.

4. **Stools** should be **monitored for evidence of blood** because ulceration of the gastrointestinal tract can occur in animals receiving corticosteroids for intracranial disease.

5. The **incision** should be **monitored daily for** signs of **infection.** A soft wrap over the incision decreases postoperative incisional edema.

III. INTRACRANIAL DISORDERS

A. **Degenerative** and **storage diseases** are uncommon. Examples include **multisystemic neuronal degeneration** (seen in cocker spaniels), **spongiform encephalopathies** (seen in Labrador retrievers, Samoyeds, silky terriers, dalmatians, and Egyptian Mau cats), and **multisystemic chromatolytic neuronal degeneration** (seen in cairn terriers).

1. **Etiology.** Storage diseases result from an inborn error of metabolism and the absence of an enzyme necessary for the breakdown of endogenous body substances. These diseases are usually breed-specific and congenital.

2. **Pathogenesis.** Poorly metabolized substances accumulate in neurons or supporting cells, resulting in dysfunction.

3. **Diagnosis**
   a. **Clinical signs** begin in young animals and are progressive.
   b. **Measurement of enzyme levels** in cells or body fluids (e.g., CSF, urine) or at necropsy is used to definitively diagnose the condition.

4. **Treatment.** There are no effective treatments for degenerative diseases. Bone marrow transplants have been used experimentally to treat fucosidosis (a storage disease) in dogs.

B. **Anomalous disorders** commonly affect the forebrain, but may also involve the brain stem and cerebellum.

1. **Hydrocephalus**
   a. **Etiology.** Hydrocephalus can be congenital or acquired as a result of obstruction of the ventricular system (e.g., by inflammation, hemorrhage, or neoplasia).
      (1) Chihuahuas, Pomeranians, and Maltese dogs have a high incidence of congenital hydrocephalus, most likely resulting from obstruction of the ventricular system during a critical stage of embryonic development.
      (2) In Siamese cats, hereditary hydrocephalus is transmitted as an autosomal recessive trait.
   b. **Diagnosis**
      (1) **Clinical signs** include mentation changes and seizures.
      (2) **Ultrasound** will reveal hydrocephalus if a fontanelle is present.
      (3) **Computed tomography** or **magnetic resonance imaging** will confirm ventricular dilation and allow for a more global view of the ventricular system.
      (4) **CSF collection** and **analysis** is used to measure intracranial pressure and to exclude inflammatory causes.
   c. **Treatment options** include therapy with corticosteroids or carbonic anhydrase inhibitors and ventriculoperitoneal shunting.

2. **Lissencephaly,** which is seen most commonly in Lhasa apso dogs, is a lack of gyri and sulci.

3. Hydranencephaly, exencephaly, and **anencephaly** are uncommon, usually present at birth, and result in neonatal or early infant death.

C. **Systemic metabolic diseases** (e.g., hepatic, renal, or pancreatic encephalopathy, hypo- or hyperglycemia, sodium, potassium, and calcium imbalances, acid–base disturbances) may alter brain function.

   1. **Diagnosis** is based on physical examination and clinical pathologic abnormalities.

   2. **Treatment** of the underlying systemic disease usually improves CNS signs.

D. **Neoplastic disease**

   1. **Primary brain tumors** include meningiomas, gliomas (i.e., astrocytoma, oligodendroglioma, ependymoma), and choroid plexus tumors. Tumors of the pituitary gland also occur.
      a. **Meningiomas** are the most common primary brain tumor in dogs and cats, especially dolichocephalic dogs.
         (1) **Source.** Meningiomas arise from the **arachnoid layer of the meninges.**
         (2) **Diagnosis**
            (a) **Clinical signs** reflect the area of the tumor, unless secondary pathophysiologic sequelae (e.g., increased intracranial pressure) have damaged additional brain areas.
            (b) **Advanced imaging studies** usually reveal an extra-axial, broad-based, contrast-enhancing mass.
            (c) **Biopsy** is necessary for definitive diagnosis.
         (3) **Treatment** options include surgical removal and radiation.
      b. **Gliomas** tend to occur in brachycephalic breeds of dogs.
         (1) **Source.** Gliomas arise from cells of the brain **parenchyma.**
         (2) **Diagnosis.** Magnetic resonance imaging is usually best for defining these types of tumors.
         (3) **Treatment options** include surgical removal, radiation, and chemotherapy (with carmustine or lomustine).
      c. **Choroid plexus tumors**
         (1) **Source.** Choroid plexus tumors arise from the cells of the **choroid plexus** and occur within or in close proximity to the **ventricular system.**
         (2) **Treatment options** include surgical removal. Radiation therapy may be less effective than with other primary brain tumors.

   2. **Secondary brain tumors** have metastasized from an extracranial primary site. Examples include hemangiosarcoma, some lymphosarcomas, and various carcinomas.

E. **Inflammatory processes**

   1. **Etiology**
      a. **Infectious diseases** that can affect the brain include:
         (1) **Viral diseases** (e.g., distemper, parvovirus, parainfluenza, herpes virus, feline infectious peritonitis, feline immunodeficiency virus, pseudorabies, rabies)
         (2) **Bacterial diseases** (e.g., *Staphylococcus, Streptococcus, Pasteurella*)
         (3) **Rickettsial diseases** (e.g., Rocky Mountain spotted fever, ehrlichiosis)
         (4) **Spirochetal diseases** (e.g., Lyme disease, leptospirosis)
         (5) **Fungal diseases** (e.g., blastomycosis, histoplasmosis, cryptococcosis, coccidioidomycosis, aspergillosis)
         (6) **Protozoal diseases** (e.g., toxoplasmosis, neosporosis)
         (7) **Parasitic diseases** (e.g., *Toxocara,* heartworm aberrant migration)
         (8) **Unclassified diseases** (e.g., protothecosis)
      b. **Noninfectious causes** (e.g., granulomatous meningoencephalitis, idiopathic encephalitides) are more common than infectious diseases.

   2. **Diagnosis**
      a. **Clinical signs** usually reflect multifocal CNS involvement.
      b. **CSF analysis** usually reveals inflammatory cells, increased protein, or both.

(1) Other structural diseases, such as brain neoplasia, may also produce CSF inflammation and should be ruled out with advanced imaging studies.

(2) Rarely, organisms are detectable in the CSF.

(3) Titers for infectious diseases can be performed on CSF to establish infectious etiologies.

3. **Treatment**

    a. If an infectious organism is found, appropriate **antibiotic therapy** is initiated.

    b. If no infectious cause can be found, **corticosteroids** are usually beneficial for reducing CSF inflammation.

    c. **Whole-brain radiation therapy** has been used to treat granulomatous meningoencephalitis with success in a small number of dogs.

F. **Idiopathic disorders**

1. **Epilepsy** for which no structural or metabolic cause is found is a common cause of seizures in young adult dogs.

2. **Narcolepsy.** Affected dogs episodically fall asleep during the day, usually during eating.

3. **Cataplexy** is similar to narcolepsy and is characterized by periods of acute muscular hypotonia. These animals, however, appear to remain conscious.

G. **Trauma** (see also Chapter 19 III A 8 b)

1. **Etiology**

    a. **Exogenous.** The brain can be traumatized exogenously by automobile injury, gunshot injury, or a blow to the head. Exogenously induced lesions are categorized as **concussions** (i.e., the result of a violent blow to the head), **contusions** (i.e., bruising of the brain), or **lacerations,** depending on the severity of the injury.

    b. **Endogenous** injury can occur from any disease affecting the brain.

2. **Pathogenesis.** Sequelae of trauma include physical injury, hemorrhage, edema, and increases in intracranial pressure.

3. **Treatment** focuses on controlling the pathophysiologic sequelae.

    a. **Decompressive surgery** may be needed to removed skull fragments or other debris.

    b. **Craniectomy** can be useful for controlling the elevated intracranial pressure.

H. **Toxins** (e.g., organophosphates, metaldehyde, strychnine, lead) and **therapeutic agents given in excessive amounts** (e.g., metronidazole) affect the brain either primarily or by altering systemic metabolic functions.

I.

Cerebrovascular disorders are uncommon causes of brain disease in animals (as compared with humans).

1. **General**

    a. **Etiology.** Thrombosis and hemorrhage can occur spontaneously; secondary to drug therapy (e.g., with L-asparaginase, anticoagulants), thrombocytopenia, or other bleeding disorders; or in association with trauma, hypertension, hypothyroidism, atherosclerosis, or systemic infection (septic emboli).

    b. **Clinical signs** are acute in onset; advanced imaging studies and angiography may aid diagnosis.

    c. **Treatment** is supportive.

2. **Feline ischemic encephalopathy** is an ischemic necrosis that occurs in the cerebral hemispheres of cats. The infarction occurs in the distribution of the middle cerebral artery.

    a. **Clinical signs** reflect unilateral forebrain disease.

    b. **Treatment** is supportive.

J. **Cerebellar diseases**

1. **Abiotrophy** results from a loss of vital substances necessary for the continued life of the neuron.
   a. **Predisposed breeds.** Abiotrophic diseases are seen most often in Kerry blue terriers, Gordon setters, rough-coated collies, border collies, and bullmastiffs. Samoyeds, Airedales, Finnish harriers, Labrador retrievers, golden retrievers, beagles, cocker spaniels, Cairn terriers, and Great Danes are less commonly affected.
   b. **Diagnosis.** Clinical signs, which are slowly progressive, usually become apparent in dogs at less than 1 year of age. In Gordon setters, a later onset of cerebellar degeneration has been described.

2. **Hypomyelination** and **dysmyelination** result in clinical signs of tremor that appear similar to the tremor of cerebellar disease.

3. **Neuroaxonal dystrophy** and **leukoencephalomyelopathy** are diseases of rottweiler dogs characterized by ataxia and hypermetria.
   a. **Clinical signs** begin in young adults and may appear similar to those of a spinal cord lesion.
   b. **Diagnosis** is usually made at necropsy; myelography and CSF analysis are normal.

4. **Congenital malformations** of the cerebellum are occasionally seen.
   a. **Caudal vermian hypoplasia** has been described in dogs; ventricular dilation (Dandy-Walker malformation) is also seen in some animals.
   b. **Cerebellar hypoplasia** has been recognized in chow chows, Irish setters, and wire-haired fox terriers. The latter two breeds may have concurrent lissencephaly.
   c. **Cerebellar hypoplasia** in cats is almost always the result of *in utero* or perinatal infection with the panleukopenia virus.

K. **Cranial nerve diseases**

1. **Cavernous sinus syndrome.** Lesions of the cavernous sinus (i.e., the venous structure that lies on the floor of the skull and encircles the pituitary) may involve cranial nerves III, IV, VI, the ophthalmic branch of V, and the sympathetic nervous system. Causes include **neoplasia** and **granulomatous disease.**

2. **Neoplasia** (e.g., **nerve sheath tumors**) rarely involves a single cranial nerve; however, cranial nerve V may be preferentially affected. **Lymphomas** and **leukemias** may involve single or multiple cranial nerves.

3. **Idiopathic neuritis** is thought to involve some cranial nerves.
   a. **Trigeminal neuritis** involves the mandibular branches of cranial nerve V, resulting in an inability to close the jaw. Clinical signs usually improve in 2–4 weeks, regardless of treatment.
   b. **Idiopathic feline vestibular disease** and **canine geriatric vestibular disease**
      (1) **Etiology.** These diseases are thought to be caused by inflammation of the vestibular nerve.
      (2) **Clinical signs** suggest a peripheral vestibular abnormality and usually improve within 2–4 weeks.

4. **Otitis media interna** can result in abnormalities of cranial nerves VII and VIII, as well as the sympathetic system (Horner's syndrome).

SELECTED READINGS

Dewey CW, Downs MO, Aron DN: Acute traumatic intracranial hemorrhage in dogs and cats. *Vet Comp Orthop Trauma* 6:153–159, 1993.

Gordon LE, Thacher C, Matthiesen DT: Results of craniotomy for treatment of cerebral meningioma in 42 cats. *Vet Surg* 23:94–100, 1994.

Kirby R: Treatment of dogs and cats with severe head injuries. *Prog Vet Neurol* 5:72–74, 1994.

Kornegay JN: Pathogenesis of diseases of the central nervous system. Edited by Slatter D. *Textbook of Small Animal Surgery,* 2nd ed. Philadelphia, WB Saunders, 1022–1037, 1993.

LeCouteur RA: Brain tumors of dogs and cats—diagnosis and management. *Vet Med Rep* 2: 332–342, 1990.

Niebauer GW, Dayrell-Hart BL, Speciale J: Evaluation of craniotomy in dogs and cats. *J Am Vet Med Assoc* 198:89–95, 1991.

Oliver JE Jr: Surgical approaches to the canine brain. *Am J Vet Res* 29:353–378, 1969.

Chapter 22
Spinal Cord and Vertebrae
Rodney S. Bagley

 SURGICAL PROCEDURES. The goal of spinal surgery is usually to decompress or stabilize the spine.

 Decompression techniques

1. **Hemilaminectomy.** The lamina (bone) on one side of the vertebrae is removed with a high-speed air drill and bur or rongeurs to provide access to the epidural space and dural tube (Figure 22–1).

   a. **Indications.** Hemilaminectomy is indicated when access to the ventral and lateral aspects of the spinal cord is necessary for decompression or exploration of the perispinal area.

   b. **Technique.** Hemilaminectomy is more easily performed in the thoracolumbar, as opposed to the cervical, region of the spine because the cervical area has more overlying musculature and care must be taken to avoid the vertebral artery, which runs laterally through the cervical vertebrae.

      (1) **Approach.** A **dorsal approach** is used. A **lateral approach** for cervical spinal decompression has also been described.

      (2) **Exposure.** The lateral epaxial musculature is elevated from the lateral dorsal spinous process and lateral lamina of the vertebrae.

      (3) **Removal of the bone.** The articular facets overlying the affected disk space are removed with rongeurs, and a laminectomy defect is created with rongeurs or a high-speed air drill and bur.

      (4) **Removal of compressive material.** Herniated disk material or tumors are gently removed by aspiration and retrieved with blunt or sharp probes or dental instruments.

      (5) **Closure.** A gelatin sponge or autogenous fat graft is placed in the laminectomy defect to prevent the formation of a "laminectomy membrane" (i.e., epaxial muscle and fibrous tissue adhesions resulting in spinal cord compression). The thoracodorsal fascia is apposed along the midline. The subcutaneous tissue and skin are apposed routinely.

   c. **Advantages.** Hemilaminectomy allows exposure of the nerve root and spinal cord without creating vertebral instability. In addition, this procedure requires only unilateral dissection of soft tissue, and it is easy to combine with adjacent disk fenestration (see I A 4).

   d. **Disadvantages** of hemilaminectomy include the necessity for accurate localization of the side of the lesion (usually via myelography), and the risks of iatrogenic trauma to the nerve roots and hemorrhage from the vertebral sinuses.

2. **Dorsal laminectomy**

   a. **Indications.** Dorsal laminectomy is used to approach lesions that are located dorsally, laterally, or ventrally in the vertebral canal (Figure 22–2); however, spinal cord manipulation may be necessary to remove lesions from the floor of the vertebral canal.

   b. **Technique.** Three types of dorsal laminectomies have been described: **Funkquist types A** and **B,** and the **modified dorsal.** Problems with laminectomy membrane formation occurred with the Funkquist type A procedure, and the lack of ventral exposure hindered the type B procedure. The modified dorsal laminectomy permits better exposure of the ventral aspect of the canal while decreasing the risk of laminectomy membrane formation.

      (1) **Approach.** A **dorsal approach** is used.

      (2) **Exposure.** Dissection and reflection of the muscle are performed on both sides of the vertebrae to expose the entire dorsal aspect.

A

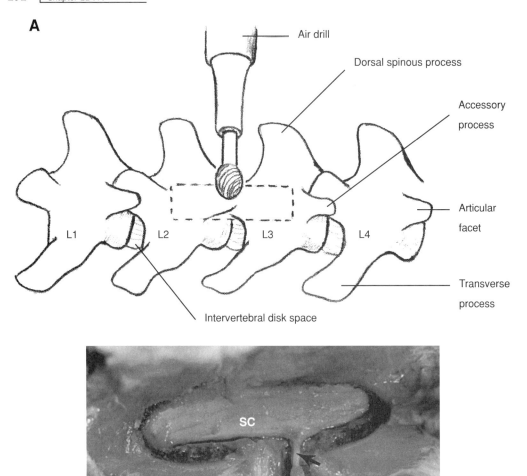

FIGURE 22-1. (*A*) Lateral schematic view of the extent of bone removal for a hemilaminectomy. The articular facets overlying the affected disk space are removed, and a high-speed air drill and bur are used to create a laminectomy defect. (*B*) Exposure of the spinal cord (*SC*) and the nerve root (*arrow*).

(3) **Removal of the bone.** A laminectomy defect is created dorsally over the affected intervertebral disk space. The caudal articular facets of the cranial vertebrae are removed during creation of this defect, but the cranial articular facets of the caudal vertebrae are left intact.

(4) **Removal of compressive material** is the same as for hemilaminectomy.

(5) **Closure** is similar to that used for hemilaminectomy.

c. **Advantages** of dorsal laminectomy include access to the dorsal and dorsolateral aspects of the spinal cord. Therefore, accurate side localization is not always necessary. There is also a reduced chance of penetrating the ventral vertebral sinuses, as compared with the hemilaminectomy procedure.

d. **Disadvantages** of dorsal laminectomy include poor exposure of the ventral aspect

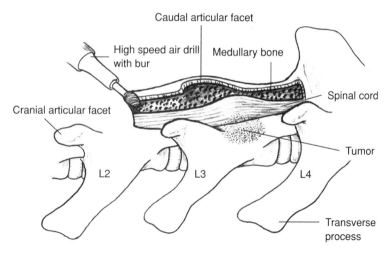

FIGURE 22–2. Dorsal schematic view showing the extent of bone removal during a dorsal laminectomy. (Redrawn with permission from Harari J, Marks SL: Surgical treatments for intervertebral disc disease. *Vet Clin North Am Small Anim Pract* 22(4):909, 1992.)

of the spinal cord, spinal instability (as compared with hemilaminectomy), the necessity for bilateral soft tissue dissection, and increased surgical morbidity leading to prolonged recovery (as compared with hemilaminectomy).

3. Ventral slot decompression

    a. Indications. Ventral slot decompression is indicated for ventral decompression in the cervical region (Figure 22–3).

    b. Technique

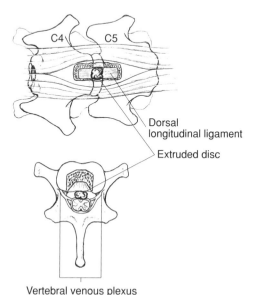

FIGURE 22–3. Ventral cervical (slot) decompression. A ventral cervical midline incision is made to expose the cervical vertebrae, and the muscles are retracted. A slot is made over the affected disk space, and the extruded disk material or abnormal structure is removed from the vertebral canal. (Redrawn with permission from Harari J, Marks SL: Surgical treatments for intervertebral disc disease. *Vet Clin North Am Small Anim Pract* 22(4):903, 1992.)

(1) Approach. The vertebrae are approached via a **ventral cervical midline incision.**

(2) Exposure. The paired sternomastoid and sternohyoid muscles are separated along the midline. The trachea, esophagus, and carotid sheath are retracted to allow access to the longus colli muscles. The longus colli muscles are separated along the midline and retracted laterally to provide access to the ventral vertebral body.

(3) Removal of the bone

    (a) A **spondylectomy** is performed over the intervertebral disk space with a high-speed air drill and bur.

    (b) The slot should be no wider than one-half of the vertebral body width and no longer than one-third of the length of each neighboring vertebral body to avoid vertebral sinus laceration and iatrogenic fracture of bone. An **inverted cone slot** has been described to lessen the chance of iatrogenic bone fracture.

(4) Decompression. Following removal of the bone, abnormal ligamentous structures (e.g., the dorsal annulus ligament, dorsal longitudinal ligament) or extruded (ruptured) disk material is removed from within the vertebral canal.

    (a) Linear traction. Material is removed from the canal as vertebrae are distracted using self-retaining instruments or gentle traction on the animal's head. This linear traction opens the intervertebral space, permitting access to the spinal canal for retrieval of tissues.

    (b) Decompression is assumed complete when the spinal cord is visualized.

(5) Closure. The longus colli muscles, sternohyoid muscles, and sternomastoid muscles are reapposed and the subcutaneous tissues and skin are closed routinely.

c. Advantages include decompression and access to the ventral aspect of the spinal cord, where disk extrusion is most commonly situated.

d. Disadvantages include hemorrhage from the ventral vertebral sinuses, spinal instability resulting from the removal of excessive amounts of the vertebral body, and, possibly, bone fracture.

4. Fenestration (nondecompressive spinal surgery) is a prophylactic procedure wherein the annulus fibrosus of the intervertebral disk space is incised and the nucleus pulposus is removed. Removal of the nucleus pulposus may prevent further extrusion of this tissue into the vertebral canal. The vertebral canal is not entered during this procedure.

a. Indications

(1) Therapy. Fenestration is indicated for animals with pain resulting from mild disk protrusion secondary to a bulging nucleus pulposus, although the therapeutic benefits are controversial.

(2) Prophylaxis. Fenestration can prevent extrusion of abnormal nucleus pulposus. Success in preventing disk extrusion with fenestration is directly proportional to how much nucleus pulposus is removed.

b. Technique. Fenestration can be performed as a primary procedure or combined with decompressive procedures.

(1) Approach

    (a) In the **thoracolumbar region,** incision of muscular insertions from the accessory process exposes the lateral disk space. The nerve roots and associated vascular structures are retracted cranially, the annulus fibrosis is incised sharply, and the nucleus pulposus is removed with a fenestration curette or dental tartar scraper.

    (b) In the **cervical region,** a similar surgical approach is used as for a ventral slot procedure.

(2) Closure. The fascia and subcutaneous tissues and skin are closed in a fashion similar to that used for laminectomy.

B. **Stabilization techniques**

1. **Indications**
   a. Stabilization of the vertebral segments is often required **following trauma** or in cases of **malformation.** In humans, stabilization is indicated when two or more of the following compartments are damaged.
      (1) The **ventral (anterior) compartment** is composed of the ventral longitudinal ligament and ventral annulus fibrosus.
      (2) The **middle compartment** includes the dorsal annulus fibrosus, the dorsal vertebral body, and the dorsal longitudinal ligament.
      (3) The **dorsal compartment** includes the articular facets and joint capsules, the ligamentum flavum, the dorsal vertebral arch and pedicle, and the dorsal spinous processes and interspinous ligaments.
   b. **Atlantoaxial** or **lumbosacral instability** and cervical vertebral malformation or malarticulation (**wobbler syndrome**) are special situations where vertebral stabilization is beneficial.

2. **Techniques**
   a. **External stabilization** (e.g., with **splints** and **bandages**) may be unrewarding as a primary treatment modality because it is difficult to rigidly stabilize the vertebral column using these devices. Splints ideally should decrease mobility above and below the unstable vertebral segments.
   b. **Internal stabilization.** A variety of **implants** have been used, including flexible or steel plates, bone screws, pins, methyl methacrylate cement, and external fixation devices (Figure 22–4).

II. CONDITIONS OF THE SPINAL CORD AND VERTEBRAE

A. **Degenerative disease**

1. **Intervertebral disk disease** most frequently affects the cervical or thoracolumbar portions of the spinal cord.
   a. **Types**
      (1) **Hansen I intervertebral disk disease** is seen in young chondrodystrophoid breeds of dogs (e.g., dachshunds, shi tzus, Pekingese, beagles).
         (a) **Pathogenesis.** Degeneration of the disk is associated with chondroid metaplasia within the disk, commonly leading to **disk extrusion.**
         (b) **Clinical signs** are usually **acute** in onset and include **paresis, plegia,** and **focal hyperesthesia.**
      (2) **Hansen type II intervertebral disk disease** is often seen in mature nonchondrodystrophoid breeds of dogs.
         (a) **Pathogenesis.** Degeneration of the disk is associated with fibroid metaplasia within the disk, leading to **disk protrusion (bulging).**
         (b) **Clinical signs** are usually **chronic** in onset and include **paresis** and **focal hyperesthesia.**
   b. **Diagnosis** is based on neurologic examination, spinal radiographs, and myelography.
   c. **Treatment** options include rest, the administration of anti-inflammatory drugs (e.g., methylprednisolone), acupuncture, fenestration, surgical decompression, or chemonucleolysis (i.e., the injection of enzymes into the disk). Electrical stimulation of the spinal cord is being used experimentally and may have future clinical implications.
   d. **Prognosis** depends on the severity, duration, and speed of onset of the disease. Delaying surgery (i.e., longer than 24–48 hours) worsens the prognosis.
      (1) The prognosis is better for animals with intact motor and sensory function.
      (2) Acutely paralyzed animals, especially those with loss of deep pain sensation,

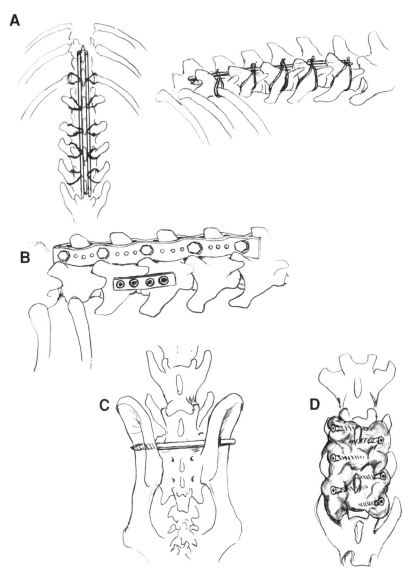

FIGURE 22–4. (*A*) Steinmann pins and orthopedic wire used to stabilize a lumbar fracture/luxation in a small- or medium-sized dog. The pins are placed around the spinous processes and the wire is secured around the transverse processes and the pin. The technique can be improved by wiring the articular processes to the pins. (*B*) Bone plates applied to the lumbar vertebrae to stabilize a fracture/luxation. A plastic dorsal spinal plate is secured with bolts placed between the spinal processes and a metal bone plate is applied to the vertebral bodies. Complications of dorsal plating include plate migration or iatrogenic fracture of the processes. (*C*) A transilial Steinmann pin used to stabilize a lumbosacral luxation. The pin is placed behind the spinous process of L7 and on top of the L7–S1 articulating facets. (*D*) Bone screws or pins are placed in the vertebral bodies and surrounded by methyl methacrylate cement (or bone) to stabilize a vertebral fracture or luxation. (*A, B,* and *C* redrawn with permission from Bojrab MJ: *Current Techniques in Small Animal Surgery,* 3rd ed. Philadelphia, Lea & Febiger, 1990, pp 644, 645, 646.)

(e.g., those that have experienced explosive disk herniation) have a worse prognosis.

2. **Degenerative myelopathy** most commonly affects middle-aged to old German shepherds; however, other large breeds may also be affected.
   a. **Etiology and pathogenesis.** The etiology of degenerative myelopathy is unknown;

histologic changes involve white matter degeneration and changes in the gray matter of the dorsal horn.

b. Diagnosis

(1) Clinical signs include slowly progressive paraparesis resulting from an upper motor neuron (UMN) lesion. No spinal pain is present.

(2) Spinal radiographs and **myelography** fail to reveal a compressive lesion.

(3) Cerebrospinal fluid (CSF) analysis (using a lumbar collection technique) may reveal normal results or increased protein.

c. Treatment includes forced exercise to maintain musculoskeletal tone, vitamin supplementation, and ϵ-aminocaproic acid therapy.

d. Prognosis is usually poor because of the progressive nature of the disease and the equivocal response to therapy.

3. **Caudal cervical spondylomyelopathy (wobbler syndrome, cervical vertebral malformation** or **malarticulation)** most commonly affects middle-aged or old Doberman pinschers and young Great Danes.

a. Etiology and pathogenesis. Caudal cervical spondylomyelopathy is often the result of vertebral malarticulation and instability. Subsequent bone deformations or hypertrophy of the ligamentum flavum or dorsal annulus fibrosus causes spinal cord compression, which occurs most frequently in the caudal cervical area (C5–C7).

b. Diagnosis. Myelography (flexion, extension, and traction views) is necessary to identify the location and nature of the lesion. Computed tomography or magnetic resonance imaging may also be helpful.

c. Treatment

(1) Mild cases can be treated with rest, anti-inflammatory drugs, and a neck brace.

(2) Lesions causing progressive motor deficits are treated with decompressive or stabilizing procedures, or both.

(a) Ventral decompression (slotting) or, less frequently, **dorsal laminectomy** is performed to treat static compressive lesions (e.g., disk herniations).

(b) Ventral decompression and **vertebral body stabilization** with a bone plate, screws, cancellous bone graft, or methyl methacrylate are performed for dynamic lesions such as annulus hypertrophy (Figure 22–5).

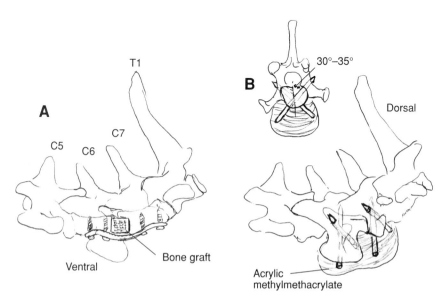

FIGURE 22–5. Ventral cervical stabilization techniques for the treatment of wobbler syndrome. (*A*) A flexible Lubra plate and cortical bone graft are used to maintain linear traction. (*B*) Methyl methacrylate cement and pins are used for distraction. (Redrawn with permission from Bojrab MJ: *Current Techniques in Small Animal Surgery*, 3rd ed. Philadelphia, Lea & Febiger, 1990, pp 582, 583.)

    d. Prognosis. The procedures are technically demanding, associated with a high degree of morbidity, and produce a fair to guarded prognosis depending on the severity of the lesions.

       (1) In general, 75% of dogs that are able to walk before surgery will experience stabilization or improvement of clinical signs following surgery.

       (2) Only 50% of animals that are unable to stand prior to surgery will experience a favorable prognosis.

4. Cauda equina syndrome (lumbosacral disease) most frequently affects middle-aged to older large-breed dogs.

    a. Etiology and pathogenesis. Cauda equina syndrome results from lumbosacral vertebral canal stenosis (e.g., by dorsal bulging of the annulus fibrosis or bone malformations). The stenotic canal compresses the terminal peripheral nerves that course caudally from the spinal cord. Neoplasia or infection in the L7–S1 region may produce similar signs.

    b. Diagnosis

       (1) Clinical signs include lumbosacral pain, fecal and urinary incontinence, tail atonia, and lower motor neuron (LMN) sciatic paraparesis as a result of compression of the terminal lumbar, sacral, and coccygeal nerves (i.e., the cauda equina).

       (2) Lumbosacral radiography and **myelography** may show the lesion if the dural tube ends caudal to the lumbosacral junction.

          (a) Epidurography and **diskography** may be helpful for visualizing the lesion.

          (b) Electromyography of the pelvic limbs, anus, and tail may reveal evidence of nerve compression and entrapment.

          (c) Computed tomography and **magnetic resonance imaging** may help identify the lesion.

    c. Treatment involves rest, anti-inflammatory drugs, and surgery to decompress and stabilize the spinal cord and vertebrae.

       (1) Dorsal decompression and **unilateral facetectomy** (i.e., excision of the articular process) or **foraminotomy** (i.e., enlargement of the intervertebral foramen) is performed to reduce dural tube and nerve root compression.

       (2) Dorsal decompression and **L7–S1 traction/fusion** are performed by some surgeons using screws, pins, and cancellous bone grafts to fix the vertebrae in a stretched position, reduce dorsal annulus compression, and open the intervertebral foramen.

    d. Prognosis is favorable for continent animals without severe motor deficits.

B. **Anomalous disorders** can affect any area of the spinal cord or vertebrae; however, the caudal lumbar area is most commonly affected.

1. Anomalous vertebral diseases include spina bifida, block vertebrae, and hemivertebrae. **Atlantoaxial instability** is a common condition affecting the first and second caudal vertebrae of young, small dogs.

    a. Etiology and pathogenesis. Spinal cord trauma and compression result from malarticulation of the C1–C2 vertebrae as a result of ligamentous abnormalities or the absence or malformation of the odontoid process.

    b. Diagnosis

       (1) Clinical signs include tetraparesis, ataxia, and cervical pain.

       (2) Cervical radiography confirms the diagnosis. Frequently, lateral view radiographs reveal a widened space between the arch of the atlas and the dorsal spinal process of the axis.

    c. Treatment

       (1) Mild cases can be treated with rest, anti-inflammatory drugs, and external support bandages.

       (2) Moderate to severe cases. Ventral surgical stabilization of the C1–C2 articulations using pins or screws is recommended for animals with moderate or severe neurologic signs.

2. Anomalous spinal diseases include spinal dysraphism, syringomyelia, meningocele, myelocele, and meningomyelocele.

   a. **Clinical signs** suggestive of a spinal problem are usually present at a young age.
   b. **Survey radiography, myelography,** and **advanced imaging** are helpful for diagnosis.

C. Neoplasia

1. **Types.** Spinal neoplasia is categorized according to the location of the tumor relative to the spinal cord and meninges.
   a. **Extradural tumors** arise external to the dura. These tumors include tumors of the **bone** (i.e., osteo-, fibro-, and chondrosarcoma), **blood vessels** (i.e., hemangiosarcoma), **bone marrow** (i.e., plasmacytoma, multiple myeloma), and **adipose tissue** (i.e., lipoma, liposarcoma), as well as **metastatic lesions** (i.e., carcinoma, lymphoma).
   b. **Intradural (extramedullary) tumors** arise within or below the dura but outside the spinal cord proper. **Meningioma** and **nerve sheath tumors** are most common.
   c. **Intramedullary tumors** arise from the spinal cord. **Astrocytoma** and **ependymoma** are most common.

2. **Diagnosis**
   a. **Clinical signs** depend on the location and the nature of the tumor. In general, intramedullary tumors produce acute, nonpainful signs.
   b. **Radiographs, myelography,** and **advanced imaging** are helpful for diagnosis.

3. **Treatment** entails surgical removal. Corticosteroids are used to reduce nervous tissue swelling and inflammation.

4. **Prognosis** depends on the type of tumor and the extent of mass excision.

D. Inflammatory processes

1. **Primary causes** of spinal cord inflammation are uncommon. **Toxoplasmosis** and **granulomatous meningoencephalomyelitis** are examples.

2. **Secondary causes** of spinal cord inflammation include **diskospondylitis,** an infection of the intervertebral disk space most often associated with a bacterial infection (e.g., by *Staphylococcus aureus, Brucella canis,* or *Escherichia coli*).
   a. **Pathogenesis.** The genitourinary, cardiovascular, or alimentary system is most commonly the source of the septic embolus.
   b. **Diagnosis**
      (1) **Clinical signs** include spinal pain, paraspinal muscle atrophy and paresis, pyrexia, and lethargy.
      (2) **Survey radiography** (which reveals bone lysis, sclerosis, and collapse), **blood** and **urine cultures,** and *Brucella* **titers** are most helpful for making a definitive diagnosis.
   c. **Treatment.** Diskospondylitis is effectively treated with long-term antibiotic therapy based on the results of antimicrobial culture and sensitivity testing. Prior to identifying the causative bacteria, cephalosporins are usually used.

E. Trauma

1. **Etiology.** Most traumatic spinal cord disorders are caused by vertebral fracture or subluxation resulting from automobile trauma or, less frequently, gunshot wounds.

2. **Pathogenesis.** Because the spinal cord is encased by bone (i.e., the vertebrae) and the spinal parenchyma is semisolid, any change in vertebral canal diameter results in spinal cord displacement and pressure.
   a. Increases in intraspinal pressure can produce **ischemia, hemorrhage,** and **edema.**
   b. **Secondary injury theory.** The ischemia, hemorrhage, and edema perpetuate the damage to the spinal cord and may be more detrimental to the spinal cord than the initial mechanical injury.
      (1) **Putative mediators** of this self-perpetuating process include **excitatory neurotransmitters, endorphins, catecholamines,** and **free radicals** released after the initial insult.

(2) Currently, **therapeutic efforts** are being directed at neutralizing the effects of these by-products of trauma. To date, attempts at counterbalancing single mediators alone have not dramatically improved treatment outcomes.

3. **Diagnosis**
   a. **Clinical signs** are usually acute in onset and may be progressive or static, depending on the severity and stability of the injury. The majority of lesions occur where the stable and movable portions of the spine meet (i.e., the atlantooccipital, cervicothoracic, thoracolumbar, and lumbosacral regions).
   b. **Survey radiography, myelography,** and **neurologic examination** are usually performed after the animal has recovered from the initial shock. Radiographs may reveal a static lesion; vertebral displacement may be reduced prior to the study.
   c. **Biopsy, resection,** or **durotomy** can provide diagnostic information and may be therapeutic as well.

4. **Treatment** involves cage rest, intravenous methylprednisolone, and surgical fixation or decompression for animals with progressive, severe, or unstable lesions.

5. **Prognosis** is favorable for animals that have intact pain sensation. Nursing care, which entails provision of padded surfaces for the animal, bladder and bowel evacuations, and physical therapy, including hydrotherapy, is critical for functional recovery.

F. **Vascular disease. Fibrocartilaginous emboli (FCE)** can affect the spinal cord. Most frequently, the cervical or lumbar intumescence is affected.

1. **Breed predisposition.** Nonchondrodystrophoid breeds of dogs are affected. An increased incidence of the disease has been noted in miniature schnauzers.

2. **Diagnosis**
   a. **Clinical signs** reflect an acute onset of spinal cord dysfunction that is nonprogressive after the first 24 hours.
      (1) Although many dogs are noted to vocalize as if in pain early in the disease, **no spinal hyperesthesia** is found during palpation.
      (2) The lack of spinal pain is helpful in distinguishing FCE from intervertebral disk extrusion or other spinal compressive diseases.
   b. **Survey radiography, myelography,** and **CSF analysis** usually are normal.

3. **Treatment.** Currently, there is no effective treatment for FCE. In animals with intact deep pain sensation, improvements are usually seen within 2 weeks of the onset of signs.
   a. **Supportive nursing care** of the plegic animal is imperative.
   b. **Corticosteroids** are often used during the acute onset of the disease, but objective evaluations of their benefit are not available.

4. **Prognosis** is based on the severity of the neurologic dysfunction.

SELECTED READINGS

Bojrab MJ (ed): *Current Techniques in Small Animal Surgery,* 3rd ed. Philadelphia, Lea & Febiger, 1990, pp 579–648.

Bracken MB, Shephard MJ, Collins WF: A randomized, controlled trial of methyl prednisolone or naloxone in the treatment of acute spinal cord injury. *N Engl J Med* 322:1405–1412, 1990.

Braund KG (ed): *Clinical Syndromes in Veterinary Neurology.* St. Louis, CV Mosby, 1994.

Carberry CC, Flanders JA, Dietze AE: Nonsurgical management of thoracic and lumbar spinal fractures and fracture/luxations in the dog and cat: a review of 17 cases. *J Am Anim Hosp Assoc* 25:43–54, 1989.

McCarthy RJ, Lewis DD, Hosgood G: Atlantoaxial subluxation in dogs. *J Comp Contin Educ Pract* 17:215–224, 1995.

McKee WM: Comparison of hemilaminectomy and dorsal laminectomy for the treatment of thoracolumbar disc protrusion in dogs. *Vet Rec* 130:296–300, 1994.

Moore MM (ed): Diseases of the spine. *Vet Clin North Am Small Anim Pract* 22(4), July, 1992.

Seim HB (ed): Nervous system. In *Textbook of Small Animal Surgery*, 2nd ed. Edited by Slatter D. Philadelphia, WB Saunders, 1993, pp 984–1121.

Selcer RR, Bubb WJ, Walker TL: Management of vertebral column fractures in dogs and cats: 211 cases (1977–1985). *J Am Vet Med Assoc* 198:1965–1968, 1991.

Toombs JP, Collins LG, Graves GM: Colonic perforation in corticosteroid-treated dogs. *J Am Vet Med Assoc* 188:145–150, 1986.

Wheeler SJ, Sharp NJ: *Small Animal Spinal Disorders: Diagnosis and Surgery.* St. Louis, Mosby-Wolfe, 1994.

Chapter 23

Peripheral Nerves and Muscles

Rodney S. Bagley

I. PERIPHERAL NERVES

A. Preoperative assessment

1. When **trauma** is the cause of the peripheral nerve disorder, attempts should be made to determine the extent of injury.
   a. **Classification of injury**
      (1) **Neurapraxia** is a functional, rather than an anatomical, interruption of peripheral nerve function.
      (2) **Axonotmesis** is more severe than neurapraxia. Axons within the nerve are separated; however, the nerve itself remains intact.
      (3) **Neurotmesis** is a complete severance of the nerve with anatomical separation of all axons.
   b. **Diagnostic evaluations.** Electromyography, nerve conduction velocity (NCV) testing, and late potentials can be used to determine the extent and location of peripheral nerve injury (see Chapter 20 II C 3).

2. When the source of peripheral nerve dysfunction is **nontraumatic,** it is important to determine the location of the disease (i.e., single versus multiple peripheral nerves) in order to successfully biopsy a nerve that is affected with, and representative of, the disease process.
   a. Assessments should be made for **underlying systemic disease** (e.g., neoplasia, insulinoma, diabetes mellitus, hypothyroidism).
   b. **Diagnostic evaluations** to determine the extent and location of peripheral nerve disease are similar to those described in I A 1 b.

B. Surgical procedures

1. **Anastomosis**
   a. **General principles**
      (1) Severed nerves heal between ends as the proximal segment sends axon sprouts to find the distal segment. Guide tubes can be placed around cut nerve ends to improve axonal channeling to the distal stump.
      (2) If there is excessive distance between the severed nerve ends or excessive tension between the nerve ends after anastomosis, regeneration will fail.
   b. **Techniques**
      (1) **Suturing.** Severed nerve ends can be sutured together in the following ways.
         (a) **Epineurial repair** is the preferred technique and provides sufficient repair in most instances. In this technique, four to six sutures are placed circumferentially around the nerve.
         (b) **Perineurial repair** is more tedious and usually requires microsurgical skill and magnification; however, it may allow for better anatomic alignment of fascicles.
      (2) **Lasers, fibrin glues,** or **clotting material** permit sutureless repair. Of these techniques, laser methods appear most promising.
      (3) **Nerve grafts.** If primary repair is not feasible because of excessive distance between the cut ends, a free autogenous nerve graft can be used to facilitate repair.

2. **Biopsy** of an affected peripheral nerve is often helpful for diagnosis of a peripheral nerve disorder and for clarification of the primary pathologic features (e.g., inflammation, degeneration, primary myelin abnormalities, primary axonal disease).
   a. **Selection of a biopsy site.** Nerves commonly biopsied include the peroneal and

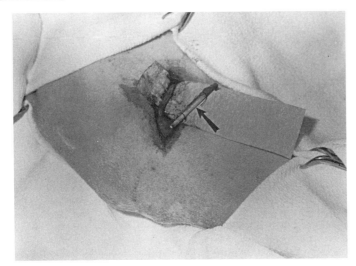

FIGURE 23–1. Fascicular nerve biopsy of the peroneal nerve. The portion of the nerve to be removed has been secured to a sterile wooden applicator stick (*arrow*).

tibial nerves of the pelvic limb and the cutaneous radial and ulnar nerves of the thoracic limb. When selecting a biopsy site, the following criteria should be met.

(1) The nerve should **perform a nonessential function.**
(2) The nerve should be **affected by the disease.**
(3) The nerve should be **constant** in its **anatomical location.**
(4) The nerve should normally be **protected from entrapment** and **recurrent trauma.**
(5) The **surgical approach should not damage nearby blood vessels, tendons,** or **joints.**
(6) The area should be **apt to heal well** after surgery.
(7) Normal quantitative **data should exist about the nerve morphology.**

b. Technique

(1) **Segmental biopsy.** If the entire nerve can be sacrificed (e.g., a sensory branch), a small segment of the nerve is removed.
(2) **Fascicular biopsy** (Figure 23–1). More commonly, a mixed nerve is biopsied. No more than one-third of the diameter of the nerve should be removed to avoid iatrogenic damage.

c. Sample analysis. Pathologic changes in peripheral nerves can be difficult to detect with routine histologic processing and evaluation. It is recommended that peripheral nerve specimens be evaluated by a pathologist experienced in microscopic evaluation of peripheral nervous tissue.

(1) **Morphometric analysis** determines the percentage of fibers of a certain diameter within the nerve using an electron microscope.
(2) **Teased-fiber analysis,** which is useful for evaluating demyelinating diseases, evaluates individual fibers in a longitudinal plane.

d. Postoperative care. The biopsy site is monitored for inflammation. Some swelling at the incisional site is expected; however, a light pressure bandage used for 1–3 days following surgery may minimize swelling.

3. Decompression

a. Hemilaminectomy or **foraminotomy** is used to decompress peripheral nerves within the spinal canal or at the intervertebral foramina that become compressed as a result of spinal cord disease. For example, hypertrophied bone, annulus fibrosis, or other ligamentous structures may compress the L7 or sacral peripheral nerves in cauda equina syndrome (lumbosacral disease).

b. Neurolysis (i.e., the surgical freeing of an entrapped nerve) may be necessary to decompress peripheral nerves entrapped by fibrous, cartilaginous, or bony tissues subsequent to bone healing or soft tissue scarring.

C. **Disorders of the peripheral nervous system (PNS)**

1. **Trauma**
   a. **Brachial plexus avulsion** most commonly occurs in a single thoracic limb following automobile trauma.
      (1) **Pathogenesis.** Nerve root contusion or separation from the spinal cord causes acute, nonpainful, nonprogressive dysfunction (i.e., monoparesis or monoplegia).
      (2) **Treatment.** With partial avulsions, **muscle tendon transpositions** or **carpal arthrodesis** can be performed. In severe cases, **amputation** may be necessary to prevent mutilation.
      (3) **Prognosis** depends on the severity of nerve injury. Loss of pain sensation in the limb indicates a poor prognosis.
   b. **Orthopedic trauma.** Peripheral nerves may be injured at the same time orthopedic trauma is sustained. For example, damage of the radial nerve has been associated with humeral fractures, and damage to the sciatic nerve, pelvic nerve, and pudendal nerve is often associated with pelvic fractures. Vertebral fractures may also cause peripheral nerve damage.
   c. **Iatrogenic trauma.** Peripheral nerves may be injured during orthopedic surgery. The sciatic nerve, for example, may be damaged by intramedullary pins used to repair a fractured femur. Treatment involves removal or redirection of the pin.

2. **Neoplasia**
   a. **Nerve sheath tumors** of the PNS include **schwannoma, neurofibroma,** and **neurofibrosarcoma.**
      (1) **Location.** Nerve sheath tumors commonly affect the nerves of the **brachial plexus.** In the **spinal cord,** they most commonly occur as **intradural, extramedullary lesions.**
      (2) **Characteristics.** Nerve sheath tumors are **locally invasive** and **slow to metastasize.**
      (3) **Diagnosis**
         (a) **Clinical signs** include **chronic, progressive lameness.** Physical examination may show **atrophy, hyporeflexia tending to areflexia,** and **axillary pain.** Occasionally, a **mass** is palpable in the axillary region.
         (b) **Electromyography** reveals evidence of **denervation** in the muscles of the limb, suggesting a neurogenic rather than an orthopedic cause for the lameness.
         (c) **Myelography** may be indicated if the tumor encroaches on the spinal cord.
         (d) **Computed tomography** or **magnetic resonance imaging** may reveal a mass in the perispinal or axillary region.
         (e) **Exploratory surgery** of the brachial plexus should be considered if there is a high index of suspicion of nerve sheath tumor.
      (4) **Treatment**
         (a) Because these tumors are usually slow-growing and locally invasive, **radical local resection** is important.
         (b) If these tumors involve nerves of the thoracic limb, **amputation** is often indicated unless the lesion is very focal and wide surgical margins can be achieved around the tumor.
         (c) If the tumor invades proximally toward or within the spinal canal, **hemilaminectomy** is often necessary to remove the portion of the tumor within the vertebral canal.
      (5) **Prognosis.** The overall prognosis is poor when the tumor invades the spinal cord.
   b. **Lymphosarcoma** may involve the nerve roots and peripheral nerves, especially in cats.

3. **Inflammatory processes**
   a. **Chronic neuritis** is idiopathic. The condition may be relapsing or self-limiting and responsive to corticosteroids.
   b. **Brachial plexus neuritis** is an idiopathic or allergic inflammation primarily involving the nerves of the brachial plexus. Signs are similar to those of a brachial plexus tumor or injury. Definitive treatments have not been established, but corticosteroids may be beneficial.
   c. **Toxoplasmosis** and **neosporosis** are infectious neuropathies. Treatment includes administration of trimethoprim sulfonamide antibiotics or clindamycin.

4. **Metabolic neuropathies.** Systemic metabolic disease [e.g., **hypothyroidism, diabetes mellitus, insulinoma,** and **hyperlipidemia** (in cats)] can alter neuronal physiology, causing neuropathy.

5. **Toxin-related neuropathies**
   a. **Heavy metals** (e.g., mercury, lead) may cause peripheral nerve damage.
   b. **Botulism** and **tick paralysis** are associated with toxins that affect the neuromuscular junction (NMJ).
   c. **Organophosphates** can cause a chronic neuropathic condition that is characterized primarily by muscle weakness.

6. **Paraneoplastic neuropathies** have been seen **in association with** systemic neoplastic diseases (e.g., **lymphoma, insulinoma,** and various **carcinomas**).

7. **Congenital or hereditary neuropathies.** Numerous peripheral neuropathies occur in young animals and are assumed to be congenital or inherited.
   a. **Hypomyelination** and **axonopathy** are seen in malamutes, dalmatians, and golden retrievers.
   b. **Giant axonal neuropathy** is seen in German shepherds.
   c. **Hypertrophic neuropathy** affects Tibetan mastiffs.
   d. **Progressive axonopathy** is seen in boxers.
   e. **Sensory neuropathy** is seen in English pointers and dachshunds.
   f. **Globoid cell leukodystrophy** occurs most commonly in West Highland and cairn terriers.

II. MUSCLE

A. **Muscle biopsy** provides diagnostic and prognostic information in a variety of congenital, degenerative, inflammatory, and metabolic muscle disorders. In addition, muscle biopsy is useful for eliminating potential causes of myopathy to arrive at a diagnosis.

1. **Indications.** An animal with **elevated creatine kinase concentrations** or **abnormal electromyographic studies** should have a muscle biopsy unless a cause for the abnormalities has already been identified.

2. **Selection of a biopsy site.** Criteria are similar to those used for selecting a nerve biopsy site (see I B 2 a).
   (a) **Biopsy** of the muscle **should not alter function.**
   (b) The muscle should be **affected by the disease.**
   (c) Normal quantitative **data should exist about the muscle morphology. Muscle groups that have not been penetrated by an electromyography needle** should be selected to avoid misinterpretation of iatrogenic muscle damage.
   (d) The muscle should be **easily approached surgically,** and if possible, the surgical **approach should allow for combined muscle and nerve biopsy.**
   (e) The site should be associated with **minimal postoperative pain.**

3. **Technique**
   a. **Approach.** The biopsy site is aseptically prepared for surgery. An incision is made in the overlying skin and fascia to expose the muscle.

b. **Excision.** A segment of muscle is grasped with forceps, and a cylinder of tissue is resected with sharp scissors or a scalpel blade.

c. **Closure.** The fascia and subcutaneous tissue are closed with absorbable suture and the skin is closed with nonabsorbable suture.

d. **Specimen preservation.** It is not necessary to maintain stretch in muscle using muscle biopsy clamps if routine histochemical analysis is to take place; however, maintaining stretch in the sample is important for electron microscopic evaluations.

4. **Sample analysis.** Muscle samples taken at biopsy are analyzed differently than other tissues. Consultation with a muscle pathologist will help the surgeon collect and submit muscle in the appropriate way.

   a. **Enzyme histochemical evaluations** for fiber type determination require fresh frozen muscle.

      (1) Refrigeration of the muscle sample is necessary to maintain its cytochemical and histochemical properties until the sample can be frozen.

      (2) Ideally, muscle should be frozen within 1 hour of collection. The muscle is quickly immersed in a container of isopentane, a preservative, that has been chilled to just above the freezing point by immersion in liquid nitrogen.

   b. **Formalin fixation** affords limited information regarding muscle pathology.

   c. **Electron microscopic analysis** requires stretching the sample and fixing it as soon after sampling as possible using glutaraldehyde.

5. **Postoperative care** is similar to that following nerve biopsy (see I B 2 d).

B. **Disorders of muscle.** Clinical signs of myopathy are primarily related to weakness.

1. **Trauma**

   a. **Infraspinatus contracture** occurs in hunting dogs and produces outward rotation of the limb and adduction of the elbow joint. Resection of the fibrous musculotendinous portion of the muscle results in full recovery.

   b. **Quadriceps contracture** is a serious consequence of femoral fracture and poor surgical repair in young dogs (Figure 23–2).

      (1) **Pathogenesis.** Adhesions between the quadriceps muscle and periosteal tissue fix the limb in extension.

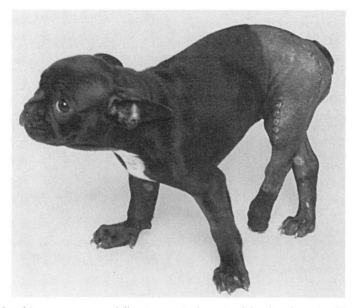

FIGURE 23–2. Quadriceps contracture following surgical repair of distal and proximal femoral physeal fractures. The limb posture is characterized by hyperextension of the stifle and hock joints. (Reprinted with permission from Hodges CC: Postoperative physical therapy. In *Surgical Complications and Wound Healing.* Edited by Harari J. Philadelphia, WB Saunders, 1993, p 401.)

    (2) Treatment. Surgical resection of fibrotic tissue is often unrewarding because of the severity and chronicity of the injury. Amputation of the limb may be necessary.

    (3) Prevention in terms of delicate surgical dissection, stable fracture fixation, flexion bandaging, and postoperative physical therapy should be routinely performed.

2. Idiopathic myopathies

    a. Fibrotic myopathy is a progressive, idiopathic muscle fibrosis that most frequently affects the semitendinosus muscles. Surgical release of affected tissues produces inconsistent results.

    b. Myositis ossificans is a non-neoplastic form of heterotopic ossification that affects fibrous connective tissue and skeletal muscle, frequently near the hip joint. Surgical resection of an encapsulated calcified mass is rewarding.

3. Inflammatory processes may be associated with infectious or noninfectious disease.

    a. Infectious diseases that affect muscle include **toxoplasmosis, neosporosis, heartworm infestation, clostridiosis, trichinosis,** and **leptospirosis** (in cats).

        (1) Clinical signs. Hyperextension of the pelvic limbs is often seen in young dogs affected with toxoplasmosis or neosporosis.

        (2) Serology is often helpful in diagnosis of infectious diseases.

        (3) Muscle biopsy may reveal the organism.

    b. Noninfectious myositis is often an immune-mediated disorder.

        (1) Polymyositis is a systemic muscle disorder.

            (a) Diagnosis

                (i) Clinical signs. Muscle pain and weakness are the most common clinical signs.

                (ii) Serology. Creatine kinase is often elevated in serum.

                (iii) Electromyography may reveal abnormalities.

            (b) Treatment. Corticosteroids may be helpful.

        (2) Masticatory (eosinophilic) myositis is a disease that primarily affects the muscles of the head. The immune reaction is thought to be specific for the type 2M muscle fibers of these muscles.

            (a) Pathogenesis. Initially, muscles are swollen and painful. In chronic cases, the muscles become fibrotic.

            (b) Treatment. Corticosteroids may be helpful.

        (3) Dermatomyositis is an immune-mediated disease affecting both skin and muscle that is most commonly seen in Shetland sheepdogs and collies.

4. Metabolic myopathies are uncommon.

    a. Lipid storage myopathy has been observed in dogs with other types of myopathy. Poorly localized myalgia, weakness, and atrophy are characteristic.

    b. Mitochondrial myopathy has been described in Old English sheepdog littermates. Episodic weakness was associated with exertional lactic acidosis.

    c. Electrolyte disturbances (e.g., hypokalemia) may result in muscle disease.

    d. Exertional rhabdomyolysis and **malignant hyperthermia** are possible causes of muscle damage.

    e. Endocrine diseases (e.g., hyperadrenocorticism, hypothyroidism) are associated with myopathy.

    f. Storage diseases (e.g., type VII glycogen storage disease) and **enzyme deficiencies** [e.g., phosphofructokinase (PFK) deficiency in springer spaniels] may be associated with myopathy.

5. Congenital or **hereditary myopathies** have been described in Labrador retrievers (**type II muscle deficiency**), golden retrievers and Irish terriers (**muscular dystrophy**), and chow chows (**myotonia**).

SELECTED READINGS

Bloomberg M: Muscles and tendons. In *Textbook of Small Animal Surgery,* 2nd ed. Edited by Slatter D. Philadelphia, WB Saunders, 1993, pp 1996–2019.

Braund KG: *Clinical Syndromes in Veterinary Neurology.* St Louis, CV Mosby, 1994, pp 376–422, 450–456.

Braund KG: Nerve and muscle biopsy techniques. *Prog Vet Neurology* 2:35–56, 1991.

Brehm DM, Vite CH, Steinberg HS: A retrospective evaluation of 51 cases of peripheral nerve sheath tumors in the dog. *J Am Anim Hosp* 31:349–359, 1995.

Cuddon PA: Feline neuromuscular diseases. *Feline Pract* 22:7–13, 1994.

Killingsworth CR: Repair of injured peripheral nerves, tendons, and muscles. In *Surgical Complications and Wound Healing in the Small Animal Practice.* Edited by Harari J. Philadelphia, WB Saunders, 1993, pp 169–202.

Rodkey WG: Peripheral nerve surgery. In *Textbook of Small Animal Surgery,* 2nd ed. Edited by Slatter D. Philadelphia, WB Saunders, 1993, pp 1135–1141.

Scott-Moncrieff JC, Hawkins EC, Cook JR: Canine muscle disorders. *Comp Contin Educ Pract Vet* 12:31–39, 1990.

Comprehensive
Exam

Directions: Each of the numbered items or incomplete statements in this section is followed by answers or by completions of the statement. Select the **one** numbered answer or completion that is **best** in each case.

1. Repair of a closed transverse femoral fracture in a healthy 2-year-old Labrador retriever would be classified in which surgical risk category?

(1) Physical status I
(2) Physical status II
(3) Physical status III
(4) Physical status IV
(5) Physical status V

2. Which one of the following suture materials is best suited for intraoral tissue closure following maxillary or mandibular surgery?

(1) Plain catgut
(2) Chromic catgut
(3) Polydioxanone or polypropylene
(4) Silk
(5) Polyamide

3. Two characteristics of second intention wound healing are:

(1) tissue necrosis and granulation tissue formation.
(2) persistent inflammation and wound drainage.
(3) epithelialization and skin contraction.
(4) fibrosis leading to cartilage formation.
(5) tissue edema and wound dehiscence.

4. Which one of the following statements regarding tracheal reconstruction is true?

(1) In dogs, no more than 10% of the trachea can be removed.
(2) In dogs, a maximum of 5 rings can be removed safely.
(3) Postoperative exercise is recommended to stimulate breathing.
(4) A split-cartilage technique is preferred to preserve lumen size.
(5) Anastomosis overlapping the cartilage rings results in a more precise anatomic alignment.

5. Which one of the following drugs can be used to stimulate appetite?

(1) Morphine
(2) Butorphanol
(3) Diazepam
(4) Acetylpromazine
(5) Yohimbine

6. Anal stenosis is a complication of which one of the following procedures?

(1) Anal sacculectomy
(2) Tumor excision
(3) Cryosurgery
(4) Deroofing and fulguration
(5) Resection and open drainage

7. Which of the following statements best characterizes aortic stenosis?

(1) It occurs most frequently in small breeds.
(2) It involves a subvalvular lesion.
(3) It causes right ventricular hypertrophy.
(4) Immediate surgical treatment is usually required.
(5) It normally requires patch grafting surgery.

8. Which one of the following is the treatment of choice for necrotizing cholecystitis?

(1) Cholecystotomy and lavage of the gallbladder
(2) Tube cholecystostomy
(3) Cholecystectomy
(4) Cholecystoduodenostomy
(5) Cholecystojejunostomy

9. Intermittent open-mouth lower jaw locking is best treated with:

(1) intralesional corticosteroid injections.
(2) partial resection of the zygomatic arch.
(3) systemic administration of corticosteroids.
(4) arthrodesis of the joint.
(5) long-term oral physical therapy.

10. A 6-year-old dog with recurrent mild gastrointestinal signs is scheduled to undergo an exploratory laparotomy for a suspected bowel obstruction. What are the minimum required presurgical tests?

(1) Electrocardiogram (ECG), urinalysis
(2) Complete blood count (CBC), urinalysis
(3) Blood chemistries, urinalysis
(4) Blood gases, urinalysis
(5) CBC, blood chemistries, urinalysis

11. Which cranial nerve is responsible for controlling facial expression, taste, and lacrimation?

(1) XI (spinal accessory)
(2) IX (glossopharyngeal)
(3) VII (facial)
(4) V (trigeminal)
(5) III (oculomotor)

12. Which one of the following is an indication for surgical repair of a pelvic fracture?

(1) A comminuted nondisplaced pubic fracture
(2) A mildly displaced sacroiliac luxation
(3) A medially displaced ilial body fracture
(4) An ischial body fracture

13. Which one of the following is a commonly used tranquilizer in veterinary medicine?

(1) Atropine
(2) Glycopyrrolate
(3) Flunixin meglumine
(4) Acepromazine
(5) Atipamezole

14. In dogs, bacterial osteomyelitis is most often caused by:

(1) *Pasteurella.*
(2) *Staphylococcus.*
(3) *Streptococcus.*
(4) *Escherichia coli.*
(5) *Proteus.*

15. Which one of the following statements regarding acute splenic torsion in dogs is true?

(1) It requires immediate intravenous antibiotic medication.
(2) It requires an upper gastrointestinal contrast study for diagnosis.
(3) It can be treated by rolling the animal.
(4) It produces a waxing and waning course.
(5) It can be life-threatening and requires

prompt administration of intravenous fluids.

16. Which of the following is the most common cause of bile duct rupture in small animals?

(1) Trauma
(2) Choleliths
(3) Choledocholiths
(4) Necrotizing cholecystitis
(5) Neoplasia

17. Which one of the following statements is true regarding fenestration?

(1) It affords spinal cord decompression.
(2) It permits evaluation of the spinal cord for prognosis determination.
(3) It prevents future disk herniations.
(4) It is used for treatment of spinal neoplasia.
(5) It requires ancillary antibiotic therapy.

18. Which one of the following statements is true regarding the nutritional support of starved, injured, or diseased animals?

(1) Mammals require less fat.
(2) The caloric density of the diet should be decreased by decreasing the fat content.
(3) Medium-chain triglycerides are preferred for ease of digestion and absorption.
(4) Long-chain triglycerides are preferred for ease of digestion and absorption.
(5) Dietary fiber should be reduced.

19. Which one of the following nerves must be avoided during a total ear canal ablation?

(1) Facial nerve
(2) Hypoglossal nerve
(3) Lingual nerve
(4) Trigeminal nerve
(5) Vestibular nerve

20. What is the most common mediastinal mass in cats?

(1) Squamous cell carcinoma
(2) Lymphosarcoma
(3) Thymoma
(4) Mediastinal abscesses
(5) Pneumomediastinum

21. A medial patellar luxation that can easily be manually reduced and causes periodic lameness would be classified as grade:

(1) I.
(2) II.

(3) III.
(4) IV.
(5) V.

22. What is the holding layer for sutures in the esophagus?

(1) Epithelium
(2) Mucosa
(3) Submucosa
(4) Muscularis
(5) Serosa

23. The most efficacious skin antiseptic agents are:

(1) isopropyl alcohol and ethyl alcohol.
(2) povidone-iodine and chlorhexidine.
(3) chlorhexidine and benzalkonium chloride.
(4) benzalkonium chloride and hexachlorophene.
(5) hexachlorophene and chlorhexidine.

24. Which of the following therapies best allows selective destruction of the zona fasciculata and reticularis?

(1) Mitotane
(2) Methimazole
(3) Propranolol
(4) Carbimazole
(5) Radioactive iodine (^{131}I)

25. Which one of the following statements regarding spinal trauma is true?

(1) It develops most frequently in static spinal regions (e.g., the thoracic vertebrae).
(2) It produces static, nonprogressive lesions.
(3) It requires immediate surgical intervention.
(4) It occurs most frequently at junctions of stable and mobile spinal segments (e.g., the cervicothoracic or thoracolumbar vertebrae).

26. Rhinotomy and turbinectomy are indicated for treatment of:

(1) nasal adenocarcinoma.
(2) nasal aspergillosis.
(3) nasal cryptococcosis.
(4) chronic unresponsive bacterial rhinitis.
(5) oronasal fistulae.

27. Hip joint pain and lameness in an otherwise healthy, young dog of a small breed are most likely associated with:

(1) aseptic femoral necrosis.
(2) septic arthritis.
(3) synovial cell sarcoma.
(4) hip dysplasia.
(5) sciatic neurapraxia.

28. Which one of the following statements regarding the use of an opioid as an induction agent is true?

(1) The opioid should be administered following preoxygenation.
(2) Cats require large doses.
(3) The opioid should be given in small doses to immature dogs.
(4) Opioids should be administered after a meal.

29. Which one of the following procedures involves suturing the uterine stump to the abdominal wall to encircle the bladder neck, thereby improving sphincter function?

(1) Vaginopexy
(2) Colposuspension
(3) Urethroplasty
(4) Cystoplasty
(5) Cystic relocation

30. When are prophylactic antibiotics used?

(1) To treat dirty wounds
(2) Immediately prior to prolonged surgery
(3) Orally for 10 days following urinary bladder surgery
(4) Orally for 2 days prior to elective procedures
(5) Topically on open wounds prior to closure

31. Chronic recurrent anal sacculitis should be treated with:

(1) colopexy.
(2) anal sacculectomy.
(3) tail amputation.
(4) enemas.
(5) rectal amputation and anastomosis.

32. Acute, life-threatening upper airway obstruction resulting from postoperative edema of the larynx and requiring immediate tracheostomy would be classified in which surgical risk category?

(1) Physical status II
(2) Physical status III
(3) Physical status IV
(4) Physical status V

33. The most common primary brain tumor of dogs and cats is:

(1) meningioma.
(2) lymphosarcoma.
(3) astrocytoma.
(4) glioma.
(5) choroid plexus tumor.

34. Which one of the following can impair weight-bearing?

(1) An acetabular fracture
(2) A pubic fracture
(3) Coccygeal vertebrae fractures
(4) Rupture of the prepubic tendon
(5) Diaphragmatic hernia

35. A rostral mandibular tumor involving the symphysis should be treated with:

(1) bilateral rostral mandibulectomy.
(2) unilateral rostral mandibulectomy.
(3) total hemimandibulectomy.
(4) partial rostral maxillectomy.
(5) segmental horizontal mandibulectomy.

36. Chronic bacterial otitis externa and media would best be treated by:

(1) pinna resection.
(2) bulla osteotomy.
(3) lateral wall resection.
(4) horizontal canal ablation.
(5) total ear canal ablation and bulla osteotomy.

37. Which suture pattern is preferred for end-to-end anastomosis of the esophagus?

(1) Single-layer inversion
(2) Double-layer inversion
(3) Single-layer eversion
(4) Double-layer apposition
(5) Single-layer apposition

38. Shoulder joint lameness in a young, rapidly growing large dog would most likely result from:

(1) bicipital tenosynovitis.
(2) synovial cell sarcoma.
(3) osteosarcoma.
(4) osteochondritis dissecans (OCD).
(5) medial luxation.

39. The most common congenital cardiac defect in dogs is:

(1) patent ductus arteriosus (PDA).
(2) persistent right aortic arch (PRAA).
(3) aortic stenosis.
(4) ventricular septal defect.
(5) pulmonic stenosis.

40. Halothane is a useful inhalation anesthetic characterized by:

(1) a minimum alveolar concentration (MAC) value less than that of methoxyflurane.
(2) a more rapid induction than methoxyflurane.
(3) its appropriateness for use in animals with intracranial pathology.
(4) its lack of myocardial sensitization.
(5) its ability to provide analgesia into the recovery period.

41. Hindlimb extension and proximal thigh muscle adhesion to the femur are characteristic of:

(1) leptospirosis.
(2) infraspinatus contracture.
(3) myositis ossificans.
(4) quadriceps contracture.
(5) fibrotic myopathy.

42. The risk of mammary tumors can be reduced to the greatest extent if ovariohysterectomy is performed:

(1) 1 year after the first estrus.
(2) 2 years after the first estrus.
(3) anytime during the dog's life.
(4) after 7 years of age.
(5) before the first estrus.

43. A 10-year-old cat with chronic liver disease characterized by hypoproteinemia, anemia, and weight loss is scheduled for a biopsy. What anesthetic agent would be most appropriate?

(1) Isoflurane
(2) Halothane
(3) Methoxyflurane
(4) Ketamine
(5) Thiamylal

44. Ataxia, dysmetria, intentional tremor, and pupillary abnormalities would suggest a lesion in the:

(1) cerebellum.
(2) cerebrum.
(3) spinal cord.

(4) brain stem.
(5) mesencephalon.

45. Which one of the following is true regarding pelvic fractures and repair?

(1) Healing times are prolonged.
(2) Open fractures are common.
(3) Medially displaced ischiatic tubercle fractures compromise the pelvic canal.
(4) Self-reduction of ischial fractures results from reduction of ilial fractures.
(5) A second surgery is required to remove acetabular plates.

46. Lateral patellar luxation is best treated with:

(1) external support (i.e., a cast) for 2 months.
(2) lateral imbricating sutures.
(3) medial relief incisions.
(4) medial imbricating sutures.
(5) lateral tibial tuberosity transposition.

47. Which one of the following is used to surgically treat hydrocephalus?

(1) Ventriculoperitoneal shunting
(2) Callosotomy
(3) Transsphenoidal pituitary removal
(4) Craniotomy
(5) Hemispherectomy

48. The energy requirement of a dog being treated for cancer is equal to:

(1) the resting energy requirement (RER).
(2) one-half of the RER.
(3) one and one half times the RER.
(4) the RER squared.
(5) two and one half times the RER.

49. In a large, heavily muscled, 2-year-old dog with a comminuted midshaft fracture of the femur, which of the following provides rigid stability and the quickest return to limb function?

(1) A splint
(2) A large intramedullary pin
(3) External skeletal fixation
(4) A bone plate and screws
(5) Bone screws and wires

50. Chronic, recurrent pericardial effusion is most effectively treated with:

(1) balloon valvuloplasty.
(2) pericardiocentesis.
(3) pericardiectomy.

(4) pericardiotomy.
(5) vagotomy.

51. A transsphenoidal hypophysectomy would most likely be performed for treatment of which one of the following conditions?

(1) Gastrinoma
(2) Insulinoma
(3) Pituitary-dependent hyperadrenocorticism
(4) Adrenocortical carcinoma
(5) Parathyroid adenoma

52. A common complication following maxillary or mandibular resection is:

(1) disfigurement.
(2) impaired vision.
(3) dysphonia.
(4) dysphagia.
(5) wound dehiscence.

53. In white cats, which neoplasm is associated with solar dermatitis of the ear tips?

(1) Squamous cell carcinoma
(2) Lymphosarcoma
(3) Mastocytoma
(4) Chondrosarcoma
(5) Leukemia

54. Which one of the following procedures is associated with a high degree of patient morbidity?

(1) Percutaneous biopsy
(2) Ultrasonographic-guided fine needle aspiration
(3) Intraoperative punch biopsy
(4) Intraoperative incisional biopsy
(5) Partial splenectomy

55. Damage to parathyroid tissue during surgery of the thyroid produces:

(1) hypercalcemia.
(2) hypocalcemia.
(3) hyperkalemia.
(4) hypokalemia.
(5) hypernatremia.

56. What is the treatment of choice for an aural hematoma?

(1) Ablation of the pinna
(2) Oral antibiotic therapy
(3) Chemotherapy
(4) Surgical drainage
(5) Bulla osteotomy

57. Which of the following treatments is recommended for benign prostatic hyperplasia?

(1) Castration
(2) Estrogen therapy
(3) Marsupialization
(4) Drainage
(5) Prostatectomy

58. Which one of the following drugs would be contraindicated in a 7-year-old cat with urinary obstruction caused by renal and cystic calculi?

(1) Acepromazine
(2) Thiamylal
(3) Halothane
(4) Isoflurane
(5) Ketamine

59. Abaxial deviation of contrast medium in dorsoventral and lateral views during myelography indicates:

(1) normal spinal cord.
(2) diskospondylitis.
(3) intramedullary swelling.
(4) dural neoplasia.
(5) osteosarcoma of the vertebrae.

60. Which one of the following statements concerning secondary wound closure is true?

(1) It is performed 24–48 hours after wounding.
(2) It is performed 5–6 days following injury.
(3) It delays wound healing.
(4) It is performed before granulation tissue forms.
(5) It requires wound drainage.

61. Which of the following suture materials is best suited for most vascular surgery?

(1) Chromic catgut
(2) Polypropylene
(3) Polydioxanone
(4) Polyglactin 910
(5) Polyglycolic acid

62. Which surgical approach provides greatest exposure of the thoracic cavity?

(1) Rib pivot thoracotomy
(2) Rib resection thoracotomy
(3) Medium sternotomy
(4) Intercostal thoracotomy

63. The most severe form of peripheral nerve damage is termed:

(1) neurapraxia.
(2) axonotmesis.
(3) neurotmesis.
(4) myelomalacia.
(5) myotonia.

64. Cranioventral displacement of pubic fractures can lead to:

(1) traumatic myocarditis.
(2) diaphragmatic hernia.
(3) sciatic neurapraxia.
(4) caudal abdominal visceral herniation.
(5) degenerative osteoarthritis.

65. Which of the following statements regarding treatment of hip dysplasia is true?

(1) Anti-inflammatory medications, exercise restriction, and weight reduction are usually ineffective.
(2) Triple pelvic osteotomy should be performed before degenerative joint changes occur.
(3) Femoral head and neck excision promotes progressive joint disease.
(4) Total hip replacement should be performed before skeletal maturity is reached.
(5) Capsulorrhaphy will prevent subluxation of the femoral head.

66. Twenty blood-soaked surgical sponges were collected during a celiotomy and bowel resection. Approximately how much fluid was lost?

(1) 100 ml
(2) 200 ml
(3) 300 ml
(4) 400 ml
(5) 500 ml

67. Which one of the following is a complication of total splenectomy?

(1) Bacterial infection
(2) Viral infection
(3) Anemia
(4) Hemorrhage
(5) Gastric torsion

68. What statement is true regarding traumatic diaphragmatic hernias?

(1) They are best diagnosed by an oral barium contrast radiographic study.
(2) They are considered a surgical emer-

gency; surgery should be performed within 24 hours.

(3) They are most commonly circumferential.
(4) They do not require repair if the animal is asymptomatic.
(5) They are best repaired via a thoracotomy.

69. Seizures, circling, behavioral changes, and contralateral hemiparesis would suggest a lesion in the:

(1) spinal cord.
(2) peripheral nervous system (PNS).
(3) musculoskeletal system.
(4) forebrain.
(5) brain stem.

70. Surgical treatment for osteochondritis dissecans (OCD) of the humeral head is:

(1) flap resection and subchondral bone curettage.
(2) joint lavage with antibiotic solution.
(3) joint lavage with steroid solution.
(4) application of a spica splint.
(5) external skeletal fixation.

71. What is the best technique for preparing the skin for surgery?

(1) Vigorous scrubbing to eradicate follicular bacteria
(2) Scrubbing with strokes parallel to the incision site
(3) Circumferential scrubbing beginning peripherally
(4) Circular scrubbing beginning at the incision and moving outward

72. Which one of the following conditions is associated with an acute, nonpainful, traumatic unilateral forelimb paresis in a 6-year-old Brittany spaniel?

(1) A spinal tumor
(2) Cervical disk herniation
(3) Brachial plexus avulsion
(4) Cervical diskospondylitis
(5) Atlantoaxial instability

73. Radiographic changes indicative of degenerative joint disease (DJD) include:

(1) subchondral bone sclerosis.
(2) subchondral bone lucency.
(3) periosteal new bone production and lysis.
(4) widening of the joint space.
(5) increased intramedullary bone density.

74. Total parenteral nutrition (TPN) would be indicated in an animal with:

(1) cardiomyopathy.
(2) urinary calculi.
(3) ectopic ureters.
(4) pancreatitis.
(5) a splenic tumor.

75. Pyothorax is best treated by:

(1) thoracic fluid drainage and antibiotics.
(2) thoracic lavage with povidone-iodophore.
(3) exercise to break down pleural adhesions.
(4) environmental humidification.
(5) chemotherapy.

76. Which one of the following statements is true regarding suturing patterns used in the small intestine?

(1) Crushing is useful for preventing leakage.
(2) Inverting is useful for preventing edema.
(3) Eversion is useful for preventing adhesions.
(4) Apposition is preferred for uncomplicated wound closure.
(5) Stapling prevents leakage and abscess formation.

77. What is the critical level of bacterial contamination that will result in wound infection?

(1) 10^1 Bacteria/g of tissue
(2) 10^2 Bacteria/g of tissue
(3) 10^3 Bacteria/g of tissue
(4) 10^4 Bacteria/g of tissue
(5) 10^5 Bacteria/g of tissue

78. What is the surgical approach for a total splenectomy?

(1) Paralumbar fossa incision
(2) Ventral abdominal midline incision
(3) Left per-rectus abdominis incision
(4) Right paracostal incision
(5) Thirteenth rib resection incision

79. Osteochondrosis of which of the following joints holds the worst prognosis for normal function?

(1) Shoulder
(2) Elbow
(3) Stifle
(4) Tarsus
(5) Carpus

80. In cats, the most common malignant renal neoplasia is:

(1) squamous cell carcinoma.
(2) tubular cell carcinoma.

(3) nephroblastoma.
(4) fibrosarcoma
(5) lymphoma.

81. Which one of the following is an advantage of total parenteral nutrition (TPN)?

(1) Catheter-related sepsis can be avoided.
(2) The nutritional requirements of a vomiting animal can be met.
(3) Metabolic complications are minimal.
(4) It is a technically simple procedure.
(5) Secretory immunoglobulin A (S-IgA) production is enhanced.

82. Intraoperative hypotension should be treated by:

(1) increasing the depth of anesthesia.
(2) using a higher vaporizer setting.
(3) inducing hypothermia.
(4) increasing the rate of intravenous crystalloid administration.
(5) administering phenothiazines.

83. Fracture and avulsion of the supraglenoid tubercle of the scapula should be treated with:

(1) tension band fixation using screws or pins and wires.
(2) ostectomy of the fragment.
(3) external skeletal fixation.
(4) Robert-Jones bandaging of the limb.

84. Which one of the following is a frequent complication of acetabular fractures and their surgical repair?

(1) Traumatic myocarditis
(2) Degenerative osteoarthritis
(3) Soft-tissue hematomas
(4) Quadriceps contracture
(5) Compromise of the pelvic canal

85. Resection without replacement of the skull is termed:

(1) craniotomy.
(2) craniectomy.
(3) durotomy.
(4) laminectomy.
(5) fenestration.

86. The most frequently used antibiotic for prevention of surgical infections is:

(1) penicillin.
(2) ampicillin.
(3) cefazolin.

(4) chloramphenicol.
(5) tetracycline.

87. The treatment of choice of splenic hemangiosarcoma in dogs is:

(1) irradiation.
(2) chemotherapy.
(3) transfusion.
(4) splenectomy.
(5) antibiotic therapy.

88. Ceruminous gland adenoma of the vertical ear canal would best be treated by:

(1) bulla osteotomy.
(2) vertical ear canal ablation.
(3) horizontal ear canal ablation.
(4) total ear canal ablation.

89. Which type of cystic calculi is most closely associated with portosystemic shunts?

(1) Magnesium ammonium phosphate
(2) Urate
(3) Cystine
(4) Silicate
(5) Calcium phosphate

90. In dogs, abdominal infections associated with gastrointestinal lesions or surgery are most often caused by:

(1) *Pasteurella.*
(2) *Staphylococcus.*
(3) *Streptococcus.*
(4) *Escherichia coli.*
(5) *Proteus.*

91. Abnormal bone healing characterized by a persistent fracture gap and excessive external callus formation is termed:

(1) secondary bone union.
(2) primary bone union.
(3) inactive union.
(4) malunion.
(5) hypertrophic nonunion.

92. Forelimb trauma in hunting dogs that produces an outward rotation of the limb and adduction of the elbow joint is:

(1) infraspinatus contracture.
(2) quadriceps contracture.
(3) biceps contracture.
(4) triceps contracture.
(5) fibrotic myopathy.

93. Traumatic elbow luxation is usually in a:

(1) medial direction because of contraction of the triceps muscle.
(2) lateral direction because of medial obstruction by the humeral condyle.
(3) cranial direction because of contraction of the biceps muscle.
(4) caudal direction because of contraction of the flexor muscles.
(5) cranial direction because of contraction of the pronator and supinator muscles.

94. Mandibular symphyseal fracture–separation in cats is best treated with:

(1) interfragmentary lag screw compression.
(2) application of cyanoacrylate.
(3) orthopedic wiring techniques.
(4) application of a "mini" bone plate.
(5) external skeletal fixation.

95. The duration of action of thiobarbiturates would be prolonged in a:

(1) greyhound.
(2) Siamese cat.
(3) Manx cat.
(4) German shepherd.
(5) dachschund.

96. Premature closure of the distal ulnar physis as a result of trauma causes:

(1) lateral deviation of the carpus.
(2) medial deviation of the carpus.
(3) internal rotation of the carpus.
(4) caudal displacement of the carpus.

97. Nasopharyngeal polyps in cats require which of the following treatments for excision of the mass and stalk?

(1) Lateral wall resection
(2) Ventral bulla osteotomy
(3) Total ear canal ablation
(4) Vertical wall ablation
(5) Pinna resection

DIRECTIONS: Each of the numbered items or incomplete statements in this section is negatively phrased, as indicated by an italicized word such as *not, least,* or *except.* Select the **one** numbered answer or completion that is **best** in each case.

---

98. All of the following statements regarding primary cleft palate in dogs are true *except:*

(1) primary cleft palate is most common in males and brachycephalic breeds.
(2) it is usually a congenital disease.
(3) it appears more often on the left side.
(4) it occurs most often as a single lesion.
(5) it is a cleft anterior to the incisive foramen.

99. Surgical ligation of a single congenital extrahepatic shunt is performed on a 1-year-old Yorkshire terrier. Portal pressure and central venous pressure before ligation are 6 cm H_2O and 2 cm H_2O, respectively. Which one of the following would *not* be an indicator for partial shunt ligation?

(1) Increased intestinal peristalsis
(2) Increased intestinal vascular pulsation
(3) Pallor and cyanosis of the pancreas
(4) Increased portal pressure to 24 cm H_2O
(5) Increased central venous pressure to 3 cm H_2O

100. All of the following decrease intracranial pressure *except:*

(1) mannitol.
(2) furosemide.
(3) corticosteroids.
(4) hyperventilation.
(5) hypoventilation.

101. All of the following statements regarding peritonitis are true *except:*

(1) the most common cause of contamination is surgical dehiscence.
(2) the most common source of contamination is the gastrointestinal tract.
(3) mortality rates are lower with open abdominal drainage than without drainage.
(4) closure of an open abdomen should be delayed until bacterial cultures are negative.
(5) intracellular bacteria seen on abdominocentesis are diagnostic for septic peritonitis.

102. Cesarean section is recommended for all of the conditions listed *except:*

(1) obstructive dystocia.
(2) primary uterine inertia causing dystocia.
(3) secondary uterine inertia unresponsive to oxytocin.

(4) nonobstructive dystocia without primary uterine inertia.
(5) mechanical dystocia.

103. Considerations when choosing a peripheral nerve biopsy site include all of the following *except:*

(1) the health of the nerve.
(2) its proximity to blood vessels.
(3) the type of nerve.
(4) the function of the nerve.
(5) the speed with which the incision site will heal.

104. Delayed colonic healing and increased morbidity after colonic resection and anastomosis result from all of the following factors *except:*

(1) the rapid rate of collagen lysis compared to synthesis.
(2) the segmental blood supply.
(3) the lack of serosa.
(4) the high bacterial content.
(5) the mechanical stress of solid feces.

105. An 11-year-old toy poodle is diagnosed with grade IV tracheal collapse. All of the following factors seriously affect or would worsen the dog's prognosis *except:*

(1) the animal's age.
(2) the degree of tracheal collapse.
(3) concurrent bronchial collapse.
(4) involvement of the thoracic trachea.
(5) concurrent laryngeal paralysis.

106. Operative management of progressive degenerative joint disease (DJD) can include all of the following *except:*

(1) arthrodesis.
(2) joint replacement.
(3) joint excision.
(4) limb amputation.
(5) joint lavage.

107. All of the following are common components of brachycephalic syndrome *except:*

(1) laryngeal paralysis.
(2) tracheal hypoplasia.
(3) elongated soft palate.
(4) stenotic nares.
(5) everted laryngeal saccules.

108. All of the following are advantages of

hemilaminectomy as compared with dorsal laminectomy *except:*

(1) precise localization of the lesion is unnecessary.
(2) reduced patient morbidity.
(3) ease of adjacent disk fenestration.
(4) preservation of vertebral stability.
(5) less soft tissue dissection.

109. Arterial blood supply to the stomach is provided by all of the following vessels *except* the:

(1) splenic artery.
(2) left gastric artery.
(3) hepatic artery.
(4) gastroduodenal artery.
(5) celiac artery.

110. All of the following statements regarding primary lung neoplasia in dogs are true *except:*

(1) it occurs most commonly in the right caudal lung lobe.
(2) it is most commonly characterized radiographically by a single nodule.
(3) it is common in older, large-breed dogs.
(4) it is diagnosed as fibrosarcoma most often.
(5) median survival time is at least 1 year if there is no metastasis to the tracheobronchial lymph nodes.

111. A critically ill cat requires all of the following amino acids *except:*

(1) arginine.
(2) taurine.
(3) leucine.
(4) lysine.
(5) glutamine.

112. Horner's syndrome is characterized by all of the following *except:*

(1) mydriasis.
(2) miosis.
(3) ptosis.
(4) enophthalmus.
(5) vasodilation.

113. Techniques for correcting pulmonic stenosis include all of the following *except:*

(1) balloon valvuloplasty.
(2) blind valvuloplasty.
(3) patch grafting.

(4) pulmonary arterial banding.
(5) valvulectomy.

114. Perianal fistulae could be treated with all of the following *except:*

(1) surgical excision and open drainage.
(2) chemical cauterization.
(3) cryotherapy.
(4) electrical cauterization.
(5) oral antibiotics and fecal softeners.

DIRECTIONS: Each group of items in this section consists of numbered options followed by a set of numbered items. For each item, select the **one** numbered option that is most closely associated with it. Each numbered option may be selected once, more than once, or not at all.

Questions 115–118
Match each application with the appropriate bandage.

(1) Carpal flexion bandage
(2) Velpeau sling
(3) Plastic or aluminum spoon splint
(4) Robinson limb sling
(5) Ehmer sling

115. Used following scapular joint injury or surgery

116. Used following repairs of hip luxation

117. Used following flexor tendon or forelimb orthopedic injuries

118. Used following repair of fractures or luxations distal to the carpal or tarsal joint

Questions 119–123
Match each pelvic fracture with the appropriate treatment.

(1) Insertion of a pin and bone screw
(2) Application of a bone plate and screws
(3) Femoral head and neck resection
(4) Tension band fixation
(5) Non–weight-bearing sling
(6) Figure-of-eight wiring

119. A highly comminuted, irreparable acetabular fracture

120. An oblique fracture of the ilium

121. A sacroiliac luxation

122. A fracture that affects the cranial two thirds of the acetabulum

123. An avulsion fracture of the ischiatic tubercle

Questions 124–128
Match each clinical presentation with the correct diagnosis.

(1) Diskospondylitis
(2) Cauda equina syndrome
(3) Atlantoaxial instability
(4) Degenerative myelopathy
(5) Caudal cervical spondylomyelopathy (wobbler syndrome)

124. A 10-year-old German shepherd with progressive upper motor neuron (UMN) hindlimb paresis but no evidence of spinal pain or compression

125. An 8-year-old Doberman pinscher with fecal and urinary incontinence, tail atonia, and lower motor neuron (LMN) sciatic paresis

126. A 4-year-old rottweiler with spinal pain; radiographs reveal bone lysis centered around the disk space

127. A 2-year-old Great Dane with cervical ventriflexion and progressive tetraparesis

128. A 3-year-old Yorkshire terrier with high cervical pain and tetraparesis

ANSWERS AND EXPLANATIONS

1. The answer is 2 [*Table 1–2*].
Repair of a closed fracture accompanied by soft tissue trauma would place the patient in classification II. Patients in class III or IV would have open or comminuted fractures with moderate to severe soft tissue trauma. Patients in class I are generally undergoing elective surgery and have no abnormalities on physical examination.

2. The answer is 3 [*Chapter 10 I G 2 f*].
Polydioxanone or polypropylene is recommended for intraoral wound closure because of the strength, durability, and nonreactive nature of these materials. Polydioxanone is absorbable, whereas polypropylene is not.

3. The answer is 3 [*Chapter 4 II B 2, 3*].
Second intention wound healing is characterized by epithelialization and skin contraction. Tissue necrosis, persistent inflammation, edema, dehiscence, and wound drainage delay wound healing. Fibrosis and cartilage formation are unrelated to soft tissue wound healing.

4. The answer is 4 [*Chapter 7 IV C*].
A split-cartilage technique is preferred for tracheal reconstruction, because it allows for anatomic reappositioning of rings and preserves lumen size better than other techniques, such as apposition of intact rings, suturing of the annular ligaments, or overlapping the cartilage rings. In dogs, 20%–60% of the trachea (8 to 23 rings) can be safely removed. Postoperatively, exercise is restricted.

5. The answer is 3 [*Chapter 5 IV B 1 b*].
Benzodiazepines, such as diazepam or oxazepam, are useful appetite stimulants. Morphine and butorphanol are opioids. Phenothiazines (e.g., acetylpromazine) are tranquilizers. Yohimbine is used as a reversal agent for α_2-adrenergic agonists.

6. The answer is 3 [*Chapter 10 V C 5 e (1)*].
Cryosurgery, which is used to treat perianal fistulae and adenomas, relies on tissue necrosis and sloughing. Swelling, malodorous discharge, and anal stenosis (occurring in up to 47% of the animals treated) are complications of cryosurgery. Recurrence is a complication

of deroofing and fulguration. Resection carries a risk of incontinence. Complications of anal sacculectomy include fistulae, incontinence, intraoperative hemorrhage, and postoperative tenesmus and dyschezia.

7. The answer is 2 [*Chapter 8 II B 3*].
Aortic stenosis is associated with subvalvular fibrocartilaginous tissue formation. It typically occurs in large-breed dogs and causes left ventricular hypertrophy. Surgical treatment is usually reserved for those dogs with systolic aortic blood pressure gradients greater than 70 mm Hg. Surgical techniques for correcting aortic stenosis include blind valvuloplasty, open arteriotomy and valvulectomy, and conduit placement. Patch grafting is not performed because animals cannot tolerate the resultant aortic valve insufficiency.

8. The answer is 3 [*Chapter 11 III E 2 e*].
Cholecystectomy is the treatment of choice for acute, chronic, and necrotizing cholecystitis. Necrotizing cholecystitis may lead to gallbladder rupture; therefore, surgical removal of the gland is preventative and less technically demanding than cholecystotomy, cholecystoduodenostomy, or cholecystojejunostomy. Furthermore, handling the gallbladder, which is required by the other surgical options, may lead to rupture and the spread of infection.

9. The answer is 2 [*Chapter 19 III C 3*].
Intermittent open-mouth lower jaw locking is associated with temporomandibular joint dysplasia, which causes joint subluxation. Subluxation of the diseased temporomandibular joint either laterally displaces the contralateral coronoid process or causes it to contact the ventral aspect of the adjacent zygomatic arch. This mechanical interference prevents the mouth from closing; therefore, partial resection of the rostroventral portion of the zygomatic arch prevents open-mouth locking jaw episodes. Corticosteroids would not resolve the anatomic discrepancy responsible for the condition. Arthrodesis would fuse the joint in a locked position and prevent mastication.

10. The answer is 5 [*Table 1–1; Table 1–3*].
Assuming that no severe systemic signs of disease are present, this dog would be classified

in physical status category III. A minimum database for a 6-year-old, class III dog includes a complete blood count (CBC), blood chemistries, and urinalysis.

11. The answer is 3 [*Table 20–1*].
The facial nerve (cranial nerve VII) is a motor nerve to the muscles of facial expression, and plays a role in taste and lacrimation. The spinal accessory nerve (cranial nerve XI) is a motor nerve to the trapezius muscle. The glossopharyngeal nerve (cranial nerve IX) plays a role in swallowing and taste. The trigeminal nerve (cranial nerve V) is sensory to the head and eye and motor to the masticatory muscles. The oculomotor nerve (cranial nerve III) influences ocular movement and pupillary constriction.

12. The answer is 3 [*Chapter 17 II C 1*].
Medially displaced ilial segments can compromise the pelvic canal and are an indication for surgical treatment. A comminuted nondisplaced pubic fracture is usually left *in situ* to heal. Fractures of the ischial body are usually associated with iliac or acetabular fractures; primary repair of these bones usually produces nearly normal realignment of the ischial segments. Therefore, surgical repair of the ischial body is rarely necessary. Mild displacement of the sacroiliac joint does not warrant surgical repair unless gross instability and lameness are present.

13. The answer is 4 [*Chapter 2 I C 2*].
Phenothiazine tranquilizers, such as acepromazine, are extremely popular as preanesthetic agents because they are inexpensive and they exert a predictable effect. Atropine and glycopyrrolate are anticholinergics that promote bronchodilation and mydriasis and counteract parasympathetically induced bradycardia. Flunixin meglumine is a potent prostaglandin inhibitor used to treat pain and inflammation associated with musculoskeletal disease. Atipamezole is used as a reversal agent for medetomidine.

14. The answer is 2 [*Table 3–4*].
Staphylococcus organisms are most often associated with osteomyelitis in dogs. *Pasteurella* is associated with soft tissue infection in cats. *Escherichia coli* is often associated with traumatic wounds or incisions near the gastrointestinal tract. *Streptococcus* infections usually involve the urogenital tract or oral cavity. *Proteus* is associated with burns and urogenital tract infections.

15. The answer is 5 [*Chapter 15 IV C 1 b*].
Acute splenic torsion requires immediate intravenous fluid resuscitation, because sequestration of blood in the spleen leads to hypovolemia. Splenic torsion is an anatomical (mechanical) problem that is not associated with infection; therefore, intravenous administration of antibiotics would not be effective. Performing an upper gastrointestinal study to arrive at a diagnosis could lead to the loss of the animal because splenic torsion, an acute, life-threatening condition in most cases, requires immediate intervention. Treatment entails direct manipulation of the spleen; rolling the animal would be inefficient and ineffective. A waxing and waning course is typical of chronic, not acute, splenic torsion, which occurs in approximately 25% of cases.

16. The answer is 1 [*Chapter 11 III D 1*].
Trauma causes 98% of bile duct ruptures; the remainder are caused by cholelithiasis. Bile stones (choledocholiths) cause only 2% of bile duct ruptures. Choleliths (gallstones) cause the majority of gallbladder ruptures. Necrotizing cholecystitis involves necrosis and rupture of the gallbladder, not the bile duct. Neoplasia may cause bile duct obstruction, but not rupture.

17. The answer is 3 [*Chapter 22 I A 4*].
Fenestration prevents future disk herniations if adequate amounts of the nucleus pulposus are removed. Spinal cord decompression or evaluation requires decompressive surgeries such as hemilaminectomy or dorsal laminectomy. Spinal neoplasia requires decompressive surgery.

18. The answer is 3 [*Chapter 5 III C–D*].
In stressed patients, medium-chain triglycerides are digested and absorbed easily, independently of pancreatic or biliary enzyme or salt digestion. Critically ill animals have an increased need for fat. Increasing the fat content of the diet increases the caloric density of the diet. Dietary fiber helps normalize intestinal motility and improves the bacterial colonization of the colon; dietary levels should not be reduced for the critically ill patient.

19. The answer is 1 [*Chapter 14 III B 2 b (2)*].
The facial nerve is located just ventral to the horizontal portion of the external ear canal and acoustic meatus. Damage to the facial nerve can lead to postoperative facial paralysis or paresis.

20. The answer is 2 [*Chapter 9 V C 1 a*].
Lymphosarcoma is the most common mediastinal mass in cats (and dogs). Thymoma is more common in dogs than cats. Squamous cell carcinoma and mediastinal abscesses are uncommon causes of mediastinal masses in cats. Pneumomediastinum does not cause a mediastinal mass per se, but it will cause distention of the mediastinum. It is an uncommon condition.

21. The answer is 2 [*Chapter 18 IV D 1 b*].
A grade II medial patellar luxation is characterized by infrequent lameness and manual or spontaneous reduction of the dislocation. These animals do not have severe clinical signs or bone deformations. Grade I luxations rarely occur and do not require manual reduction. Grade III luxations occur frequently and require manual reduction. Grade IV luxations cause persistent lameness and the patella cannot be relocated in the trochlear groove. Grade V luxations do not exist.

22. The answer is 3 [*Chapter 10 II B 2 b (1) (a)*].
The submucosa is the major holding layer for sutures in the esophagus and other gastrointestinal organs.

23. The answer is 2 [*Chapter 3 II B 2 b; Table 3–2*].
Povidone-iodine and chlorhexidine are the most efficacious and frequently used antiseptic agents. Povidone-iodine and chlorhexidine kill 99% of accessible bacteria within 30 seconds of application; they have varying effectiveness against spores, viruses, protozoa, and fungi. When used alone, the aliphatic alcohols are slightly less effective than povidone-iodine and chlorhexidine, but combinations with either increase the efficacy of alcohol. Hexachlorophene and benzalkonium chloride are of limited use as skin antiseptics; hexachlorophene is not recommended for use as a preoperative skin antiseptic and benzalkonium chloride is recommended for the cleaning of nonsterile areas only.

24. The answer is 1 [*Chapter 13 I B 1 d (1); II B 2 d*].
Mitotane is used for selective destruction of the adrenal cortex as a treatment for hyperadrenocorticism to reduce excessive glucocorticoid synthesis. Methimazole, carbimazole, and radioactive iodine block thyroid hormone synthesis. Propranolol blocks the effect of excessive thyroid hormones on the heart.

25. The answer is 4 [*Chapter 22 II E 3 a*].
Spinal trauma occurs most frequently where stable and mobile spinal segments meet (e.g., the cervicothoracic or thoracolumbar regions). Spinal trauma produces lesions of variable severity and reversibility. Immediate surgical intervention is not always warranted.

26. The answer is 4 [*Chapter 9 III C 1 c (1)*].
Chronic bacterial rhinitis that is unresponsive to antibiotic therapy often requires rhinotomy and turbinectomy. Chronic fungal rhinitis, such as that caused by *Aspergillus* or *Cryptococcus,* is treated with systemic or topical antifungals. Rhinotomy is only indicated for these conditions when a diagnosis is unattainable or it is necessary to establish drainage; turbinectomy is not indicated. Nasal adenocarcinoma is most effectively treated with radiation; occasionally surgical debulking is necessary. Oronasal fistulae are corrected by creating a gingival/buccal mucosal flap or a mucoperiosteal flap, or both.

27. The answer is 1 [*Chapter 16 V B 6*].
Aseptic necrosis of the femoral head (Legg-Calvé-Perthes disease) causes bone destruction and subsequent pain and lameness in young small dog breeds. Infection or neoplasia would not be common in a young, healthy dog, and hip dysplasia occurs more frequently in large, rapidly growing dogs. Sciatic neurapraxia is associated with pelvic or femoral fractures or improper pinning of a femoral fracture.

28. The answer is 1 [*Chapter 2 II A 5*].
Opioids produce respiratory depression; hence, preoxygenation is recommended prior to opioid induction. Large doses of opioids produce excitement and delirium in cats. Opioids may not be the agent of choice in young, healthy dogs because large doses are required to facilitate endotracheal intubation, and even then, intubation may not be successful. No preanesthetic or anesthetic agent should be administered after a meal if at all possible, because of the risk of regurgitation and aspiration pneumonia.

29. The answer is 2 [*Chapter 12 IV B 3 e (2) (a) (i)*].
Colposuspension is used to increase urethral pressure by suturing the uterine stump to the abdominal wall and encircling the bladder neck to increase urethral pressure and improve incontinence. In vaginopexy, the vagina

is sutured to the abdominal wall. In urethroplasty, the urethra is encircled by fascial
slings. Cystoplasty and cystic relocation involve the bladder, but not the uterus.

30. The answer is 2 [*Chapter 2 III A 1; Table 3–3*].
Prophylactic antibiotics are usually given intravenously prior to prolonged procedures (i.e.,
those lasting longer than 2 hours). Dirty
wounds are already infected with bacteria;
therefore, the antibiotics used to treat them
would be "therapeutic," not "prophylactic."
There is no evidence that continuing antibiotic therapy for extended periods following
surgery decreases the incidence of wound infection. Elective procedures do not routinely
involve antibiotic prophylaxis; oral dosing for
2 days prior may produce resistant strains or
inconsistent tissue levels by the time of surgery. Topical delivery does not produce adequate serum and tissue levels at the time of expected contamination.

31. The answer is 2 [*Chapter 10 V C 4*].
Anal sacculitis that is unresponsive to medical
therapy requires resection (i.e., sacculectomy)
and drainage of diseased, infected tissues. Rectal amputation and anastomosis is indicated
for necrotic, friable, severely edematous pro-
lapses. Tail amputation may be indicated for
perianal fistulae. Colopexy is indicated for
chronic, recurrent rectal prolapse.

32. The answer is 3 [*Table 1–2*].
A life-threating condition such as upper airway obstruction resulting from postoperative
edema of the larynx would place the patient
in category IV ("E" denotes that the surgery
was performed as an emergency). Classifications II and III indicate a mild to moderate systemic disturbance. Classification V is reserved
for moribund or comatose patients.

33. The answer is 1 [*Chapter 21 III D 1 a*].
Meningiomas are the most common primary
brain tumors in small animals. Gliomas,
which include astrocytomas, tend to occur in
brachycephalic dogs. Choroid plexus tumors
occur within or in close proximity to the ventricular system and are less common than meningiomas and gliomas. Lymphosarcoma may
metastasize to the brain.

34. The answer is 1 [*Chapter 17 II C 1 a, E 3*].
The acetabulum plays an important role in

pelvic limb weight-bearing. The pubis is the
site of attachment for abdominal muscles; rupture of the prepubic tendon can lead to caudal abdominal herniation. The coccygeal vertebrae provide tail support. A diaphragmatic
hernia may affect cardiopulmonary and gastrointestinal functions.

35. The answer is 1 [*Chapter 10 I G 2 f*].
A bilateral rostral mandibulectomy is indicated for resection of tumors involving the
mandibular symphysis.

36. The answer is 5 [*Chapter 14 III B–C*].
Chronic bacterial otitis externa and media require resection of external canal tissues (ablation) and curettage and drainage of the bulla.

37. The answer is 4 [*Chapter 10 II B 2 b*].
A double-layer simple interrupted appositional closure is preferred for end-to-end anastomosis of the esophagus. This type of closure
facilitates healing, tissue approximation, and
wound strength. Inversion and eversion techniques are rarely used for esophageal closure.

38. The answer is 4 [*Chapter 16 V B 3*].
Osteochondrosis of the humeral head is a
common cause of shoulder joint lameness in
large, rapidly growing dogs. Synovial cell sarcoma and osteosarcoma more frequently
occur in older, mature dogs. Bicipital tenosynovitis occurs in mature dogs, often as a se-
quel to untreated osteochondritis dissecans
(OCD). Medial luxation of the shoulder occurs as a congenital lesion in small, toy
breeds.

39. The answer is 1 [*Chapter 8 II B 1*].
Patent ductus arteriosus (PDA) is the most
common congenital cardiac defect in dogs.
Pulmonic stenosis is the second most common, aortic stenosis the third, and persistent
right aortic arch (PRAA) the fourth most common. Ventricular septal defect is the most
common congenital cardiac defect in cats.

40. The answer is 2 [*Chapter 2 II B 4 c; Table 2–4*].
Halothane produces a more rapid induction
and recovery than methoxyflurane because of
its low solubility. The minimum alveolar concentration (MAC) is an indicator of potency;
halothane, with a MAC of 0.87, is less potent
than methoxyflurane, with a MAC of 0.23.
Methoxyflurane, not halothane, may provide
analgesia into the recovery period. Halothane,

a potent cerebral vasodilator, is contraindicated for use in animals with intracranial pathology. Halothane, like all inhalation anesthetics, sensitizes the myocardium to some degree.

41. The answer is 4 [*Chapter 23 II B 1 b*].
Quadriceps contracture produces hindlimb extension as a result of fibrous adhesions among the femur, periosteum, and quadriceps muscles following trauma or surgery. Infraspinatus contracture is seen in hunting dogs and is characterized by outward rotation of the limb and adduction of the elbow joint. Myositis ossificans is a non-neoplastic form of heterotopic ossification that affects fibrous connective tissue and skeletal muscle, frequently near the hip joint. Fibrotic myopathy most frequently affects the semitendinosus muscles. Leptospirosis causes muscle pain in cats.

42. The answer is 5 [*Chapter 12 V D 1*].
Ovariohysterectomy performed before the first estrus has the maximum effect of reducing mammary gland neoplasia development. This protective effect is lost after subsequent estrous cycles. Tumor development is, thus, hormone (estrogen) dependent.

43. The answer is 1 [*Chapter 2 II B 4 d*].
Isoflurane is the most potent and inert inhalation anesthetic. It is exhaled unchanged; therefore it does not undergo hepatic metabolism. In addition, isoflurane maintains hepatic blood flow better than halothane or methoxyflurane. Halothane, methoxyflurane, ketamine, and barbiturates, such as thiamylal, all require hepatic metabolism and therefore would be inappropriate for this animal.

44. The answer is 1 [*Chapter 20 I A 2 b*].
The cerebellum controls the rate, range, and force of movement. Therefore, lesions in this area can produce clinical signs of ataxia, dysmetria, tremors, and pupillary changes. Lesions of the supratentorial structures (e.g., the cerebrum) are characterized by normal pupillary light reflex activity and normal cranial nerve VII function accompanied by contralateral loss of the menace response, hemiparesis, seizures, behavioral abnormalities, circling, head-turning, and head-pressing. Brain stem lesions, which include those of the mesencephalon, are most often manifested as disturbances of the functions of cranial nerves III–XII. Spinal cord lesions commonly produce paresis or plegia.

45. The answer is 4 [*Chapter 17 I A 1; II D 1–2*].
Because of the box-like structure of the pelvis, fractures rarely affect only one bone in the pelvic girdle, and stabilization of the cranial segments usually brings the other fragments into alignment. Therefore, reduction and stabilization of ilial fractures help reduce displaced ischiatic fractures. Pelvic fractures generally heal quickly because the area is well vascularized and supported, and cancellous bone is abundant. Medially displaced fractures of the ilium or acetabulum, not the ischiatic tubercle, can compromise the pelvic canal. Implants are not routinely removed after the bone heals because the low incidence of associated problems usually does not warrant a second invasive surgery. Most pelvic fractures are closed because of the extensive muscular coverage of the area.

46. The answer is 4 [*Chapter 18 IV D 1 d (2)*].
Treatment appropriate for a lateral luxation of the patella includes lateral relief incisions and medial tightening or imbrication to realign the patella. External immobilization with a cast is not done following treatment for patellar luxation. Lateral imbricating sutures and tibial tuberosity transposition are used for medial patellar luxation.

47. The answer is 1 [*Chapter 21 II B 2*].
Ventriculoperitoneal shunting is used to treat hydrocephalus. Ventriculoperitoneal shunting transfers excess cerebrospinal fluid (CSF) to the abdominal cavity, where it is absorbed. Callosotomy (i.e., longitudinal division of the corpus callosum) may eliminate recalcitrant seizures by removing a potential conduit for seizure generation. Transsphenoidal pituitary removal is used to treat pituitary tumors. Craniotomy only involves removal of a portion of the skull and would not be effective for treating hydrocephalus. Hemispherectomy involves removal of one cerebral hemisphere.

48. The answer is 3 [*Chapter 5 III A 3; Table 5–2*].
The illness energy requirement (IER) is calculated by multiplying a factor that represents the severity of the disease by the resting energy requirement (RER). These factors range from 1.25–2; for cancer patients, the RER is usually multiplied by a factor ranging from 1.35–1.5.

49. The answer is 4 [*Chapter 16 V A 7 b*]. A bone plate and screws would provide the greatest stability and quickest return to function in repair of a femoral fracture. The percutaneous intermuscular insertions required by external fixators may limit postoperative patient mobility. An external splint or intramedullary pin cannot stabilize these bone fragments because of the distractive forces associated with the limb muscles. Bone screws and wires do not provide adequate fracture stability; they are ancillary implants used in combination with plates or pins.

50. The answer is 3 [*Chapter 8 III A 4 b*]. Pericardiectomy is useful to reduce production of pericardial effusion and cardiac tamponade. Pericardiocentesis is not effective for chronic recurrent pericardial effusion because recurrence of the effusion is likely. Pericardiotomy is a technique that only incises the pericardium; this is likely to close or to adhere to the myocardium, and hence is ineffective. Balloon valvuloplasty and vagotomy are techniques that are not related to the pericardium.

51. The answer is 3 [*Chapter 13 I B 1 e (2)*]. A transsphenoidal hypophysectomy is used to remove the pituitary in pituitary-dependent hyperadrenocorticism. An oral approach is used to incise the soft palate and sphenoid bone. The aim is to remove the source of excessive adrenocorticotropic hormone (ACTH) production. Abdominal surgery is used for gastrinomas, insulinomas, and adrenal carcinomas. Parathyroid tumors are treated by surgical excision of the glands from the neck.

52. The answer is 5 [*Chapter 10 I G 2 f*]. Wound dehiscence occurs frequently following mandibular or maxillary surgery. Excessive tension, improper suture placement, use of electrocautery, concurrent use of radiation and chemotherapy, tumor location, and tumor recurrence are all contributing factors. Dehiscence is seen in 60% of animals undergoing preoperative radiation, 42% undergoing postoperative radiation, and 100% undergoing chemotherapy and radiation therapy. Eighty percent of dehiscences were associated with caudal maxillectomies. Fifty percent of dehiscences were associated with local tumor recurrence.

53. The answer is 1 [*Chapter 14 III A 2 c*]. Squamous cell carcinoma is associated with solar dermatitis in white cats. Lymphosarcoma

and chondrosarcoma are tumors of the mediastinum and rib cage, respectively.

54. The answer is 1 [*Chapter 15 III A 1*]. Percutaneous biopsy of a splenic abscess may lead to rupture, peritonitis, and sepsis. Ultrasonographic-guided fine needle aspiration of an enlarged spleen is technically easy and reduces the risk of morbidity and mortality. Biopsy, via an incision or a punch, is relatively free of postoperative complications. Partial splenectomy, because it is an open procedure, is more direct and associated with less patient morbidity.

55. The answer is 2 [*Chapter 13 II B 2 e (1)*]. Damage to parathyroid tissue affects production of parathyroid hormone (PTH) leading to a fall in plasma calcium and a rise in phosphate levels. In these patients, calcium and vitamin D supplementation is necessary until parathyroid gland function returns. Potassium and sodium levels are not affected unless underlying functional kidney disease is also present.

56. The answer is 4 [*Chapter 14 III A 1*]. Surgical drainage evacuates an aural hematoma (i.e., the excessive collection of blood within fractured auricular cartilage) and prevents recurrence. Bulla osteotomy is indicated for otitis media resulting from chronic inflammatory, infectious, or neoplastic lesions.

57. The answer is 1 [*Chapter 12 VI C 1 d (2)*]. Benign prostatic hyperplasia can be treated by castration to reduce the effects of testosterone. Estrogen therapy can cause metaplasia and prostatic enlargement. Marsupialization, drainage, and prostatectomy are not necessary because castration is effective and simpler to perform.

58. The answer is 5 [*Chapter 2 II A 4*]. Cyclohexylamines, such as ketamine, are contraindicated in animals with renal disease because an inability to excrete active metabolites of the drug prolongs recovery from anesthesia. Acepromazine, thiamylal, halothane, and isoflurane can be used safely because they are excreted via the lungs or hepatic metabolism.

59. The answer is 3 [*Chapter 20 II C 2 a (2)*]. Intramedullary lesions produce swelling and abaxial deviation of contrast medium during myelography in both the dorsoventral and lateral views. A normal myelogram rarely shows the subarachnoid spaces as two parallel contrast lines. Diskospondylitis is an extradural vertebral disease centered around the disk space. Dural neoplasia would most often produce an intradural, extramedullary myelographic pattern. Osteosarcoma of a vertebrae would result in an extradural myelographic pattern.

60. The answer is 2 [*Chapter 4 II C*].
Secondary wound closure, or third intention wound healing, is performed following formation of granulation tissue at least 5–6 days after wounding. Healing is not delayed in these wounds. Rather, it is enhanced because the wound is in the reparative phase of wound healing—the inflammatory phase has already occurred. Because of the open and granulating nature of these wounds, bacterial infection is reduced, dead space or fluid accumulation does not develop, and, therefore, wound drainage is not required.

61. The answer is 2 [*Chapter 8 IV C 1 c (2)*].
Polypropylene is a useful vascular suture material because it is nonabsorbable, inert, monofilament, and has reduced thrombogenic potential compared to other sutures. Chromic catgut, polydioxanone, polyglactin 910, and polyglycolic acid are all absorbable suture materials and, therefore, are unsuitable. Chromic catgut is absorbed quickly and induces an inflammatory reaction. Polyglactin 910 is a multifilament suture with considerable tissue drag; hence it could be damaging to the endothelium.

62. The answer is 3 [*Chapter 9 III C*].
A median sternotomy provides access to the entire thoracic cavity. Rib resection and rib pivot thoracotomy provide greater access to the thoracic cavity than an intercostal (lateral) thoracotomy, but they provide less exposure than a median sternotomy.

63. The answer is 3 [*Chapter 23 I A 1 a*].
Neurotmesis is complete severance of the nerve and disruption of all axons. Neurapraxia is a functional, rather than an anatomical, disruption of the nerve function. In axonotmesis, axons within the nerve are severed, but the nerve itself remains intact. Myelomalacia is softening and necrosis of the spinal cord parenchyma. Myotonia is increased muscular irritability and contractility.

64. The answer is 4 [*Chapter 17 I B; II E 5 b*].
Cranioventral displacement of pubic fractures associated with prepubic tendon rupture can lead to caudal abdominal visceral herniation. Because the pelvic girdle is well protected by musculature, it is safe to assume that an injury leading to fracture of these bones is fairly substantial. In fact, most pelvic fractures involve vehicular trauma or significant falls, and concurrent soft tissue injuries (e.g., diaphragmatic hernia, traumatic myocarditis) are common. Because the sciatic nerve courses medially and caudally to the acetabulum, pelvic fractures are frequently associated with sciatic neurapraxia, which usually resolves on its own within 2–3 weeks of the injury. Degenerative osteoarthritis is a common sequela to acetabular fractures that are inadequately stabilized.

65. The answer is 2 [*Chapter 18 IV B 1 e*].
Triple pelvic osteotomy to rotate the acetabulum is performed as a treatment for hip dysplasia in young dogs that have no radiographic or palpable evidence of degenerative joint disease. Conservative therapy, including medication and weight and exercise restrictions, may be useful in mildly affected or geriatric animals. Femoral head and neck excision produces a false joint, or pseudarthrosis, to eliminate discomfort from the disease. Total hip replacement is reserved for mature animals with lameness and pain not controlled by other treatments. Capsulorrhaphy, or tightening of the joint capsule, may be effective for acute traumatic luxations of normal hips. The shallow acetabula that are characteristic of hip dysplasia would not be able to support the femoral head no matter how tightly the joint capsule is closed.

66. The answer is 2 [*Chapter 1 IV A 1 a (1) (c)*].
Blood-soaked surgical sponges contain approximately 10 ml of fluid; therefore, this animal lost approximately 200 ml of fluid during the surgical procedure.

67. The answer is 4 [*Chapter 15 III D*].
Hemorrhage resulting from inadequate ligation of splenic vessels or tissue may occur following splenic surgery. Production of red blood cells and white blood cells by the bone marrow is unaffected by splenectomy; therefore, bacterial or viral infection and anemia are not complications. Because splenectomy does not involve manipulation of the stom-

ach, gastric torsion is an unlikely complication. However, gastric torsion is sometimes an indication for splenectomy.

68. The answer is 3 [*Chapter 9 V F 1 b, c*]. Traumatic diaphragmatic hernias are most commonly associated with circumferential tears in the diaphragm, and less commonly associated with radial tears. Oral barium studies are associated with a high rate of false-negative results; positive- or negative-contrast peritoneography or ultrasound is a more reliable method of diagnosis. Traumatic diaphragmatic hernias are considered a surgical emergency only when the stomach is herniated and distended with gas, or in the presence of bowel incarceration, obstruction, or rupture, or ongoing hemorrhage. In nonemergency situations, surgery should be delayed until the animal has been stabilized. Herniorrhaphy is usually performed via a midline celiotomy; the incision may be extended through the xiphoid and sternum if necessary.

69. The answer is 4 [*Chapter 20 I A 1 b*]. Lesions of the supratentorial (forebrain) structures (i.e., the cerebrum, basal nuclei, diencephalon, and rostral mesencephalon) produce seizures, circling, hemiparesis, and behavioral changes. These structures are associated with conscious functions, such as movement and sensation.

70. The answer is 1 [*Chapter 16 V B 3 d*]. Surgical treatment for osteochondritis dissecans (OCD) of the humeral head is cartilage flap resection and subchondral bone curettage to stimulate fibrocartilage filling of the defect. Joint lavage with antibiotics or steroids would not have any effect on the cartilage flap or underlying bone. An external fixator or spica splint is unnecessary; joint immobilization does not improve healing.

71. The answer is 4 [*Chapter 2 II B 2 c*]. Preoperative scrubbing should be gentle, using circular strokes directed away from the incision site. Vigorous scrubbing brings follicular bacteria to the surface, where they may infect abrasions introduced by the scrubbing. Scrubbing should always be directed away from the incision site, toward the peripheral margins.

72. The answer is 3 [*Chapter 23 I C 1 a*]. A brachial plexus avulsion injury produces a unilateral, nonprogressive, nonpainful fore-

limb paresis or plegia. A tumor in the cervicothoracic region of the spinal cord can produce bilateral signs and would not be associated with an acute traumatic injury. Cervical diskospondylitis would produce neck pain and bilateral lesions and would not be associated with trauma. Atlantoaxial instability produces severe bilateral forelimb signs in young toy breeds following ventriflexion of the neck.

73. The answer is 1 [*Chapter 18 II A 3 b*]. Degenerative joint disease (DJD) is characterized radiographically by subchondral bone sclerosis, narrowing of the joint space, and periarticular osteophyte formation. Subchondral bone lucency may be indicative of avascularity, cysts, or neoplasia. Periosteal bone production and lysis are characteristic of neoplasia or infection. Increased intramedullary bone density may result from inflammation or sepsis.

74. The answer is 4 [*Chapter 5 V A 2 b*]. Pancreatitis would be an indication for total parenteral nutrition. By infusing nutrients intravenously, it is possible to avoid adverse stimulation of pancreatic digestive enzymes.

75. The answer is 1 [*Chapter 9 V B 4*]. Pyothorax should be treated initially with thoracic fluid drainage and appropriate antimicrobial therapies. Surgical exploration and possible lobectomy are indicated for chronic, recurrent, or unresponsive pyothorax. The addition of antimicrobial agents, such as povidone-iodophore, to lavage solution is not recommended. Pleural adhesions are a complication of chylothorax; exercise would likely exacerbate symptoms of significant respiratory compromise. Environmental humidification is not indicated because viscous airway secretions are not a problem. Chemotherapy is not indicated because pyothorax is not a neoplastic disease.

76. The answer is 4 [*Chapter 10 IV B 1 c (1) (a)*]. An appositional suture pattern is preferred over crushing, inverting, and everting techniques to promote intestinal healing. Crushing suture patterns and mucosal eversion techniques tend to cause necrosis and inflammation, delaying healing. Eversion also promotes adhesion formation. Inversion decreases the intestinal lumen diameter and compromises the blood supply, resulting in edema, necrosis, and delayed mucosal healing. Early postoperative complications of stapling include leakage and abscess formation.

77. The answer is 5 [*Chapter 3 I A 1*].
Wound infection results when bacterial contamination reaches the critical level of 10^5 bacteria/g of tissue. When normal body defenses are inhibited (e.g., in the presence of necrotic tissue or foreign material), the threshold for infection is lower.

78. The answer is 2 [*Chapter 15 III C*].
A ventral midline approach to the abdomen provides access to the spleen. A paralumbar fossa, left per-rectus abdominis, right paracostal, or thirteenth rib resection approach does not provide direct access to the spleen.

79. The answer is 4 [*Chapter 18 IV A 4*].
Osteochondrosis of the tarsus has the worst prognosis because of joint instability resulting from the lesion and from surgery. Because of the location of the lesion on the medial or lateral trochlear ridges of the talus, the tarsal joint may become unstable. Surgical excision of the cartilage flap also creates instability. This condition has not been described in the carpus.

80. The answer is 5 [*Chapter 12 I C 3 a (2)*].
Lymphoma is the most common renal malignancy. Squamous cell carcinomas, nephroblastoma, and fibrosarcomas occur less frequently than lymphoma in cats. In dogs, tubular cell carcinoma is the most frequent malignancy. Primary renal tumors are uncommon in both dogs and cats.

81. The answer is 2 [*Chapter 5 V A 3–4*].
Total parenteral nutrition (TPN) can be delivered to vomiting animals or animals with diarrhea. Sepsis, metabolic disturbances, and impaired secretory immunoglobulin A (S-IgA) production are complications associated with TPN. In general, enteric feeding is preferable to TPN whenever circumstances permit it. Technical complications such as catheter occlusion, displacement, or disconnection are common.

82. The answer is 4 [*Chapter 2 II C 1 b*].
Intraoperative hypotension requires fluid resuscitation with intravenous crystalloid administration. A higher vaporizer setting would increase the depth of anesthesia, which is undesirable in this situation. Hypothermia is a common cause of prolonged recovery from

anesthesia; inducing hypothermia is not recommended. Phenothiazines decrease blood pressure and would not be indicated.

83. The answer is 1 [*Chapter 16 V A 2 c (3)*].
Acromion and supraglenoid tubercle fractures of the scapula are best stabilized using a tension band technique. Stabilization is necessary to counteract the pull of the biceps brachii muscle. Ostectomy would remove the point of insertion of the shoulder muscles. External fixation is too cumbersome and would not adequately stabilize the bone fragment. Bandaging would not permit secure fixation of the distracted bone segment.

84. The answer is 2 [*Chapter 17 II E 3 a (1)*].
Degenerative osteoarthritis can occur secondary to injury and inadequate stabilization or reconstruction of acetabular fractures. Degenerative osteoarthritis results from trauma to the cartilage from the initial injury or during surgical repair, or postoperative trauma resulting from incongruency of the articular surface.

85. The answer is 2 [*Chapter 21 II B 1*].
During craniectomy, a portion of the skull is removed but not replaced following surgery. Craniectomy allows room for the brain to swell, which often occurs postoperatively. During craniotomy, the resected portion of the skull is replaced. Durotomy involves incision of the dura, in either the intracranial area or spinal cord. Laminectomy and fenestration are spinal surgeries.

86. The answer is 3 [*Chapter 3 II B*].
Cephalosporins such as cefazolin are used most frequently for prevention of surgical wound infection because of their bactericidal nature and spectrum of activity. Cefazolin has 99% in vitro activity against *Staphylococcus* and 90% activity against *Escherichia coli,* the most frequently cultured bacteria from wounds in small animal surgical patients.

87. The answer is 4 [*Chapter 15 IV A 2 a–b*].
Hemangiosarcoma is best treated by total splenectomy. Irradiation, chemotherapy, transfusion, or antibiotic therapy would have no effect.

88. The answer is 2 [*Chapter 14 III B 1 b*].
Vertical canal ablation permits complete removal of the vertical canal, including masses (e.g., ceruminous gland adenoma). Total canal ablation is indicated for irreversible hy-

perplastic lesions, chronic bacterial infections, or neoplastic lesions (e.g., carcinomas, sarcomas) that cause ear canal occlusion and pain. Bulla osteotomy is indicated for chronic otitis media.

89. The answer is 2 [*Chapter 12 III C 1 a (2) (d)*].
Urate stones in the bladder are associated with portosystemic shunts. Inadequate liver function associated with portosystemic shunt leads to high blood levels of uric acid and ammonia, which can cause urate calculi formation. Magnesium phosphate calculi (struvite) can be associated with bacterial infections. Cystine stones result from an inability to absorb cystine in the proximal tubules of the kidney. Silica uroliths are associated with diets high in corn gluten or soybean hulls. Calcium phosphate crystals are associated with excessive calcium in the urine.

90. The answer is 4 [*Table 3–4*].
Escherichia coli is most frequently associated with gastrointestinal or abdominal surgical infections. *Pasteurella* is associated with soft tissue infections in cats. *Staphylococcus* is associated with bone infections. *Streptococcus* and *Proteus* are associated with urogenital infections.

91. The answer is 5 [*Chapter 16 III A, B, C 3 a*].
Hypertrophic nonunion is characterized by inadequate fracture healing with peripheral callus formation in an attempt to bridge unstable fragments. Nonunion may be inactive; inactive nonunions show no callus formation and sclerosis of the bone ends. Primary bone union is characterized by direct formation of bone under conditions of rigid stability; the gap between the fractured ends is minimal. Secondary bone union is associated with gaps and motion at the fracture site, but the callus formed during the repair phase is eventually replaced by bone. Malunion is nonanatomic fracture healing that causes functional or cosmetic defects.

92. The answer is 1 [*Chapter 23 II B 1 a*].
Infraspinatus contracture is a traumatic injury to the shoulder joint that causes external rotation and adduction of the limb. Hunting dogs are most often affected. Quadriceps contracture is a serious complication of poor surgical repair of femoral fractures in young dogs. Traumatic contractures of the biceps

and triceps muscles have not been routinely described and would not cause external rotation and adduction of the limb. Fibrotic myopathy affects the hind limbs.

93. The answer is 2 [*Chapter 18 V C 2*].
Traumatic elbow luxation is usually in a lateral direction. Obstruction by the large medial aspect of the humeral condyle prevents medial luxation. Muscular contractions do not cause bone displacement because of the natural stability of the joint associated with humeroulnar articulation and regional tendons and ligaments.

94. The answer is 3 [*Chapter 19 III A 3 a (1)*].
Orthopedic wiring techniques (e.g., circumferential wiring) are useful for stabilizing mandibular symphyseal fracture–separations in cats. Interfragmentary lag screw compression may be indicated for large animals or in the presence of excessive tissue loss. Application of cyanoacrylate, a "mini" bone plate, or an external skeletal fixation device would be excessive for this type of fracture.

95. The answer is 1 [*Chapter 2 II A 1 a (3) (c)*].
The duration of action of thiobarbiturates in sight hounds, such as greyhounds, is longer than in mixed or other breeds of dogs. The long duration of action contributes to the prolonged and rough recovery from thiobarbiturate-induced anesthesia that is common in sight hound breeds. For this reason, methohexital, an oxybarbiturate, is often used as an alternative induction agent.

96. The answer is 1 [*Chapter 16 V A 4 c*].
Premature closure of the distal ulnar physis causes carpus valgus (i.e., lateral deviation of the carpus due to continued radial growth). Medial deviation and internal rotation of the carpus would be caused by closed distal radial physes and continued growth of the distal ulnar physis. Caudal displacement of the carpus may occur with traumatic carpal injuries, not growth deformities.

97. The answer is 2 [*Chapter 14 III C 1 b*].
A ventral bulla osteotomy permits resection of the epithelial base of the polyp in the bulla and nasopharyngeal mass and stalk extraction.

98. The answer is 4 [*Chapter 7 III E 1*].
Primary cleft palate (i.e., a cleft anterior to the incisive foramen) is most likely to be seen in

combination with a cleft of the secondary palate, rather than as an isolated lesion. Primary cleft palate is a congenital condition; male and brachycephalic dogs are affected most often. The left side appears to be affected more often than the right.

99. The answer is 5 [Chapter 11 III G 5 b]. Partial ligation of shunts is indicated when systemic signs of portal hypertension, such as increased peristalsis, visceral cyanosis, and increased intestinal vascular pulsation, are present. Portal pressure should not exceed a maximum of 9–10 cm H_2O over baseline (preligation) pressure. In animals with poorly developed intrahepatic portal vasculature, the central venous pressure decreases upon complete shunt ligation because of decreased cardiac return.

100. The answer is 5 [Chapter 21 I B 1]. Hypoventilation increases the arterial carbon dioxide partial pressure, causing cerebral vasodilation and increasing cerebral blood flow. Conversely, hyperventilation reduces the arterial carbon dioxide partial pressure, causing cerebral vasoconstriction, reducing cerebral blood flow, and lowering the intracranial pressure. Diuretic therapy with mannitol and furosemide decreases brain edema, lowering intracranial pressure. Corticosteroids may lower intracranial pressure by decreasing cerebral edema. In addition, corticosteroids have anti-inflammatory properties. Attempts must be made to lower intracranial pressure prior to surgery to minimize the incidence of brain trauma during surgery.

101. The answer is 4 [Chapter 10 IV C 8]. Most open abdomens have positive bacterial cultures at the time of closure. Closure is performed when the quantity of fluid decreases, the quality of fluid changes to sanguineous or serosanguineous, and the cells become less toxic. The most common cause of peritonitis is dehiscence of gastrointestinal wounds. Intracellular bacteria are indicative of septic peritonitis. The mortality rate is 33%–48% with open abdominal drainage and 68% without it.

102. The answer is 4 [Chapter 12 V C 5 c (1)–(2)]. Nonobstructive dystocia without primary uterine inertia can be treated with oxytocin to stimulate uterine contractions, and fluid and electrolyte support. Obstructive dystocia, primary uterine inertia, secondary uterine inertia

unresponsive to oxytocin, and mechanical dystocia require cesarean section.

103. The answer is 3 [Chapter 23 I B 2 a]. The type of nerve to be biopsied is not really a consideration when selecting a nerve biopsy site. If the entire nerve can be sacrificed, a small segment of the nerve is removed. If the entire nerve cannot be sacrificed, a fascicular biopsy is performed on a mixed nerve. More important, the surgeon must consider whether the nerve is affected by the disease he or she is trying to diagnose, the presence of nearby blood vessels, tendons, or joints that may be damaged by the surgical approach, the function of the nerve (i.e., it should be nonessential), and the ability of the incision site to heal well.

104. The answer is 3 [Chapter 10 IV B 1 d (2)]. The esophagus, not the colon, lacks a serosal covering, which enhances wound healing. Collagen lysis exceeds synthesis for 3–4 days after surgery, increasing the risk of dehiscence. The segmental blood supply, mechanical stress from solid feces, and high bacterial content (primarily anaerobic gramnegative rods) result in higher morbidity and mortality rates following colonic resection and anastomosis.

105. The answer is 1 [Chapter 7 IV A]. Tracheal collapse is a disease of middle-aged and older miniature and toy-breed dogs; however, age has no bearing on the prognosis. The prognosis is poorer for animals with greater than grade II collapse, bronchial collapse, laryngeal paralysis, or involvement of the thoracic trachea (versus the cervical trachea). Fifty percent of dogs with tracheal collapse have some degree of bronchial collapse.

106. The answer is 5 [Chapter 18 II A 4 b]. Progressive degenerative joint disease (DJD) can be treated by joint fusion, resection, replacement, or limb amputation to alleviate patient discomfort. Joint lavage, together with systemic antibiotics, may be useful in treatment of inflammatory septic arthritis. Lavage of the joint environment does not stop the progression of joint deterioration that is characteristic of DJD.

107. The answer is 1 [Chapter 7 III A]. The three major components of brachycephalic syndrome include stenotic nares, elongated soft palate, and everted laryngeal saccules. Tracheal hypoplasia is also present in most cases. Laryngeal paralysis is not a common concurrent condition; rather, laryngeal collapse is seen as the disease progresses.

108. The answer is 1 [*Chapter 22 I A 1 c–d*]. Hemilaminectomy requires precise localization of the lesion because a hemilaminectomy exposes only the ventral and lateral aspects of the spinal cord, as compared with a dorsal laminectomy, which exposes the dorsal and dorsolateral aspects of the spinal cord. However, hemilaminectomy requires unilateral dissection (as opposed to bilateral dissection) and associated patient morbidity is reduced. With dorsal laminectomy, there exists the risk of causing vertebral instability. The approach used for hemilaminectomy facilitates adjacent disk fenestration.

109. The answer is 4 [*Chapter 10 III A 1*]. The stomach is supplied by the three branches of the celiac artery: the left gastric, hepatic, and splenic arteries. The gastroduodenal and gastrosplenic veins drain gastric blood into the portal vein.

110. The answer is 4 [*Chapter 7 IV D 2 a*]. Adenocarcinoma and alveolar carcinoma, not fibrosarcoma, are the most common primary lung tumors in dogs. Primary lung neoplasia is most common in older, large-breed dogs. Radiography usually reveals a single nodule in the right caudal lung lobe. Prognosis, based on wide excision and no evidence of metastatic disease, is good, with a median survival time of at least 1 year.

111. The answer is 4 [*Chapter 5 III C 3*]. Lysine is not required by critical care patients. All critical care patients require arginine for wound healing, glutamine as an energy source, and leucine for nitrogen retention. Taurine supplementation is necessary in cats, especially if diets formulated for humans are being used for extended periods of time.

112. The answer is 1 [*Chapter 20 I B 2 b (2)*].
Horner's syndrome is characterized by miosis, ptosis, enophthalmos, and vasodilation resulting from lower motor neuron (LMN) damage of the sympathetic nerves in the cranial thoracic spinal cord segments (i.e., T1–T3). Mydriasis is not part of the syndrome. Horner's syndrome is a common sign associated with a variety of nervous system diseases. It may also be a complication of surgeries involving a ventral approach to the cervical vertebrae.

113. The answer is 4 [*Chapter 8 II B 2 c (2)*]. Pulmonic stenosis can be treated with percutaneous balloon valvuloplasty, blind valvuloplasty through the myocardium, open valvulectomy, or patch grafting with natural or synthetic material. Pulmonary arterial banding would only increase the resistance to flow in the pulmonary artery and hence exacerbate the condition.

114. The answer is 5 [*Chapter 10 V C 5 d*]. Perianal fistulae can be treated by surgical excision, cryosurgery, chemical cauterization, or electrical cauterization (i.e., deroofing and fulguration). Antibiotics, at best, would provide temporary relief, whereas stool softeners may worsen local tissue infection. Selection of a treatment modality is based on the extent of disease and the potential for complications.

115–118. The answers are: 115-2 [*Chapter 6 I C 3 a (2) (e)*], **116-5** [*Chapter 6 I C 3 c*], **117-1** [*Chapter 6 I C 3 a (2) (f)*], **118-3** [*Chapter 6 I C 3 a (2) (b)*].
The Velpeau sling, which maintains the forelimb in a flexed position close to the thorax, is used following scapular joint injury or surgery.

An Ehmer sling is applied to the pelvic limb to internally rotate and abduct the femur following repairs of hip luxation.

A carpal flexion bandage is used to prevent weight-bearing following repair of flexor tendon or forelimb orthopedic injuries.

Plastic or aluminum spoon splints are applied to the palmar or plantar aspect of the bandage to treat fractures or luxations distal to the carpal or tarsal joint.

119–123. The answers are 119-3 [*Chapter 17 II E 3 b (3)*], **120-2** [*Chapter 17 II E 2 a (3)*], **121-1** [*Chapter 17 II E 1 a*], **122-2** [*Chapter 17 II E 3 a, b (2)*], **123-4** [*Chapter 17 II E 4 b*].
Femoral head and neck resection, which produces a pseudarthrosis, is useful for the treatment of irreparable, comminuted acetabular fractures.

A laterally applied bone plate and screws are usually used to stabilize ilial body fractures, most of which are oblique. Alternatively, intramedullary pins or wiring can be used in small dogs and cats.

Sacroiliac luxations are stabilized with a pin and bone screw (two-point fixation and compression).

Because the cranial two-thirds of the acetabulum are crucial for weight-bearing, surgery is recommended over conservative therapy. A dorsally applied reconstruction or acetabular plate is used.

Avulsion fractures of the ischiatic tubercle causing lameness require tension band fixation. Fractures of the ischial body usually do not require primary surgery.

124–128. The answers are 124-4 [*Chapter 22 II A 2 b*], **125-2** [*Chapter 22 II A 4 b (1)*], **126-1** [*Chapter 22 II D 2 b*], **127-5** [*Chapter 22 II A 3 b*], **128-3** [*Chapter 22 II B 1 b*]. Degenerative myelopathy occurs most frequently in German shepherds. Clinical signs include progressive paraparesis. Spinal pain is not evident upon examination, and radio-graphs and myelography fail to reveal a compressive lesion.

Fecal and urinary incontinence, tail atonia, and lower motor neuron (LMN) sciatic paresis are signs of cauda equina syndrome (lumbosacral disease). Compression of the sciatic nerve roots produces hindlimb motor and sensory deficits.

Diskospondylitis is a blood-borne bacterial infection of the vertebral end-plates and associated disks. Clinical signs include pain, pyrexia, and bone lysis on radiographs.

Caudal cervical spondylomyelopathy (wobbler syndrome) produces progressive tetraparesis and ventriflexion of the neck as a result of spinal cord compression. Middle-aged to old Doberman pinschers and young Great Danes are most often affected.

Atlantoaxial instability occurs in young, small dogs and is characterized by high cervical pain as a result of spinal cord compression and distraction of the C1–C2 vertebrae.

Index

Note: Page numbers in *italic* indicate figures; those followed by t indicate tables; those followed by Q indicate questions; and those followed by E indicate explanations.

A

Abdomen
  infections of, *Escherichia coli* and,
    320Q, 333E
  palpation of, in preoperative
    assessment, 4
  pendulous, in hyperadrenocorticism,
    181
Abdominocentesis, in urinary bladder
    rupture, 166
Abiotrophy, 288
Ablation
  of scrotum, 179
  of vertical ear canal, for ceruminous
    gland adenoma, 320Q,
    332E–333E
Abscess(es)
  liver, 147
  lung, 81
  pancreatic, 190–191
Acepromazine, 314Q, 325E
  as preanesthetic agent, 11, 12t
Acetabulum, fractures of, 234–235,
    234, 254
  complications of, 320Q, 332E
  highly comminuted, treatment of,
    323Q, 335E–336E
  treatment of, 323Q, 335E–336E
  and weight-bearing, 316Q, 327E
Acid–base balance, restoration of, in
    preoperative patient stabilization,
    8
Adherent dressings, 53
Adrenalectomy
  for hyperadrenocorticism, 182
  for pheochromocytoma, 183
Adrenal glands, 181–183
  anatomy of, 181
  disorders of, 181–183
  hyperadrenocorticism of, 181–183
  pheochromocytoma of, 183
Adrenergic agonists, as preanesthetic
    agents, 11, 12t
Age, wound healing and, 37
Airway(s), upper, obstruction of, 77,
    78
  risk category of, 315Q, 327E
  tracheostomy for, 77, *78*
Airway management, postanesthetic,
    21
Alimentary system, 115–142. *See also*
    specific organ, e.g., Oropharynx
  esophagus, 121–124
  intestines, 130–138
  oropharynx, 115–121
  rectum and anus, 138–142
  stomach, 125–130
Aliphatic alcohols, antisepsis and, 25t,
    26
Allodynia, 13

Allograft(s), cortical, for bone grafting,
    213
Amikacin, for treatment of wound
    infections, 29t
Amino acids
  for critically ill cats, 322Q, 335E
  supplementation of, 43
Amoxicillin-clavulanate, for wound
    infections, 29t
Amphiarthrosis, 237
Ampicillin, for wound infections, 29t
Amputation
  for degenerative joint disease, 240
  forelimb, for neoplasia, 225
  hindlimb, for neoplasia, 225
  limb, for patellar luxation, 251
  for peripheral nervous system
    neoplasia, 305
  rectal, 139
Analgesia
  in physical therapy, 57
  postoperative, 21–22, 21t
    opioids used for, dosages, 21t
  preemptive, 13
Anal sacculectomy, 139
  for chronic recurrent anal sacculitis,
    315Q, 327E
Anal sacculitis, 140
  chronic recurrent, treatment of,
    315Q, 327E
Anal stenosis, cryosurgery and, 313Q,
    324E
Anastomosis
  end-to-end, of esophagus, suture
    pattern for, 316Q, 327E
  of esophagus, 122
  of intestines, 131–132, *132*
  for peripheral nerve injury, 303
  Pott's, for tetralogy of Fallot, 92
  split-cartilage, for tracheal
    reconstruction, 77–78
  ureteral, for ureteral obstruction, 163
  for urethral trauma, 169
  vascular, vascular disorders and, 100
Anesthesia/anesthetics, 11–22
  for cesarean section, 174
  induction of, 13–20
  inhalation, 16–20, 18t, 19t. *See also*
    Inhalation anesthesia
  for intracranial disease, 280
  intraoperative monitoring, 20
  intravenous, 13–16. *See also*
    Intravenous anesthesia
  machines and circuits for, 17–18, 18t
  postoperative considerations, 21–22,
    21t. *See also* Postoperative
    considerations, anesthesia
  preanesthetic considerations, 11–15.
    See also Preanesthetic
    considerations

preoperative considerations,
    respiratory, 64
  in all animals, 64
  in brachycephalic breeds, 64
  risks associated with, 4–5, 5t
  for skull trauma, 261
  for traumatic diaphragmatic hernias,
    111
Angiography
  contrast, for peripheral arteriovenous
    fistulae, 99
  in intracranial disease, 275
  positive contrast, for cardiac
    neoplasms, 95
  radionuclide, for aortic
    thromboembolism, 98
  selective, in patent ductus arteriosus
    (PDA), 85
Antibiotic(s)
  for hepatobiliary surgery, 145
  for osteomyelitis, 223–224
  prophylactic use of
    indications for, 315Q, 327E
    and infection control, 27–28, 27t
    administration of, 27–28
    indications for, 27, 27t
    selection of, 27
    surgical procedures requiring, 27t
  for pyothorax, 319Q, 331E
  for skull and jaw fracture repair, 261
  for wound infection, 29, 29t
Anticholinergic(s), as preanesthetic
    agents, 11, 12t
Anti-inflammatory drugs, nonsteroidal
    (NSAIDs), for degenerative joint
    disease, 239
Antisepsis, skin, in surgical site
    preparation, 24–26, 25t
Antiseptic agents, for skin, 315Q, 326E
Antithyroid drugs, for thyroid tumors,
    186
Anus, 138–142
  anatomy of, 138
  conditions related to, 139–142
  congenital anomalies of, 139
  fecal incontinence and, 142
  neoplasia of, 141
  perianal fistulae of, 140–141
  perineal hernia of, 141–142
  surgical procedures for, 138–139
    general considerations, 138–139
Aortic arteriotomy, for aortic
    thromboembolism, 98
Aortic stenosis, 84t, 88–89
  described, 313Q, 324E
  treatment of, 89
Aortic thromboembolism, 97–98
  in cats, 97–98
  in dogs, 97
  treatment of, 98

Subchondral bone curettage, for osteochondritis dissecans, 319Q, 331E
Subchondral bone sclerosis, in degenerative joint disease, 319Q, 331E
Substrate phase, in wound healing, 35
Sulcoplasty, trochlear, for patellar luxation, 250, *250*
Supplementation
  amino acid, 43
  protein, 43
Suppurative prostatitis, 176
Supracondylar fractures
  of femur, 219
  of humerus, 215
Supratentorial structures, of intracranial nervous system, described, 271, *272*
Surgical drainage, for aural hematoma, 317Q, 329E
Surgical gastrostomy, 47
Surgical pain, preemptive analgesia for, 13
Surgical risk, assessment of, 4–7, 4t–6t
  anesthetic risk, 4–5, 5t
  obesity in, 6
  organ system involvement in, 5–6
  presurgical screening, 6–7, 6t
Surgical site, preparation of
  asepsis and, 24–27, 25t
  draping, 26–27
  hair removal, 24
  scrubbing, 26
  skin antisepsis, 24–26, 25t
Surgical technique
  proper, nosocomial infections and, 31
  wound healing and, 36
Surveillance routine, nosocomial infections and, 30–31
Survey radiography
  for diaphragmatic hernias, 110, 112, *113*
  in respiratory preoperative evaluation, 63
Suture(s)
  for cranial cruciate ligament injuries, 255
  fabellar, for patellar luxation, 249, *250*
  labial retraining, for vaginal prolapse, 173
  materials for, 313Q, 318Q, 324E, 330E
  medial imbricating, for lateral patellar luxation, 317Q, 328E
  patterns of
    for end-to-end anastomosis of esophagus, 316Q, 327E
    for small intestine surgery, 319Q, 331E–332E
  for peripheral nerve injury, 303
  placement of, in esophagus, 315Q, 326E
Synarthrosis, described, 237
Synovial cell carcinoma, 241
Synovial fluid, described, 237
Synovial fluid culture
  findings indicative of disease, 238t
  for immune-mediated arthritis, 241
  for infectious arthritis, 242
Synovial joint
  anatomy of, 237
  described, 237

T

Tape
  elastic adhesive, for bandaging, 54
  porous, for bandaging, 54
Tape muzzle, for mandibular body fractures, 261–262
Tarsal(s)
  fractures of, 257, 323Q, 335E–336E
  injuries to, 257
  luxation of, 257, 323Q, 335E–336E
Tarsus, osteochondrosis of, 244
  prognosis of, 319Q, 332E
Teeth
  canine, intraoral dental bonding of, for mandibular body fractures, 264
  conditions related to, 117
  extraction of, 117
Telazol, indications, induction, and precautions, 14t, 15–16
Temporomandibular joint
  abnormalities of, 267
  luxation of, 267
Tendon(s)
  flexor, injury to, bandages for, 323Q, 335E–336E
  resection of, for hip dysplasia, 245
Tension band fixation
  for ischial fractures, 235, *235*
  for scapular fractures, 320Q, 332E
Testis(es)
  described, 175
  surgical removal of, 178–179
    for cryptorchidism, 176
  tumors of, 177–178
Tethering, for temporomandibular joint luxation, 267
Tetralogy of Fallot, 84t, 91–92, *91*
  dog breeds predisposed to, 84t
  treatment of
    medical, 91
    surgical, 92
T fractures, 252
  of humerus, 215
Thermography, for aortic thromboembolism, 98
Thiamylal, indications, induction, and precautions, 13, 14t
Thiobarbiturate(s)
  duration of action of, 321Q, 333E
  indications, induction, and precautions, 13–14, 14t
Thiopental, indications, induction, and precautions, 13, 14t
Thoracic cavity, 101–113
  air or fluid in, postoperative ventilation and, 102
  anatomy of, 101
  auscultation of, in preoperative assessment, 3
  chylothorax of, 107–108, 108t
  conditions related to, 107–113
  diaphragmatic hernias and, 110–113, *112, 113*
  exposure of, during surgery, 318Q, 330E
  mediastinal masses of, 109
  mesothelioma and, 110
  pneumomediastinum and, 109–110
  pre- and postoperative considerations, 101–102
  pyothorax of, 108–109
  surgical approaches to, 102–105
Thoracic fluid, drainage of, for pyothorax, 319Q, 331E

Thoracic wall, 101–113
  anatomy of, 101
  conditions related to, 105–107
  congenital malformations, 105
  neoplasia of, 106–107
  pre- and postoperative considerations, 101–102
  trauma to, 105–106
Thoracostomy
  for lung disease, 80, *80*
  tube, for pyothorax, 109
Thoracostomy tube, for traumatic diaphragmatic hernias, 111
Thoracotomy
  and assisted ventilation, 101
  exploratory, for pyothorax, 109
  lateral (intercostal), 102–103, 102t, *103*
  for lung disease, 79
  positive intrathoracic pressure during, 101
  rib pivot, 103–104
  transsternal, 105
Thorax, radiography of, in presurgical screening, 6
Thromboembolism, aortic, 97–98. See *also* Aortic thromboembolism
Thrombolytic agents, for aortic thromboembolism, 98
Thyroidectomy
  for thyroid tumors in cats, 186
  for thyroid tumors in dogs, 185
Thyroid gland, 183–186
  anatomy of, 183, *184*
  surgery of, hypocalcemia and, 317Q, 329E
  tumors of
    in cats, 185–186, *185*
    in dogs, 183–185, *184*
Tibia, fractures of, 219–220
  distal, 220
  proximal, 219
  shaft, 219–220, *220*
Tibial crest transposition, for patellar luxation, 249–250
Ticarcillin, for wound infections, 29t
Tissue perfusion, and skull trauma, 260–261
Tongue
  conditions related to, 116–117
  eosinophilic granulomas of, 116–117
  neoplasia of, 117
  trauma to, 116
Tonsil(s)
  conditions related to, 120
  enlargement of, 120
Tonsillectomy, 120
Total hip replacement, for hip dysplasia, 246–247
Total parenteral nutrition, 48–51, *50–51*
  advantages of, 48, 320Q, 332E
  basic solution
    composition of, 49
    supplements to, 49
  catheter placement, 49
  complications of, 51
  disadvantages of, 49
  indications for, 48, 319Q, 331E
  mixing of, 49
  protein and energy requirements, calculation of, 49, *50–51*
Toxin(s)
  and brain, 287
  and neuropathy, 306
Toxoplasmosis, 306